Surgical principles

Surgical principles

Edited by

IRVING TAYLOR MD ChM FRCS

David Patey Professor of Surgery,
Head of Department of Surgery,
University College London Medical School, London, UK

STEPHEN J KARRAN MD MA MChir FRCS FRCS (Ed)

Reader in Surgery, University of Southampton,
Honorary Consultant Surgeon, Southampton University Hospitals Trust,
Royal South Hampshire Hospital, Southampton, UK

A member of the Hodder Headline Group
LONDON • SYDNEY • AUCKLAND
Co-published in the USA by Oxford University Press, Inc., New York

First published in Great Britain 1996 by
Arnold, a division of Hodder Headline PLC,
338 Euston Road, London NW1 3BH

© 1996 Arnold

Co-published in the United States of America by
Oxford University Press Inc.,
198 Madison Avenue, New York, NY 10016
Oxford is a registered trademark of Oxford University Press

Whilst the advice and information in this book is believed to be true and
accurate at the date of going to press, neither the author[s] nor the publisher
can accept any legal responsibility or liability for any errors or omissions
that may be made. In particular (but without limiting the generality of the
preceding disclaimer) every effort has been made to check drug dosages:
however, it is still possible that errors have been missed. Furthermore,
dosage schedules are constantly being revised and new side-effects
recognized. For these reasons the reader is strongly urged to consult the
drug companies' printed instructions before administering any of the drugs
recommended in this book.

British Library Cataloguing in Publication Data
A catalogue record for this book is available from the British Library

Library of Congress Cataloging-in-Publication Data
A catalog record for this book is available from the Library of Congress

ISBN 0 340 61379 3 (pb)

1 2 3 4 5 95 96 97 98 99

Typeset in 10/11 Times by
J&L Composition Ltd, Filey, North Yorkshire
Printed and bound in Great Britain by
The Bath Press, Bath, Avon

Contents

Contributors

Lesley Bromley FRCA MHM
Academic Sub Department of Anaesthetics, Department of Surgery, University College London School of Medicine, London, UK

SE Clamp FRCS
Clinical Information Science Unit, University of Leeds, Leeds, UK

AW Clark MBBS MS FRCS (Eng)
Consultant Surgeon, Royal Sussex County Hospital, Brighton, UK

Mair Davies FRCA
Academic Sub Department of Anaesthetics, Department of Surgery, University College London School of Medicine, London, UK

JW Dawson FRCS
Lecturer in Surgery, University College London Medical School, London, UK

Tom Diamond BSC MD FRCS FRCSI
Senior Lecturer in Surgery, Institute of Clinical Science, The Queen's University Belfast, Belfast, N Ireland, UK

FT de Dombal† MA MD FRCS
Clinical Information Science Unit, University of Leeds, Leeds, UK

Allen Edwards FRCS
Senior Registrar, Department of Surgery, University Hospital Wales, Cardiff, Wales, UK

Keith Harding
Director, Wound Healing Research Unit, University Hospital of Wales, Cardiff, Wales

Stephen J Karran MA MChir FRCS (Eng) FRCS (Ed)
Reader in Surgery, University of Southampton, Honorary Consultant Surgeon, Southampton University Hospitals Trust, Southampton, UK

Victor Jaffe MA MChir FRCS
Consultant Surgeon, Chase Farm Hospital, Middlesex, UK

David Leaper MD ChM FRCS
Professorial Unit of Surgery, University of Newcastle Upon Tyne, North Tees General Hospital, Stockton-On-Tees, Cleveland, TS19 8PE, UK

Brendan J Moran MS FRCS I
Consultant Surgeon, The North Hampshire Hospital, Basingstoke, UK

MS Nathan MS FRCS D Urol
Associate Lecturer, Department of Minimally Invasive Therapy, United Medical and Dental Schools of Guy's and St Thomas's, London, UK

Daniel E Porter BSC MB ChB FRCS
Orthopaedic Registrar, Nuffield Orthopaedic Centre, Oxford, UK

Graeme J Poston MS FRCS (Eng) FRCS (Ed)
Consultant Surgical Oncologist, Royal Liverpool Hospital, Liverpool, UK

Brian J Rowlands MD FRCS FACS
Professor of Surgery, Department of Surgery, The Queens University Belfast, Belfast, N Ireland

MJ Sampson MD MRCP
Consultant Physician, Norfolk and Norwich Hospital, Norwich, UK

Maurice Slapak MChir FRCS (Eng) FRCS (Can) FACS
Wessex Regional Transplant Unit, St Mary's Hospital, Portsmouth, UK

JAR Smith FRCS (Eng) FRCS (Ed)
Consultant Surgeon, Northern General Hospital, Sheffield, UK

† Deceased

Elizabeth H Smyth MB ChB FRCS
Surgical Research Fellow, MRC Human Genetics Unit, Edinburgh, UK

Irving Taylor MD ChM FRCS
Professor of Surgery, Head of Department of Surgery, University College London Medical School, London, UK

DA Tomalin
Clinical Audit Co-ordinator, Royal Sussex County Hospital, Brighton, UK

Chris Vickery FRCS
University Department of Surgery, Southmead Hospital, Bristol, UK

Bruce P Waxman BMedSc MB BS(Monash) FRACS FRCS FACS
Associate Professor, Director, Monash University Academic Surgical Unit, Dandenong Hospital, Melbourne, Australia

Robert K Webb MB BS(Syd) FANZCA
Director, Australian Patient Safety Foundation, Adelaide, Australia

JEA Wickham MS MD BSC FRCS FRCP FRCR
Honorary Consultant and Senior Research Lecturer, United Medical and Dental Schools of Guy's and St Thomas's, London, UK

John HR Winstanley MD FRCS(Eng) FRCS(Glas)
Consultant Surgical Oncologist, Royal Liverpool Hospital, Liverpool, UK

Howard Young ChM FRCS
Consultant Surgeon, Department of Surgery, University Hospital Wales, Cardiff, Wales, UK

JS Yudkin MD FRCP
Professor of Medicine, University College London Medical School, Whittington Hospital, London, UK

Foreword

Surgical training and education in the United Kingdom are passing through a long overdue vigorous period of reform. Similar changes are occurring in many other parts of the world. In the United Kingdom the common core of surgical knowledge and technical expertise needed by all surgeons will be obtained and assessed in the first two years of post-intern work. Thereafter, specific specialty training will take five to six years leading to the award of a Certificate of Completion of Specialist Training. Current textbooks do not fit this pattern of education. They tend either to be too specialized for basic trainees, or do not contain sufficient speciality knowledge, especially basic science, for advanced training. This book describes the basic knowledge required by all trainees. It should be read and learnt during basic (common trunk) training, and re-read, together with the relevant specialist books, throughout advanced specialist training. It covers the essential core of clinical and surgical knowledge required by all surgeons, together with the basics of operating room and instrument design, robotics, audit, economics, information technology and molecular genetics.

Irving Taylor and Stephen Karran have assembled a group of top class teachers who have presented their knowledge and understanding of the fundamental principles common to all forms of surgery in a stimulating, absorbable and attractive way. They have covered everything that contributes to the success of an operation, patient support, wound healing, sepsis, essential organ failure and resuscitation, the special problems presented by cancer and concomitant medical disease such as diabetes, together with the principles of operating room safety and efficiency. There can be no doubt that this volume will be a great success for it contains 'the facts that all surgeons should know'. It will become required reading for all trainee surgeons worldwide, because all surgeons, wherever they work, must have a comprehensive and profound understanding of the principles and practice of surgery-in-general with which they can develop their advanced speciality expertise.

Sir Norman Browse

Preface

In the face of massive changes occurring in all branches of surgical practice and technology, it is easy to forget, or choose to ignore, the basic surgical principles which underpin the infrastructure for all our surgical expertise. Undoubtedly this aspect may appear less glamorous, but very often, as far as the patient is concerned, it is of paramount importance; there is little point, for example, in performing a technically brilliant operation if the patient dies in the postoperative period due to electrolyte imbalance. Colleges of Surgeons and assessment boards throughout the world have reviewed and revised all aspects of surgical curricula and training but throughout have maintained and encouraged better understanding and appreciation of the important basic principles of surgical science practice. Accordingly, they remain an integral part of the format for fellowship examinations at all levels.

In this book we have attempted to bring together important aspects of surgical science which should be understood by all surgeons in whatever specialty they practice. As far as the candidate presenting himself for the membership and fellowship examinations is concerned, we hope much of the required up-to-date information necessary to satisfy the examiners at both basic and higher surgical trainee level is provided. In addition, it may well be that established consultants will find revision of these principles of value.

The reviews cover basic aspects such as resuscitation, molecular genetics and fluid and electrolyte balance, as well as more practical aspects of pre-operative assessment, anaesthesia, renal failure and diabetes. We have also included global topics such as the design and safety of operating theatres, instrumentation, clinical audit and information science.

We are most grateful to all our reviewers for providing such comprehensive and valuable contributions.

Irving Taylor
Stephen J Karran

PART I

General principles

CHAPTER 1

Physiological responses to surgery and fluid and electrolyte balance

JAR SMITH

Introduction

In practice, all cells including those in the kidney, function adequately provided there is a sufficient supply of oxygen and nutrients and the fluid, electrolyte and acid-base milieu does not show extreme variation from normal. The range of pH compatible with normal activity is between 7.3 and 7.6, and a 0.3 variation represents a 50% reduction or doubling of the hydrogen ion concentration. A minority – the elderly, the very young and those with cardiac or renal pathology – are more demanding as regards their tolerance of fluid and electrolytes. However, if it is remembered that 60% of body weight is attributable to water and the fluctuation of body weight is no greater than 1–2% per day, it is clear that control is normally very effective.

The responses to surgical trauma are obligatory but protective, except where the severity of the trauma or the development of complications such as sepsis produce exaggerated and uncontrolled hormonal responses.

ANTI-DIURETIC HORMONE (ADH)

Following surgery there is a reduction in the renal output of sodium and water.[1] The latter effect is caused by an increased production of ADH in the supraoptic nuclei. It is now recognized that ADH is in fact arginine vasopressin, an octapeptide, stored in and released from the posterior pituitary gland. Osmoreceptors sensitive to relatively gross, i.e. 1–2%, changes in plasma osmolality are identified in the hypothalamus and more sensitive receptors probably exist in the liver and in contact with the cerebrospinal fluid.

An increase in ADH secretion is found in a variety of conditions – pneumonia, tuberculosis and neurological disease.[2] Ectopic secretion of ADH may complicate oat cell carcinoma, and secretion can be stimulated by drugs such as cyclophosphamide. In surgical practice, anaesthesia,[3] fasting and anxiety[4,5] all stimulate ADH release.

The effect of ADH may be potentiated by carbamazepine or chlorpropamide. On the other hand, the direct correlation between ADH levels and falling arterial pressure is made less sensitive by the effect of morphine in the postoperative period.[6] Pain and the extent of operative trauma influence ADH levels so that cardiac procedures and laparotomy cause higher levels than other operations.[7,8] Other factors which influence ADH secretion are osmolality, extracellular fluid (ECF) volume, nausea, pregnancy, hypoglycaemia and both alcohol and nicotine intake.[2] Relatively small changes in plasma osmolality, e.g. 1%, are sufficient to stimulate ADH production and to increase the reabsorption of water from the collecting tubules.

ALDOSTERONE

Aldosterone is produced in and released from the zona glomerulosa in the adrenal cortex. Both production and release are stimulated by angiotensin II, the active end product of the renin–angiotensin system.

The main stimulus of the angiotensin mechanism is sympathetic. Any fall in blood volume is detected by baroreceptors situated in the aortic arch, the cardiac atria and the carotid sinus. It is probable that baroreceptors also exist within the juxtaglomerular apparatus itself to allow local control of function. Furthermore it is possible that the relative local concentration of sodium and potassium perfusing the renal cortex also stimulates renin production. The

overall mechanism is best described diagrammatically (Fig. 1.1).

Aldosterone itself causes the active absorption of sodium (and therefore of water) at the distal convoluted tubule. The active absorption of sodium from cell to interstitial fluid space results in a concentration gradient so that sodium passes from the lumen into the cell in exchange for either potassium or hydrogen ions. As acid-base balance has a higher priority than electrolyte control the actual relative concentrations exchanged depend on the hydrogen ion available.[9]

ATRIAL NATRIURETIC PEPTIDES (ANPS)

Various ANPs have been identified (α1, β and γ) of which α-ANP has been studied most. It has a half-life of between 2 and 9 minutes. The peptide consists of 28 amino acids. The effect of α-ANP administered intravenously to healthy volunteers is a rapid (less than 30 minutes) increase in output of water and sodium in the urine, sufficient to induce hypotension. There are no associated changes in plasma levels of renin, ADH or aldosterone but urinary excretion of phosphate, calcium and magnesium is increased. It is believed the ANPs activate the renin–angiotensin system as salt restriction reduces the above effects of α-ANP.

Plasma ANPs are not found in normal health. There appears to be a direct relationship between ANPs and

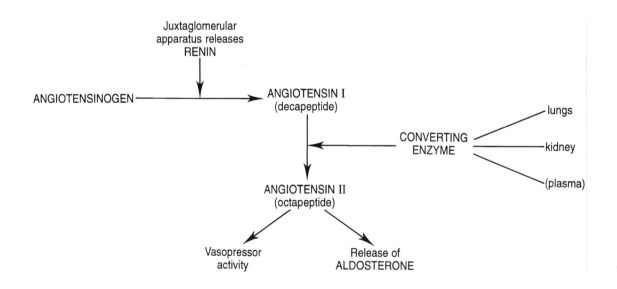

Fig. 1.1 The renin–angiotensin system.

the ECF volume in children with chronic renal failure.[10,11] Highest levels have been reported in congestive cardiac failure but the fact that there is no resulting diuresis confirms the reduced potency of ANPs when the renin system is stimulated.

OTHER FACTORS

Kinins and prostaglandins also affect sodium absorption. A sodium transport inhibitor (ouabain-like factor) has also been identified.[2]

RENAL CONTROL

Extreme changes in electrolyte concentrations are influenced by renal function. If an increased quantity of salt is filtered by the glomerulus there will be an increase in sodium being absorbed and excreted in the proximal tubule. As a rule of thumb, the proximal tubule is the site of major changes and the distal tubule that of finer control of electrolytes. Similar finer adjustments of water occurs in the collecting ducts.

It is important to remember that for the kidney to control the concentration of urine the preservation of medullary osmolality and the counter-current mechanism in the collecting tubules is vital.

THIRST

Osmoreceptors in the hypothalamus also stimulate thirst. Hypovolaemia results in an increase in oncotic pressure within the renal bed and produces increased absorption of sodium and water. It is likely that ADH and/or angiotensin II have an effect on the hypothalamus to stimulate thirst and the oral intake of salt. The overall effect is to *conserve* the available salt and water.

the synovium and within the eye, the total being about 1 litre However in the gut, for example, there are considerable variations in the course of each day, with 5–8 litres being secreted and reabsorbed. The distribution of water between the various compartments is dictated by a number of factors.

CELL MEMBRANE

The energy requiring ATPase sodium pump on the cell membrane actively expels sodium from the cell, with consequent retention of potassium as the major intracellular cation. This mechanism is also vital to limiting intracellular water content.

THE CAPILLARY MEMBRANE

The movement of fluid between the interstitial fluid (ISF) and plasma occurs across the capillary membrane. The factors involved are:

1. the hydrostatic pressure which falls from 35 mmHg to 15 mmHg from the arterial to venous end of the capillary bed (in muscle, though in other organs particularly kidney and intestine these pressures differ widely causing either formation of urine or absorption of fluid into the gut);
2. the plasma oncotic pressure, attributed to albumin: this is about 25 mmHg but is higher at the venous end because of the passage of water across the capillary at the arterial end;
3. the hydrostatic (5 mmHg) pressure in the ISF;
4. the oncotic ISF pressure (5mmHg) encouraging the passage of fluid into this space.

In maintaining this balanced relationship the role of the lymphatic drainage system to remove fluid and particulate matter from the ISF and to return it to the plasma is vital.

Normal body water

Water represents 75% of lean body mass. The greater fat content in women means that 50% of total body weight in females and 60% in men is due to water. Two-thirds of the total water is intracellular. Extracellular fluid is separated into interstitial water (14% of body weight); plasma (5%) and transcellular water (1%). The latter is present in pleura, the gut lumen,

The electrolytes

SODIUM

Sodium is the cation in the ECF space and as it is always present in hydrated form it is responsible for preservation of ECF and plasma volume. The normal plasma sodium is 140 mmol/l and in other transcellular fluids varies from 6 mmol/l in sweat to 150 mmol/l in bile. The normal daily requirement is 100 mmol. Total body sodium is 4000 mmol, of which 73% is exchangeable; 39% of the total sodium is found in bone.

As indicated, sodium is the primary influence on ECF volume and therefore indirectly on intracellular volume also. It is involved in acid-base buffers. However, it is important to remember the contribution of sodium levels to excitability, permeability and membrane permeability.

POTASSIUM

Because potassium is the main intracellular cation, accurate measurement is difficult. Isotope dilution techniques indicate the total potassium concentration to be 3500 mmol. Only 3% of this is extracellular. The intracellular concentration is 150 mmol/l of intracellular water and virtually all potassium is exchangeable, albeit over a 48-hour period. It should be remembered that only 60% of total body sodium is exchangeable. The normal daily requirement of potassium varies from 60 to 90 mmol.

Potassium is therefore important as regards the intracellular osmotic pressure and volume. Because of its role in the control of membrane permeability it is involved in the contractility and excitability of neuromuscular tissue. As will be seen, abnormalities of potassium levels are manifest particularly in myocardial function.

CALCIUM AND MAGNESIUM

Both these cations are involved in neurological and muscle function but neither have a specific role in fluid and electrolyte balance and will not be considered further.

Catabolic response to surgery

The seminal work of Cuthbertson[12,13] is now well established, although recent evidence has begun to question some of the conclusions drawn. This response is also protective, at least initially, in providing an endogenous source of energy and amino acids following trauma.

Cuthbertson described a resting or *ebb* phase, corresponding with the duration of hypovolaemia and mediated by the central nervous system (CNS) and a *flow* phase of hypercatabolism mediated by the CNS and cytokines. In the latter phase first glycogen and

then muscle protein is broken down to provide glucose as the obligatory energy source, especially for red cell, brain and neurological tissue. By a similar mechanism muscle protein is broken down to provide amino acids for synthesis and gluconeogenesis repair. The net result of tissue breakdown is the release of potassium from cells. Under normal circumstances hyperkalaemia may cause cardiac dysfunction but as a result of aldosterone production a mechanism exists to avoid significant increases in serum potassium by the route described above.

Abnormalities of fluid and electrolyte balance

Of the three main homeostatic mechanisms, electrolyte control, acid-base balance and control of effective circulating blood volume, the latter has the highest priority.[14]

SODIUM

Of the 30% of the body sodium found in bone, only 60% is exchangeable. The main site of excretion is in urine with only small quantities being lost in sweat or faeces. The reabsorption rate of sodium in the kidneys is over 99%. Oral intake varies according to taste but daily requirements are about 100 mmol. Abnormalities of sodium may occur alone or with associated changes in water.

SODIUM EXCESS ALONE

This is the least common abnormality and is usually caused by the intravenous infusion of excessive quantities of hypertonic saline, or in dehydration as a consequence of loss of water in the presence of a normal sodium concentration. High levels of ECF sodium result in loss of water from the intracellular compartment with consequent impairment of cell function and eventually disruption of subcellular and cell membranes. As a result potassium is also lost into the extracellular fluid. It is important to replace water and potassium in the treatment regimen.

EXCESS OF SODIUM AND WATER

This combination usually results in increase in ECF volume and most commonly is iatrogenic, i.e. excessive infusion despite impaired renal function. The hormonal responses described in the immediate postoperative period encourage retention of salt and water but renal disease may also contribute to the problem.

Primary excesses of aldosterone as in Conn's syndrome produces hypokalaemia and hypertension. However, excess sodium is excreted and abnormal accumulations of ECF does not result in oedema. The most common cause of secondary hyperaldosteronism is hypoalbuminaemia. This reduces the reabsorption of ISF at the venous end of the capillary bed and increases the volume escaping at the arterial end. The consequent reduction in venous return results in a fall in cardiac output so that the renin–angiotensin mechanism is stimulated. This produces inappropriate retention of both salt and water and an increase in ECF volume.

SODIUM DEFICIENCY

In surgical practice, the most common cause of sodium deficiency is inadequate replacement of losses or excessive infusion of water, i.e. of 5% dextrose. As ECF volume is normal but the fluid hypotonic there is movement of water into the cells and impaired cellular function, especially in the nervous system and in the kidneys. This means that the ability to respond to therapy is reduced.

It has been shown that after surgery there is a fall in plasma sodium concentration which is inversely proportional to the preoperative plasma sodium concentration. The extent of the fall was related both to the severity of the surgery and the volume of fluids infused but the fall occurred even when dilution as a cause could be excluded.[15] Furthermore, it was felt that the plasma sodium concentration could be used to monitor progress in the postoperative period and that hyponatraemia might well indicate the presence of sepsis, ischaemia or some other complication, prior to clinical presentation of the problem.

If the hyponatraemia is mild, infusion of normal saline will usually be sufficient therapy. If there are more serious deficiencies dialysis will be required.

DEFICIENCY OF BOTH SODIUM AND WATER

This combination results in depletion of ECF volume and is one of the most common fluid problems in surgical practice: It may result from:

1. excessive losses from the alimentary tract – vomiting, diarrhoea or a high output fistula;
2. sequestration of fluid, for example, in intestinal ileus or peritonitis;
3. skin losses in severe burns;
4. excessive renal losses with osmotic and other diuretics, or due to mineralocorticoid deficiencies.

Renal disease such as chronic pyelonephritis or salt-losing nephropathy also results in loss of sodium and water.

Volume depletion results in:

1. sympathetic nervous stimulation with a tachycardia and chronotropic stimulation of cardiac output;
2. stimulation of the renin–angiotensin system: the resultant renal retention of salt and water produces concentrated urine of small volume and low sodium levels;
3. increased production of ADH and stimulation of the thirst centre.

The total deficit can be calculated:

$$\text{Deficit (mmol)} = \text{body weight in kg} \times (140 - \text{plasma Na}) \tfrac{60}{100}$$

assuming that the total body water is 60% of body weight.

Potassium

Potassium is the predominant intracellular cation, the average being 160 mmol/l. About 5–10 mmol per day are lost in each of faeces and sweat but in the kidney, where there is major control of balance, the losses are proportional to the daily intake. It is important to remember that catabolism results in release of intracellular potassium and that even if there is potassium deprivation about 50 mmol is lost daily. As potassium is a low threshold substance any elevation in ECF levels above 5 mmol/l results in an increased renal loss. The main control of potassium excretion is by aldosterone.

Potassium is indirectly responsible for the control of intracellular volume and osmotic pressure. As it is responsible for the control of cell membrane permeability it is involved in the contractility and excitability of neuromuscular structures.

Hyperkalaemia

The main danger of hyperkalaemia is for the myocardium, beginning at ECF levels of 7 mmol/l. As levels continue to rise (Fig. 1.2) characteristic changes in the T-waves, P-waves and QRS complexes are identified.

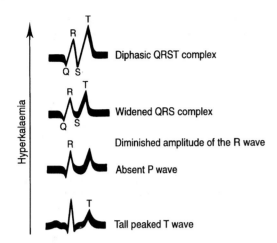

Fig. 1.2 Progressive effects of hyperkalaemia on the ECG trace.

Where levels exceed 8.5 mmol/l there is a major risk of *diastolic* cardiac arrest.

Hyperkalaemia is found:

- in acute renal failure;
- by excessive intravenous administration;
- in a combination of the two.

Treatment may be:

1. by infusion of 10% dextrose and 10 units of Actrapid insulin: the potassium passes into the cell with the glucose;
2. rectal administration of calcium or sodium resonium exchange resin;
3. where either of the above fail, some form of renal dialysis is required.

Hypokalaemia

Potassium deficiency results from excess loss or inadequate replacement. Mucus has a high content of potassium so that a rectal villous tumour may present with, or be complicated by, hypokalaemia. In pyloric stenosis the loss of gastric juice, which also contains mucus, results in low serum potassium. In dehydration, fluid is lost from the cell to replace ECF volume. This results in loss of potassium from the cells and the ECF threshold is exceeded. As a consequence the loss of potassium in urine is increased. A similar phenomenon occurs in the catabolic response to surgery.

If high levels of aldosterone are present sodium is retained at the expense of potassium. Hypokalaemia is a common complication of thiazide diuretics.

In metabolic alkalosis fewer hydrogen ions are available to exchange for sodium in the distal tubule so that relatively larger quantities of potassium are lost in the urine. Cellular dehydration is a complication of ketosis but an additional reason for hypokalaemia is the extra passage of glucose into cells accompanied by potassium. It must be remembered that when insulin is used to treat the ketosis more potassium will enter the cells and at least initially will produce another fall in ECF potassium.

Hypokalaemia produces:

- neurological disturbance – confusion, apathy and drowsiness;
- muscle weakness, including alimentary ileus and urinary retention;
- characteristic changes in electrocardiograph (ECG) and in cardiac function (Fig. 1.3).

When correcting hypokalaemia it must be remembered that the measurable serum levels do not reflect accurately the whole body picture and repeated estimations are required throughout the period of therapy for full correction of any deficiency.

Acid-base balance

Regulation of the pH compatible with both extracellular and intracellular viability depends on a number of mechanisms.

BUFFER SYSTEMS

The main role of buffers is to minimize any change in pH by donating or accepting protons. They may be either:

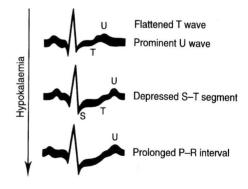

Fig. 1.3 Progressive effects of hypokalaemia on the ECG trace.

Table 1.1 Changes in pH and arterial carbon dioxide tension ($PaCO_2$) in acid-base disturbances

	Plasma pH	Plasma $PaCO_2$
Metabolic acidosis	↓	↓
Metabolic alkalosis	↑	↑
Respiratory acidosis	↓	↑
Respiratory alkalosis	↑	↓

- the weak acid and the salt of the acid with a strong alkali, or
- a weak alkali with the salt of the alkali and a strong acid.

The Henderson–Hasselbalch equation indicates that the pH depends on the *ratio* of the buffer ion to undissociated acid. The important body buffers are bicarbonate, phosphate, haemoglobin and plasma proteins. Organic acids have a very small overall contribution as their quantity is small.

The intracellular pH is acid (6.8–7.0) while the ECF pH is around 7.4. This discrepancy must be remembered when correcting disturbance of acid-base balance.

RESPIRATORY SYSTEM

Respiratory disturbance *per se* may produce changes in acid-base balance (Table 1.1.) but metabolic changes stimulate respiratory compensation.

*Hypo*ventilation follows metabolic alkalosis. The resultant retention of carbon dioxide produces a fall in pH and minimizes the shift to alkalosis. In a similar way acidosis produces stimulation of the respiratory centre, increased ventilation, increased expiration of carbon dioxide and a rise in pH.

RENAL SYSTEM

The final control – by excretion of excess acid or alkali – is the responsibility of the kidney. It is a normal function of the kidney to secrete the acid load which results from a normal diet (50–100 mmol H^+/day). It is impossible to achieve a urinary pH lower than 4.5 and mechanisms other than the simple excretion of acid are required to cope with acidosis.

REABSORPTION OF FILTERED BICARBONATE

This energy-requiring process has the net result of acidifying urine but for complete balance would mean the absorption of about 4700 mmol/day. Therefore an additional mechanism is required.

EXCRETION OF TITRATABLE ACID

This contributes 20–40 mmol/day and requires phosphate as the main buffer. The system is exhausted at a urinary pH of 4.5.

AMMONIA PRODUCTION

This is the most important method to excrete an acid load. Ammonia is produced by the deamination of glutamine within the renal cell. It then passes by diffusion into the lumen and there accepts a hydrogen ion to form an ammon*ium* ion. In response to demand ammonia production can be increased but the time to maximize production is quite long (4–6 days). At maximum production 200–300 mmol of H^+ ion per day can be buffered.

DISTURBANCES OF pH

It is traditional to consider metabolic and respiratory alkalosis and acidosis but in surgical practice the metabolic variants are more common (Table 1.1).

Metabolic *alkalosis* is most commonly seen in pyloric stenosis where there is also hypokalaemia and hypochloraemia. The loss of potassium is by vomiting of gastric juice and mucus followed by an increased renal loss at the distal tubule in view of the lack of availability of hydrogen ions in the response to aldosterone.

Metabolic *acidosis* is found as a consequence of tissue hypoxia but is also seen in severe diarrhoea, renal failure and in patients with diabetic keto-acidosis.

Correction of acid-base imbalance must include treatment of the underlying cause. In calculating what fluid infusion is required it is assumed that the normal plasma bicarbonate is 26 mmol/l and that the ECF volume is 20% of lean body weight.

To correct the *ECF* deficit the bicarbonate required is:

$$\text{weight (kg)} \times \tfrac{20}{100} \times (26 - \text{actual measured bicarbonate}).$$

In actual fact this is about half the requirement for complete correction but it is better to achieve partial correction, retest and repeat the calculation above. It is important to avoid too rapid correction to prevent paradoxical changes within the cell. As correction of the ECF pH begins, the respiratory compensation is reduced and thus more carbon dioxide is retained. Carbon dioxide enters the cell with a reduction in pH while the ECF pH is increasing. Slower-equilibration occurs within the cerebrospinal fluid.

Practical fluid and electrolyte balance

Maintenance of circulating plasma volume, acid-base balance and fluid electrolyte balance are, in order of priority, the most important components of homeostasis.[14] The responses to trauma described aim to:

- *minimize* the obligatory results of trauma;
- provide energy and building blocks for repair of damaged tissue;
- encourage recovery.

Understanding of the mechanisms discussed facilitates the practicalities required.

TWENTY-FOUR HOURS AFTER SURGERY AND BEYOND

It is standard practice in the current 24 hours to replace the fluid lost in the previous 24-hour period. It is also necessary to give the normal daily requirements and to monitor carefully the response to replacement by measuring blood pressure, pulse, urine output and serum urea and electrolytes.

To the actual measured losses must be added 600–1000 ml for the insensible losses from skin, respiratory tract and sweat. The daily need for sodium (100–125 mmol) is given as 1 litre of normal saline. Potassium is given as a supplement within the infused fluid, doses of 60–90 mmol/day being normal. Having calculated the total volume to be replaced, the balance is administered as 5% dextrose and water. The dextrose serves to render the solution isotonic *not* to provide a source of calories.

Pyrexia results in an increase fluid loss from skin, sweat and respiratory tract. Abnormal gastrointest-inal losses from nasogastric tube, fistula, diarrhoea, etc. must be replaced *in addition* to daily requirements. As the fluid lost is rich in electrolytes, normal saline with potassium supplements is the solution of choice. In practice 2.5 litres, split into 1 litre of normal saline and 1.5 litres of 5% dextrose in water, with potassium supplements, is a common starting prescription.

FIRST 24 HOURS

It is assumed that intraoperative losses of blood and of fluid from exposed surfaces have been replaced during surgery itself.

By the responses described it will be necessary to prescribe a lower total volume of fluid and a lower proportion of saline. No potassium is required in the early postoperative period. Thus 2 litres of fluid to 0.5 litres normal saline and 1.5 litres of 5% dextrose in water is the norm.

AT RISK PATIENTS

In critically injured patients more careful prescription and monitoring is essential. As regards tolerance of volume, urine volume is measured hourly and monitoring by central venous pressure (CVP) or pulmonary wedge pressure (PWP) may be required. Measurements can be made hourly or 4-hourly, the volume infused being that lost in the previous time period. Serum urea and electrolytes can be measured 4-hourly or urine losses of urea and electrolytes can be measured and specific losses replaced.

Much has been spoken about osmolality. It is particularly important to compare plasma and urine osmolality in the period of recovery after acute renal failure when the ability to concentrate urine is the first function to recovery. In practice it is not often that osmolality is measured but the *effective* osmolality can be calculated from serum concentrations of glucose and urea and this used to make therapeutic decisions.[16]

References

1. Lequesne LP, Lewis AAG. Postoperative water and sodium retention. *Lancet* 1953; **i**: 153–8.
2. Swaninathan N. Disorders of body fluids. *Surgery* 1994; **12**: 117–119.
3. Haas M, Glick SM. Radioimmuno-assayable plasma vasopressin associated with surgery. *Arch Surg* 1978; **113**: 597–600.

4. Viinimaki O, Kanto J, Maniskka M, Langas L. ADH concentration and premedication. *Br J Anaesthes* 1981; **53**: 1009–10.

5. Wu WH, Zbuzek UK. Vasopressin and anaesthesia in surgery. *Bull N Y Acad Med* 1982; **58**: 427–42.

6. Woods WGA, Forsling ML, Lequesne LP. Plasma arginine vasopressin levels and arterial pressure during open heart surgery. *Br J Surg* 1989; **76**: 29–32.

7. Moran WH, Miltenberger FW, Shu'Ayd WA, Zimmerman B. Relationship of antidiuretic hormone to surgical stress. *Surgery* 1964; **62**: 99–108.

8. Moran WH, Zimmerman B. Mechanism of antidiuretic hormone (ADH) control of importance to the surgical patient. *Surgery* 1967; **56**: 639–44.

9. Guyton AC. *Human Physiology and Mechanisms of Disease*. Philadelphia: WB Saunders, 1983.

10. Jones NF. Aspects of renal physiology. In: Marsh F (ed.) *Post Graduate Nephrology*. London: William Heinemann, 1985; 21–45.

11. Sagnella GA, McGregor GA Atrial natriuretic peptides. *Quart J Med* 1990; **77**: 101–7.

12. Cuthbertson DP. The disturbance of metabolism produced by bony and non-bony injury, with notes on certain abnormal conditions of bone. *Biochem J* 1930; **24**: 1244–63.

13. Cuthbertson DP. The metabolic response to injury and other related explorations in the field of protein metabolism: an autobiographical account. *Scot Med J* 1982; **27**: 158–71.

14. Clark RG. Fluid and electrolyte replacement. In: O'Higgins N, Chisholm GD, Williamson RCN (eds) *Principles of Surgical Care*. London: Butterworth-Heinemann, 1991: 29–37.

15. Guy AJ, Michaels JA, Flear CTG. Changes in the plasma sodium concentration after minor, moderate and major surgery. *Br J Surg* 1987; **74**: 1027–30.

16. Gennari FJ. Serum osmolality: uses and limitations. *Int Crit Care Digest* 1985; **4**: 41–4.

CHAPTER 2

Nutritional support in general surgery

BRENDAN J MORAN, STEPHEN J KARRAN

In all maladies those who are fat about the belly do best; it is bad to be thin and wasted. In every illness an eager application to food is good. The reverse is bad.

Hippocrates *c.* 460–370 BC

Introduction

General surgery is difficult to define but, with increasing subspecialization, is now predominantly surgery of the gastrointestinal tract. It is therefore not surprising that general surgeons have long had an interest in nutrition, as the gastrointestinal tract is responsible for assimilating the nutrients which are essential for survival. Indeed, general surgeons have been to the forefront in practically all the major developments in nutritional support through the ages. In 1790, John Hunter first described the use of a tube to feed a patient enterally in a paper entitled 'A case of paralysis of the muscles of deglutition cured by an artificial mode of conveying food and medicine into the stomach'. Almost a century later, the first successfully performed surgical gastrostomy was reported in 1876.[1] Whilst these were historic landmarks, another century

elapsed before the concept of 'nutritional support' was popularized. Nutritional support, as we know it today, has really emanated from the demonstration of the first successful use of total intravenous nutrition by Dudrick and colleagues in 1968.[2] This historic description of total parenteral nutrition (TPN) resulted from a realization that hypertonic nutrient solutions were best given into a large central vein. Whilst TPN has been a major advance (particularly in the management of seriously ill surgical patients) and is now widely available, the benefits of TPN are not universally accepted. The perceived cost and complications (including occasional mortality) have resulted in considerable doubt in some people's minds about the overall benefits of nutritional support, but in particular that of TPN. Whilst TPN is generally considered the 'flagship' of nutritional support, there are other aspects of nutrition which are of greater importance for the vast majority of patients. Nutritional support involves a whole range of activities, from prescribing oral intake of specialized (usually liquid) enteral feeds, to providing access to the available, functioning, gut (by enteral tubes and stomas) and by bypassing the intestinal tract in patients with intestinal failure using TPN. In this context the concept of 'intestinal failure' is useful. This is defined as a 'reduction in functioning gut mass below the minimum necessary for the adequate digestion and absorption of nutrients'.[3] The only absolute indication for TPN is intestinal failure and all other patients should be fed enterally, though this may require ingenious methods to gain access to the functioning gastrointestinal tract.

The fundamental aspects of nutritional support may be categorized into three specific areas:

1. determining which patients require nutritional support and whether they have a functioning gastrointestinal tract;
2. selection of the appropriate substrate;
3. obtaining and maintaining access for delivery of the substrate to the patient.

Selection of patients in need of nutritional support

The selection of patients for intervention has, in many ways, been the most contentious aspect of nutritional support. Indeed, little progress has been made in refining the selection criteria.

At the centre of the controversy lies the search for the optimal method(s) of nutritional assessment. The methods used to measure malnutrition fall into three broad groups:

1. methods to assess body composition, or anthropometric measurements;
2. methods which attempt to measure body function;
3. clinical assessment techniques.

Some of the methods used are outlined in Table 2.1. Whilst many of these can serve as indices of malnutrition, they may not necessarily indicate the need for adjuvant nutritional support, nor do they permit ready appraisal of the efficacy of any such nutritional therapy. Despite recent enthusiastic, though subsequently unsubstantiated, claims for individual techniques such as bioelectrical impedence analysis, the selection of candidates for nutritional support and the assessment of their nutritional status remains largely a clinical decision. This decision-making process has been called 'subjective global assessment' by Detsky and colleagues.[4] A more simplistic Southampton term which we have coined is the 'end-of-the-beddo-gram'. However, all clinical techniques entail the physician being aware of:

1. the symptoms and signs of malnutrition; though difficult to define, the obvious one is weight loss (though there can be a gross underestimation, in the presence of oedema and ascites, of the loss of

body cell mass) along with loss of muscle mass and muscle power.[5–8]
2. the prevailing disease and the likely effects of treatment;
3. the available methods and techniques for nutritional therapy.

Thus, when conclusions are made that clinical methods are best for nutritional assessment, it should be appreciated that these conclusions have been drawn by clinicians already possessing an awareness and interest in nutritional support. Any mechanism which helps to identify patients in need of nutritional support is to be encouraged, provided the limitations of any technique are recognized.

Another major unresolved issue has been the concept of perioperative nutritional support in the form of preoperative and/or postoperative feeding. It is generally acknowledged that grossly malnourished patients do not tolerate surgery well, and this has been noted in several studies since Studley[9] observed in 1936 that patients with > 20% weight loss had a 33% mortality following gastrectomy for peptic ulcer, compared with 3% in those with less than 20% weight loss. Common sense suggests that improving the nutritional status of malnourished individuals, ought to improve outcome following major surgery, but scientific evidence to confirm this has, to date, largely been lacking.

Perioperative TPN

A recent major study attempted to address the issue of the putative benefits of perioperative nutritional support in a randomized prospective study of 7–10 days preoperative TPN in malnourished patients who were undergoing either major abdominal or non-cardiac thoracic surgery.[10] The initial entry criteria excluded 3% of the patients who had an absolute requirement for TPN (i.e. they already had prolonged intestinal failure). Following randomization of 395 patients, approximately 5% were classified as being 'severely malnourished', and these patients appeared to derive benefit from TPN. In the remaining 95% who were less severely malnourished, however, TPN resulted in an increase in major complications, mainly infectious in nature, compared with controls. Not surprisingly, these data have been presented as suggesting that perioperative TPN has an unproven role and may even be detrimental.[11] However, this conclusion is misleading, as patients with intestinal failure in whom TPN was essential were, as mentioned, excluded. Furthermore, those with an intact functioning gastrointestinal tract (presumably practically all of those randomized) could (and should) have been more appropriately nourished with enteral nutrition.

Table 2.1 Some methods used for nutritional assessment

Anthropometric/body composition studies

1. Body weight – compared with *usual* for individual, or *ideal*
2. Muscle stores – mid-arm muscle circumference (MAMC)
3. Fat stores
   skinfold thickness
   triceps skinfold (TSF) thickness
   bioelectrical impedence analysis
4. Research methods (expensive and impractical)
   in vivo neutron activation analysis
   isotopic labelling studies

Functional tests

1. Muscle function
   grip strength
2. Immune function
   lymphocyte count
   delayed skin hypersensitivity

Biochemical markers

1. Albumin
2. Transferrin
3. Retinol binding protein
4. Thyroxin binding prealbumin

Clinical assessment

1. Dietary history
   dietary recall/prospective
2. History and examination by an experienced clinician

Suggested first choice for nutritional assessment

1. Body weight/height – baseline and weekly
2. Written documentation of intake and losses
3. Simple functional tests such as grip strength
4. Clinical examination – awareness of the presence or possibility of development of malnutrition
   i.e. 'End-of-the-beddogram'

Complex combination formulae such as the Prognostic Nutritional Index (PNI)[12] have not established themselves in general practice although they have value in research projects.

A realistic analysis of this study suggests that TPN is life saving in patients with intestinal failure and in addition improves the outcome in those who are severely malnourished. In borderline-to-severe malnutrition, however, the risks of TPN usually outweigh the benefits particularly in non-specialist units. As it was the risks of TPN that influenced the risk–benefit ratio, these results suggest that routine preoperative and perioperative enteral nutrition (being cheaper, safer and metabolically superior to TPN) may well prove beneficial. Again, however, evaluation is awaited. From a practical point of view though, TPN has the advantages of ease of control and monitoring nutritional input, whereas this is notoriously difficult for enteral nutrition.

Nutritional intervention-improving outcome

There is certainly evidence that enteral supplementation postoperatively can improve outcome. The study by Bastow *et al.* in 1983[13] looked at the effects, following surgical treatment of fractured neck of femur, in elderly malnourished women who were given 1000 ml (1000 kcal) per day of a liquid feed postoperatively via a fine-bore nasogastric tube as part of a randomized prospective study. In the supplemented group, there were significant improvements in the time to rehabilitation and the time to discharge from hospital.

A similar study by Delmi *et al.* simplified the method of nutrient administration.[14] They looked at the effects of an oral nutritional supplement (250 ml, 20 g protein, 254 kcal) for a mean of 32 days in a randomized prospective study of 59 elderly patients with femoral neck fractures. The median duration of hospital stay was significantly shorter in the supplemented group (24 vs 40 days). Clinical outcome was also significantly better in the supplemented group (59% favourable course vs 13% in the controls) during the stay in the convalescent hospital. The rates of deaths and complications were also significantly lower in supplemented patients (44 vs 87%) and these differences in morbidity and mortality were maintained at 6 months (40 vs 74%).

A recent study[15] looked at the effects of supplementing patients recovering from abdominal operations to ascertain if the beneficial results achieved in orthopaedic patients could be reproduced in general surgical patients. A total of 54 patients who were scheduled to undergo predetermined moderate-to-major gastrointestinal surgical procedures entered the study. They were randomly assigned to receive a normal ward diet postoperatively or the same diet supplemented *ad libitum* by an oral nutritional sip feed. The study period commenced when the surgical team indicated that the patient could have 'clear fluids'. Supplemented patients maintained their preoperative weight, whereas control patients had lost a significant amount of their preoperative weight by study day 3 (4.5 $\pm$ 1.2 kg), and by the time of discharge (4.7 $\pm$ 1.2 kg, p < 0.02). Preoperative muscle function, as evidenced by grip strength dynamometry decreased to a greater extent in the control than in the treatment group by study day 3 (14.6 $\pm$ 2.2 kPa vs 2.8 $\pm$ 2.4 kPa, p < 0.03) and by discharge (10.4 $\pm$ 3.1 kPa vs 0.1 $\pm$ 1.9 kPa, p < 0.03). There was a tendency towards fewer complications in the supplemented group but the small numbers did not allow definitive conclusions.

Nutritional intervention

The criteria for a nutritional intervention/surgical outcome study are outlined in Table 2.2. If one addresses these criteria, it can be seen why general surgical patients may be difficult to study compared with other groups of patients. The magnitude and extent of the surgical intervention varies considerably in general surgical patients and may, for example, be highly dependent on the skill of the surgeon, and the age of the patient. By contrast, patients with fractured neck of femur are generally elderly and commonly malnourished, have a relatively standard

Table 2.2 Criteria for nutritional intervention/surgical outcome study

1. Surgery with high morbidity/mortality
   Reduction clinically important
   Reduction statistically demonstrable
2. Malnutrition can be measured
   Objective measurements
   Measurements correlate with outcome
3. Patients free of non-nutritional factors increasing operative risk (e.g. skill of the surgeon)
4. Regimen of sufficient duration and intensity to alter measurements of nutrition-related risk
5. Acceptable
   Patients – acceptable discomfort/complications
   Administrators – cost
   Surgeon – delay/interference with surgery
6. Accurate recording
   Nutrient intake/retention
   Clinical outcome/complications

traumatic insult and a relatively standard surgical intervention that does not interfere directly with the gastrointestinal tract. Furthermore, time to rehabilitation (for example time to walking following surgical fixation of a fracture) is a more readily defined outcome measure than many of the measures which have been used to assess morbidity and mortality. General surgical patients suffer from different types and severity of disease, many of which interact in a complicated way with nutritional variables. The low mortality and morbidity following most general surgical procedures have resulted in difficulty in demonstrating clinical and statistically significant differences following any intervention. Furthermore, the difficulties in assessing patients' nutritional status have already been alluded to. Problems with accurately recording intake and retention have resulted in an overemphasis on TPN with its inherent cost and complications. Thus the fact that there is a paucity of scientific evidence to support perioperative nutritional intervention more likely reflects methodological problems rather than the absence of genuine benefit in carefully selected patients.

Selection of the appropriate substrate

The appropriate substrate for nutritional support depends primarily on the function of the gastrointestinal tract. Patients with prolonged intestinal failure require intravenous nutrients and it is now possible to maintain individuals indefinitely on parenteral nutrition in the form of home TPN. The past decade has seen an explosion of interest in the formulation of nutritional substrates and we are in the era of 'disease-specific nutrients' with, in general, excessive and unsubstantiated claims for their efficacy in clinical practice. This concept of 'disease-specific nutrients' extends to both enteral and parenteral feeds and much research has been channelled into the study of this area.

ENTERAL NUTRIENTS

All companies in the enteral nutrition market now produce a range of liquid enteral feeds. Enteral feeds can be used to completely nourish a patient (often via an enteral feeding tube), or may be used to supplement an inadequate oral intake (often by oral voluntary intake, or what is commonly referred to as 'sip feeding'. Enteral feeds may be broadly categorized by their composition into:

- polymeric or 'whole protein' feeds;
- elemental (also called predigested or 'chemically defined';
- disease-specific;
- modular or supplemental.

The polymeric, elemental and disease-specific feeds are 'complete' feeds containing a reasonable balance of macronutrients (protein, carbohydrate and fat) and micronutrients (vitamins and trace elements). In sufficient quantities, these feeds can be used as the sole nutrient intake for indefinite periods. Modular, or supplemental, feeds are incomplete and often are composed of one macronutrient only, such as carbohydrate, and thus should only be used to supplement and not replace a normal dietary intake.

POLYMERIC FEEDS

These feeds are made from whole protein (approximately 5 g nitrogen /l), usually contain 1 kcal /ml and are practically all lactose and gluten free. Thus 2.5 litres /day contains 2500 kcal and 12.5 g nitrogen. Variations containing 1.5–2 kcal /ml allow adequate nutrient intake in fluid-restricted patients. Similarly, polymeric feeds containing fibre are now available and have paradoxically been found to be useful in patients with either constipation or diarrhoea. Polymeric feeds are cheaper and relatively palatable compared with other feeds. They are available in various flavours and are the most acceptable type for oral consumption.

ELEMENTAL FEEDS

Elemental or 'chemically defined' feeds contain predigested protein in the form of oligopeptides or amino acids. These feeds are vigorously promoted by nutritional companies for use in patients with reduced absorptive capacity, such as patients with short bowel syndrome, and patients with pancreatic or small bowel mucosal disease. However, studies have shown that the majority of patients will absorb whole protein feeds.[16] There is some evidence, however, to support their use in a small proportion of patients such as those with severe pancreatic or Crohn's disease. The disadvantages of such feeds are their expense, their unpalatability (which almost invariably limits their use to tube feeding) and their increased osmolarity due to an increase in the number of particles per unit volume. This latter factor contributes to an increased incidence of complications such as abdominal bloating or diarrhoea.

DISEASE-SPECIFIC FEEDS

The production of disease-specific feeds stems from theoretical principles of nutrient metabolism and requirements in specific diseases or specific organ dysfunctional states. The majority of these feeds contain (with notable exceptions such as the respiratory specific feed) variations in both the type and amount of the amino acid content. Thus branched chain amino acid (BCAA) enriched solutions have been utilized in liver disease and trauma due to the reduced plasma levels of BCAA noted in individuals who were traumatized or had liver disease. These theoretical advantages, however have not been confirmed in clinical practice with conflicting and inconclusive evidence of nutritional benefits.[12] Current enthusiasm relates predominantly to the use of glutamine, and, to a lesser extent, arginine.

GLUTAMINE

Glutamine is considered a non-essential amino acid and is the most abundant amino acid in the free amino acid pool of the body. Glutamine plays an important role in the transport of nitrogen between tissues and is essential for renal ammoniagenesis. It is also the essential energy substrate for enterocytes, lymphocytes and other rapidly dividing cells.[18] Thus, glutamine-enriched solutions may be beneficial in practically any seriously ill patient. Indeed, it has been hypothesized that glutamine-enriched solutions might reduce the incidence of multiple organ failure which may be related to bacterial translocation from the intestinal lumen in patients immunocompromised by severe illness. Glutamine was not, until recently, included in TPN formulations due to its instability in solution. Research continues into both enteral and parenteral supplementation with glutamine-enriched solutions, but the early enthusiasm arising mainly from animal experimentation has not been substantiated by subsequent clinical studies. Other modulations of amino acid solutions, by arginine supplementation or the utilization of essential amino acid solutions (particularly in patients with renal disease) continue to generate interest. Clinical trials to date, however, have not demonstrated major advantages for these nutrients, individually or in combination.

PARENTERAL NUTRIENTS

The use of parenteral nutrients to nourish an individual totally is new and continues to undergo modification. The main constraints in intravenous nutritional support remain the hypertonicity of the nutrient solutions resulting in injury to the vein wall, and the chemical interactions involved when nutrients are mixed prior to infusion. Advances in venous access techniques have largely solved the former problem, though continuing research into the nutrient formulation itself has also helped to reduce venous thrombophlebitis. Nevertheless, chemical and pharmaceutical constraints continue to limit the supply of intravenous nutrients. A typical example is the amino acid glutamine, which, as mentioned, is unstable in solution, and therefore has not been added to intravenous solutions. Recent studies suggest that ill patients may have very large glutamine requirements which are vastly in excess of the patient's ability to synthesize glutamine endogenously. For this reason, attempts are currently being made to supply glutamine for TPN either as free glutamine added just prior to infusion, or as glutamine dipeptides. This approach has not yet been proven in clinical practice.

Other areas of interest include the use of medium chain triglycerides (MCT) which have theoretical advantages over conventional long chain triglyceride solutions in that MCT hydrolysis is not dependent upon lipoprotein lipase, and MCT metabolism is also independent of carnitine. Here again no clear clinical benefits have as yet been shown with these solutions.

METABOLIC MANIPULATION

It is now well established that nutrient provision in the severely ill, metabolically stressed patient may reduce but does not prevent body protein breakdown and nitrogen loss. A useful summary of the role of nutritional support is as a 'damage limitation' exercise. The metabolic response to injury and illness can be modified through cytokine manipulation and by hormonal therapy. Indeed, nutrients such as alternative fat solutions can alter both the cytokine and hormonal response. To date, however, no readily available nutrient manipulations have been shown to have obvious benefits in clinical practice. A recent area of interest has been the use of growth hormone to promote protein synthesis and considerable research is currently in progress.

CONCLUSION

The theoretical advantages and anecdotal reports of benefits of alterations in nutrient manipulations have, by and large, not been confirmed in clinical practice. The majority of individuals who require nutritional support are adequately treated with readily available standard enteral and parenteral substrates. Although selected patients may require specialized substrates, the indications for many of these expensive compounds are poorly defined.

Access techniques

The limiting factor in nutritional support of the vast majority of patients is the attainment and maintenance of safe access, whether it be to the venous system for TPN, or to the gut for enteral nutrition. General surgeons are commonly the most appropriately trained in the various technical skills of enteral and parenteral access.

Access routes for enteral nutrition

There have been three important developments in enteral access techniques during the past 20 years:

- fine-bore nasoenteral feeding tubes;
- needle catheter jejunostomy;
- percutaneous endoscopic gastronomy (PEG) (and jejunostomy).

FINE-BORE NASOENTERAL FEEDING TUBES

Although the term 'enteral feeding' usually refers to nasogastric feeding, feeding tubes can be passed nasally into the duodenum and jejunum. There is little justification for using a Ryles nasogastric (NG) tube for prolonged nutritional support, though an indwelling Ryles tube may be used for a short time (no more than a week).

Fine-bore polyurethane tubes are superior to Ryles tubes, because they are better tolerated by the patient, less likely to cause gastro-oesophageal reflux or ulceration and are easier to pass. They therefore can be inserted by patients themselves for supplemental overnight feeding. In addition, they can be positioned accurately by being passed over a guidewire, either under fluoroscopic or endoscopic control into the stomach, duodenum or upper jejunum.

The position of the tube should always be checked before starting feeding. In a patient who is alert and fully orientated this may be possible by injection of air and auscultation over the epigastrium. Aspiration of gastric contents and confirmation of acid pH provides further clinical evidence of correct positioning. If a patient has altered consciousness or has an impaired gag reflex an X-ray is needed to check the position of the tube.

Nasojejunal feeding may be successful in some instances where NG feeding has failed, for example in ventilated intensive care patients. Despite the advantages of fine-bore tubes they are still subject to most of the general complications of any feeding tube (Table 2.3).

There is a variety of tube designs. The tip of the tube may be modified by altering the shape of the opening or by adding weights, though manufacturers' claims for several of these design modifications have not been substantiated in clinical practice.[16]

Due to recent evidence that gastric stasis often prevents enteral feeding, particularly in the postoperative period, double lumen tubes are now available whereby one lumen is positioned in the stomach for nasogastric decompression and the distal lumen is positioned in the upper jejunum for feeding.

NEEDLE CATHETER JEJUNOSTOMY

In 1973 Delaney and colleagues[19] described a technique to obtain access to the jejunum via a catheter inserted at operation into the proximal jejunum. The catheter is tunnelled subserosally for several centimetres (using techniques similar to that for tunnelling a central venous catheter) prior to entering the lumen. A needle catheter jejunostomy is recommended for patients who are undergoing major upper gastrointestinal surgery e.g. oesophagectomy, gastrectomy or pancreatic surgery as these may be complicated postoperatively by a leaking gastrointestinal anastomosis. Such patients may require prolonged nutritional support and this is an ideal way to provide it.

A second laparotomy for complications of a primary procedure is another indication as postoperative nutritional support is essential.

The main complications of these catheters are tube displacement, intraperitoneal leakage and small bowel perforation, but these complications are minimized with modern catheter kits. Jejunostomy tubes can, however, only be inserted at laparotomy and their use, therefore, is limited.

PERCUTANEOUS ENDOSCOPIC GASTROSTOMY

Surgical gastronstmy has been one of the most common methods of providing long-term enteral support, but surgical techniques have recently been superceded. In 1980, Gauderer and Ponsky described the technique of percutaneous endoscopic gastrostomy (PEG) for performing a gastrostomy without a laparotomy.[20]

PEG technique

The gastroscope is passed into the stomach with the patient sedated and the patient is then rotated into the

Table 2.3   Complications

General complications of enteral or parenteral access

1. Failure to obtain access
2. Misplacement of the access device
3. Displacement
     partial resulting in extravasation
     total resulting in loss of access
4. Tube blockage
5. Tube fracture
6. Infection
     localized
     generalized

Common complications of enteral feeding tubes

1. Tube blockage – reduce incidence by flushing
     before and after the administration of medication
     before and after institution of intermittent feeding
     The optimal flushing solutions are:
         alcohol (e.g. 20 ml of sherry or whiskey) or
         carbonated mineral water (e.g. Coca-cola)
2. Tube displacement – especially nasoenteral tubes

Common complications of central venous catheters

1. Insertion
     failure (approx. 5–10% but generally underreported)
     malposition
     pneumothorax (approx 5% overall for subclavian lines)
     arterial stab (usually of no consequence if recognized and pressure applied)
2. In-use complications
     line sepsis reduced incidence by
         experienced insertor
         dedicated TPN line
         nursing protocols

supine position. The stomach is inflated with air and the light of the endoscope is directed anteriorly to transilluminate the anterior abdominal wall. Once transillumination is visualized, the area is infiltrated with local anaesthetic down to the lumen of the stomach. A cannula is passed through the skin into the inflated stomach and a thread or guidewire is passed through the cannula. The thread is grasped with a biopsy forceps or a snare, and the gastroscope, biopsy forceps and thread are then retrieved out of the mouth. The thread is used to pull the gastrostomy tube down the oesophagus into position. All current PEG kits contain detailed instructions which should be studied prior to commencing the procedure. Several variations of the original technique have been described including a radiological technique and all are detailed in a recent review.[21]

PERCUTANEOUS ENDOSCOPIC JEJUNOSTOMY

It is possible to pass a tube through the positioned PEG and guide the tube into the upper jejunum, a technique referred to as percutaneous endoscopic jejunostomy (PEJ). Jejunostomy is indicated for patients who suffer reflux resulting in aspiration pneumonia, which occurs in approximately 5% of patients with a PEG.

The main indications for PEG include:

1. acute neurological events (e.g. stroke or severe head injury) which necessitate supplemental feeding for prolonged periods;
2. chronic neurological diseases (e.g. multiple sclerosis and motor neurone disease) which affect swallowing;

3. patients with head and neck cancer (to facilitate surgery or radiotherapy), and
4. patients with growth failure or anorexia (e.g. cystic fibrosis and scleroderma).

There are few complications with PEG. A failure rate of 5% has been reported due to an inability to transilluminate the stomach, but this is usually in patients with previous extensive upper gastrointestinal surgery or patients with extreme obesity.[21]

It is often impossible to predict survival of the patient, but, as a general rule, a PEG should only be used if it is anticipated that enteral feeding will be required for at least 3 weeks. Other patients may best be treated with a fine-bore nasogastric tube, but the option of a PEG for even short-term palliation should not be completely ruled out. There have been recent reports of the use of skin-level gastrostomies or gastrostomy buttons in patients who require long-term gastrostomy feeding and already have an established gastrostomy tract. They are cosmetically more acceptable but are more difficult to utilize and require more expensive giving sets.

Parenteral access

Parenteral nutrition, by definition, involves intravenous feeding and therefore requires venous access. Indeed the historic breakthrough in the successful use of TPN resulted from an appreciation by Dudrick and Rhoads in 1968[2] that central venous access was required to infuse the hypertonic nutrients. More recently, however, there has been a shift in emphasis away from central access with renewed interest in peripheral vein parenteral nutrition. The peripheral route was strongly advocated by Blackburn and others in the 1970s for situations where full TPN may not have been required, or for temporary intravenous nutrition.[22]

PERIPHERAL VENOUS ACCESS

Novel solutions, with a lower osmolality, continue to be developed to allow peripheral TPN, which is certainly now feasible for 7–10 days and much longer in some institutions. However, some patients will be unsuitable for any form of peripheral vein feeding due to the unavailability of suitable peripheral veins. In those patients with suitable veins, the main limitation remains the hypertonicity of the solutions, caused particularly by the amino acid solutions, but also by the glucose required to provide a cost-effective energy supply. Recent changes in TPN practice such as the recognition of lower calorie requirements than were previously considered necessary, together with the availability of lipid emulsions and the use of all-in-one mixtures contained in a 3-litre bag, have all facilitated peripheral vein feeding. There have also been several recent reports of techniques to prolong the life of the peripheral vein. In order of clinical significance these are:

1. The use of very fine paediatric venous catheters which are threaded into a peripheral vein. These catheters have been very succesful when used by experts, but serious complications of TPN infusion (e.g. thrombophlebitis and infection) may still occur. Modern fine catheters are manufactured from either polyurethane or silicone, with polyurethene now being the preferred material.[23] An infusion pump is required to reduce the risk of blockage.
2. The application of glyceryl trinitrate (GTN) patches distal to the infusion site has been shown to prolong significantly the peripheral catheter infusion time. Side-effects from the GTN occasionally occur, such as dizziness and nausea.
3. Rotation of the site of the infusion every 24 – 48h is effective, but costly in terms of consumables, patient discomfort and medical and nursing time.
4. The addition of low dose heparin to the infusion at a concentration of 1000 units /l.
5. The use of both local and systemic anti-inflammatory agents, including low dose steroid additions to the infusion. Despite theoretical advantages, benefits in clinical practice have been disappointingly few.

These techniques can be combined to produce further prolongation of catheter life. A major continuing problem with peripheral parenteral nutrition is its lack of 'credibility' compared with central venous TPN. Unfortunately, medical and nursing staff do not apply the same degree of attention to detail in the care of a peripheral line. The best results are achieved in units with a multidisciplinary nutrition team where meticulous attention to protocols for TPN lines is applied. Thus, the peripheral cannula should be inserted under sterile conditions by an individual experienced with the technique, and should be cared for using protocols similar to those used in the care of central venous TPN catheters. The peripheral cannula should be used exclusively for TPN and carefully observed for the early signs of thrombophlebitis with replacement as necessary. Undoubtedly peripheral venous cannulation is safer than central venous cannulation, and peripheral parenteral nutrition is likely to form an increasing proportion of parenteral nutrition. Often more than 10 g nitrogen and 1500 kcal can be provided by peripheral vein feeding per 24 hours.

CENTRAL VENOUS ACCESS

Currently, central venous access is the optimal route for prolonged effective TPN. Techniques themselves have varied little, with the main routes being subclavian and internal jugular, by a direct cutdown or increasingly (even in children) by a blind percutaneous technique. An excellent review of the various techniques, and complications thereof, is to be found in the venous access section of a recent textbook.[24] It is salutary to note that the cumulative insertion complication rate for 12 987 catheters, in 14 large recently reported series, was approximately 10% with failure to cannulate, misplacement, pneumothorax and arterial puncture being the most common.

There is controversy as to whether percutaneous subclavian or jugular vein cannulation is safer and better. Subclavian catheters are easier to tunnel, more comfortable for the patient and have a lower incidence of catheter tip infection. The incidence of pneumothorax is, however, higher with subclavian catheters than with jugular cannulation.

Catheter sepsis in most institutions is unacceptably frequent in the absence of a dedicated nutrition team. In the hands of an experienced clinician the complication rate of subclavian catheters can be reduced significantly and this is therefore the preferred route, particularly for prolonged intravenous nutrition.

Techniques for central venous access have also been improved by recent developments such as new catheter materials, percutaneous catheters which incorporate a Dacron cuff together with the increasing use of double- and triple-lumen catheters for TPN.

CATHETER MATERIAL

Silicone and polyurethane are the only two materials suitable for prolonged central venous access. Polyurethane is stronger and has been reported to be less thrombogenic than silicone. Polyurethane catheters have a much larger lumen compared with the external diameter ratio (i.e. thin walled) and these facilitate percutaneous insertion and also reduce the amount of intravascular foreign material.

CATHETERS INCORPORATING A DACRON CUFF

A significant advance in central venous access for chemotherapy or prolonged TPN was the development and use of a catheter which incorporates a Dacron cuff by Hickman and colleagues in 1979 (still referred to as the 'Hickman' catheter). There have been several modifications of the cuffed silicone catheter, including the description of techniques for percutaneous insertion under local anaesthetic, and the family of such catheters is now referred to as 'Hickman–Broviac' catheters. The Dacron cuff is located subcutaneously and becomes incorporated in fibrous tissue which keeps the catheter in place and may reduce catheter infection.

The difficulty in attaching a Dacron cuff to polyurethane has recently been overcome with a report of the first clinical trial of prolonged use of a cuffed polyurethane catheter.[25]

Cuffed catheters are not required in most patients, however, and their use has generally been reserved for patients receiving chemotherapy or home parenteral nutrition.

MULTILUMEN CATHETERS FOR TPN

There is increasing interest in the use of multilumen catheters for TPN. Whilst this may be essential in some patients, such as small children undergoing intensive treatment with cytoxic chemotherapy, and advantageous in others, our own practice has generally been to avoid and indeed discourage the use of multilumen lines for TPN. Recent reports indicate that the incidence of infection may be greater with catheters possessing more than one lumen. Recent cumulative evidence from a review of 15 publications[24] indicated an increased incidence of sepsis in triple-lumen lines (168 cases in 1910 triple-lumen lines, compared with 56 cases in 1482 single-lumen lines, $p < 0.0001$).

However, this observation may be because the patients in whom multilumen catheters are generally used are invariably at greater risk of infection, due to more severe disease and because of greater immunosuppression. Furthermore, the requirement for, and frequency of, line usage is greater in patients with such multilumen lines. If these factors are taken into account, there may be no difference in the actual complication rates of single and multilumen lines. In either case, strict adherence to protocols minimizes the risk of infection.

HOME TPN

The principles of venous access for home TPN are similar to those for short- or medium-term venous access. In general, catheters which incorporate a Dacron cuff (Hickman–Broviac or the novel cuffed polyurethane catheter) are used and some centres advocate the use of subcutaneous implantable systems (such as those used for prolonged chemotherapy). Venous access is crucial in these patients and the complications of venous access are the leading cause of morbidity and mortality in this group of home TPN patients.

Conclusion

Nutritional support is now an essential part of the practice of general surgery.[26] Controversy continues as to the cost–benefit ratio of nutritional support, particularly for TPN. There are considerable difficulties in designing studies which can prove the assumed benefits, and many of the reported studies suffer from major flaws in study design. An explosion of interest in novel substrates has diverted attention from one of the key issues, which is the precise selection of patients who will actually benefit from adequate nutritional support.

All techniques for obtaining access to either the venous system or the gut have complications and some of these complications can be fatal. Operator experience minimizes but never abolishes such risk. Undoubtedly, a multidisciplinary nutritional support team plays a key role in the selection of patients for nutritional support, choosing appropriate substrates, deciding on the route of access, and then in the safe provision of maintenance and monitoring of enteral and parenteral feeding.

References

1. Gauderer MWL, Stellato TA. Gastrostomies: evolution, techniques, indications and complications. *Curr Probl Surg* 1986; **13**: 661–719.
2. Dudrick SJ, Wilmore DW, Vars HM, Rhoads JR. Long term total parenteral nutrition with growth, development and positive nitrogen balance. *Surgery* 1968; **64**: 134–42.
3. Fleming CR, Remington M. Intestinal failure. Nutrition and the surgical patient. In: Hill GL (ed.) *Clinical Surgery International*. Edinburgh: Churchill Livingstone, 1981: 219–35.
4. Detsky AS, McLoughlin JR, Baker JP *et al.* What is subjective global assessment of nutritional status? *J Parent Ent Nutrit* 1987; **11**: 8–13.
5. Klidjian AM, Archer TJ, Foster KG *et al.* Detection of dangerous malnutrition. *J Parent Ent Nutrit* 1982; **6**: 119–21.
6. Windsor JA, Hill GL. Weight loss with physiological impairment – basic indicator of surgical risk. *Ann Surg* 1988; **207**: 290–6.
7. Moore FD, Olesen KH, McMurrey JD *et al. The Body Cell Mass and its Supporting Environment.* Philadelphia: WB Saunders Co., 1963.
8. Shizgal HM. The effect of nutritional support on body composition. In: Karran SJ, Alberti KGMM (eds) *Practical Nutritional Support.* London: Pitman Medical, 1980: 190–200.
9. Studley HO. Percentage of weight loss: a basic indicator of surgical risk in patients with chronic peotic ulcer. *JAMA* 1936; **106**: 458–60.
10. Buzby GP. The Veterans Affairs Total Parenteral Nutrition Co-operative Study Group. Perioperative total parenteral nutrition in surgical patients *N Engl J Med* 1991; **325**: 525–32.
11. Detsky AS. Parenteral nutrition: is it helpfull? *N Engl J Med* 1991; **325**: 573–5.
12. Buzby GP, Mullen JL, Matthews DC *et al.* Prognostic Nutritional Index in gastrointestinal surgery. *Am J Surg* 1980; **139**: 160–1.
13. Bastow MD, Rawlings J, Allison SP. Benefits of supplementary tube feeding after fractured neck of femur: a randomized controlled trial. *Br Med J* 1983; **287**: 1589–92.
14. Delmi M, Rapin CH, Bengoa JM *et al.* Dietary supplementation in elderly patients with fractured neck of femur. *Lancet* 1990; **335**: 1013–16.
15. Rana SK, Bray J, Menzies–Gow J *et al.* Short term benefits of post-operative oral dietary supplements in surgical patients. *Clin Nutr* 1992; **11**: 337–44.
16. Payne-James J, Silk DBA. Enteral nutrition: background, indications and management. *Ballières Clin Gastroenterol* 1988; **2**: 825–47.
17. Morgan MY. Branched chain amino acids in the management of chronic liver disease. Facts and fantasies. *J Hepatol* 1990; **11**: 133–41.
18. Dudrick PS, Souba WW. The role of glutamine in nutrition. *Curr Opin Gastroenterol* 1991; **7**: 306–11.
19. Delaney HM, Carnevale NJ, Garvey JW. Jejunostony by a needle catheter technique. *Surgery* 1973; **73**: 768–80.
20. Gauderer MWL, Ponsky JL. Izant RJ. Gastrostomy without a laparotomy: a percutaneous endoscopic technique for feeding gastrostomy. *J Pediatr Surg* 1980; **15**: 872–5.
21. Moran BJ, Taylor MB, Johnson CD. Percutaneous endoscopic gastrostomy: a review. *Br J Surg* 1990; **77**: 858–62.
22. Karran SJ, Alberti KGMM. *Practical Nutritional Support.* London: Pitman Medical, 1980.
23. Everitt NJ, Madan M, Alexander DJ, McMahon MJ. Finebore rubber and polyurethane catheters for the delivery of complete intravenous nutrition. *Clin Nutr* 1993; **12**: 261–5.
24. Grant JP. *Handbook of Total Parenteral Nutrition,* 2nd edn. Philadelphia, London: WB Saunders, 1992.
25. Moran BJ, Sutton GLJ, Karran SJ. Clinical evaluation and long-term usage of a new cuffed polyurethane catheter for central venous access. *Ann Roy Coll Surg Engl* 1992; **74**: 426–9.
26. Moran BJ, Jackson AA. Perioperative nutritional support. *Br J Surg* 1993; **80**: 4–5.

CHAPTER 3

Wound and tissue healing and sutures

CHRIS VICKERY, KEITH HARDING, DAVID LEAPER

Historical note

Interest in wound healing and its management has been well documented. The book written by Guido Majno, *The Healing Hand: Man and Wound in the Ancient World*, is a remarkable reference book of past concepts and rituals.[1] Forrest has made a similar in-depth study of the development of wound treatments used during the rise of our civilization.[2]

The fossil record has revealed that 'patients' survived skull trepanation (presumably undertaken for some rite or other) as there is clear evidence of post 'operative' healing. Some of the first written documents describe that the Assyrians, Egyptians, Greeks and Romans were well versed in wound care (again usually post-traumatic). Sutures, topical antimicrobials and salves have all been described with working protocols. Hippocrates advocated the use of wine and vinegar to cleanse open wounds and clearly understood the value of delayed primary closure to prevent infection. Celsus introduced a scientific

approach to healing and described the 'calor, rubor, dolor et tumor' of inflammation. His close contemporary Galen taught, however, that localization of infection heralded a healing response ('pus bonum et laudabile') which was misinterpreted by many as meaning that suppuration needed to be induced in all wounds before they could heal. John Hunter, many centuries later, believed that there were two types of inflammation – adhesive, which was the key to healing after surgery, and suppurative which led to infection.

The middle part of the last century recognized, with the development of microscopy, the cellular basis of healing and the host response to infection,[3] and the cause of infection through the work of Semmelweis, Pasteur and Lister. The advent of antiseptic surgery soon gave way to modern aseptic surgery. Lister and Moynihan helped develop the early catgut sutures and laid down many of the foundations of modern surgery. They, and Halstead in the United States, preached the need for meticulous technique in operative surgery. The advent of antibiotics has helped to remove infection as a scourge of surgery, particularly in their use as prophylaxis to protect wounded tissues from infection when the host defence has not been mobilized – the decisive period.[4] The optimal moist wound environment for healing has also been described,[5] and there are increasing numbers of dressings and devices available which help to promote this.

Wound healing

In our evolution we have had to pay a price for our specialization in that we cannot regenerate most organs or appendages after damage. More primitive life forms, such as amphibia, can regenerate whole digits or limbs from totipotent cells which form in the wound.[6] The highly developed mammals, including man, require rapid restoration of defects caused by wounding. This cannot be achieved by regeneration but by repair. We can regenerate epithelial surfaces but not connective tissues. The repair sequence fills connective tissue defects by scar tissue, principally collagen, which produces poor quality connective tissue compared with unwounded tissues. Any damaged tissue, except teeth, can heal by repair.

It has been recognized that wounds inflicted on a mammalian fetus can heal without a scar. It has been suggested that this is because the fetus is in a protected environment and therefore does not require rapid healing. Following the need for rapid healing the price to be paid is an increase in scar formation. To identify the genetic codes, recombinant DNA techniques may allow control of healing by regeneration in the adult. This would have obvious benefit for tissues where scar tissue causes clinical complications.

Sequence of events following wounding

Following trauma a clotting cascade follows which involves formation of thrombin and fibrin through both the intrinsic and extrinsic pathways of coagulation.[7] At the same time the imbalance of platelet thromboxane A_2 and vessel intimal prostacyclin I_2 following exposure of Type IV and V collagen through wounding leads to platelet coagulation. Combined with vessel contraction mediated by release of serotonin, histamine and kinins, together with neural reflexes, haemorrhage may be controlled with the formation of clot. Other important plasma proteins, particularly fibronectin, appear in the coagulum of the wound.

The fibrinolytic, clotting and complement cascades lead to the acute inflammatory response. There is an increased vascular permeability at the edge of the wound with exudation of plasma constituents. Polymorphonuclear neutrophils (PMNs) marginate in adjacent vessels with adherence to the endothelial cell walls, and pass into the wound space by diapedesis within minutes of wounding. This chemotaxis is mediated by many factors, including the acute inflammatory protein fibronectin,[8] serotonin and arachidonic acid metabolites (prostaglandins) and complement-mediated cytokines.[9,10] Macrophages also appear in the wound by the second or third day after wounding. In time the macrophages further stimulate the repair sequence through release of cytokine mediators (principally interleukins IL-1, IL-2, IL-6, IL-8 and tumour necrosis factor [TNF]).[11] Many growth factors are released by macrophages, lymphocytes and activated platelets.[12,13] The most important are platelet-derived growth factor (PDGF),[14] fibroblast growth factor (FGF), epidermal growth factor (EGF),[15] transforming growth factor (TGF-α[15] and β[16]) and insulin-like growth factor (IGF-1 and 2). The response to cytokines and growth factors is a complex cascade and is mediated at very low concentrations.

Polymorphonuclear neutrophils (through release of free radicals and enzymes), lymphocytes (through B- and T-cell effector mechanisms), together with non-specific opsonization begin to exert microbicidal activity if there is contamination in the wound.

The cytokines and growth factors stimulate the formation of granulation tissue which is the precursor of tissue repair.[17] Through angiogenic factors endothelial sprouts grow from capillaries adjacent to the wound which later canalize to bring oxygen and nutrients to the wound edge. A further stimulus for this is the hypoxia of the dead space in the wound (the hypoxic drive to healing). The vascularity of a healing open wound is clear to the naked eye but several experimental models have been devised to study this in detail, and under direct vision e.g. the chick allantoic membrane, rabbit ear chamber, hamster cheek pouch and corneal pocket.

Fibroblasts are similarly stimulated by feedback mechanisms of the cytokines and growth factors (which act as mitogens) to divide and mature. They produce the proteins and fibres of the extracellular matrix. On electron microscopy, fibroblasts can be seen to produce contractile fibrils which are made up of proteins such as actin and myosin. These fibrils aid in wound closure by wound contraction, and the specialized cell producing them has been called the myofibroblast. The exact mode of action is still being debated in that fibroblasts become modified to become myofibroblasts that contract, or, by the use of contracting filaments and active locomotion of the fibroblasts, contraction occurs. This contraction can be directly visualized if fibroblasts are seeded on to a collagen lattice where the rate of contraction can be measured. Wounds healing by secondary intention are closed to a large extent by this process of contraction and can result in more functional and cosmetically acceptable scars (compared with thin split thickness skin grafts). Tensile strength (a traditional method for measuring healing) begins to increase rapidly by the fourth or fifth day after wounding in animal models. At the same time damaged extracellular matrix and collagen is broken down by collagenases and other proteinases in the wound area. Fibroblasts in the wound begin to synthesize collagen and extrude the high proline and hydroxyproline-containing collagen protein.[17,18] The three peptide α-chains of collagen form a triple helix and begin to cross-link to achieve a greatly increased tensile strength. The balance of collagen lysis and synthesis in some healing tissues is a fine one (in the colon for example) and the risk of wound failure (such as anastomotic leak) has to be avoided by the use of appropriate suture or staple closure during this latent period. The fibroblasts also secrete other proteins and fibres important in the formation of the extracellular matrix. Following the rapid ingrowth of blood vessels there is regression of angiogenesis as the scar matures and the scar tissues turn white and become relatively avascular.

Epithelialization also has a part to play in wound closure. Cytokines and growth factors mediate the response of an initial mitotic activity in the basal epithelial cells adjacent to the wound.[9] Collagen and fibronectin stimulate IL-1, EGF, PDGF and TGF-α and β to mediate cell division and growth, then migration across the healing connective tissue defect beneath. In a sutured wound this migration is minimal and ceases when migrating cells meet in the centre of the wound. Cells then adhere to the basement membrane zone.

Abnormal healing

Excessive scar tissue can cause complications, but in some instances can be beneficial. Harold Ellis regarded peritoneal adhesions as 'the surgeon's friend' if they prevented anastomotic leakage. Excessive fibrosis caused by ischaemia and infection may lead to contractures (in burns, or in Dupuytren's contracture which has an obscure aetiology). Persistent damage in the liver from toxins or alcohol may lead to excessive formation of fibrous tissue (cirrhosis) following healing, with the complication of compromise of the portal vascular system and portal hypertension. Excessive fibrous adhesions in the peritoneum can obstruct or strangulate bowel and may cause stenosis after healing of an anastomotic leak. Fibrotic capsulation of a breast implant or tendon repair are further examples of problems of excessive fibrotic tissue forming as a response to healing.

Hypertrophic scars appear in skin as heaped-up vascular scar tissue which does not extend beyond the wound edge. Keloid scars may have a similar aetiology but extend beyond the scar and are difficult to treat as excision may worsen the extent of the keloid. The abnormal response is comprised of increased numbers and altered function of cells. The extracellular matrix has an increased metabolic activity, and there is failure of normal tissue remodelling. There may be cosmetic implications and symptomatic complications. The number of treatment options, including topical steroids, radiotherapy and pressure (which may all improve keloids), testifies to the fact that few are completely effective.

Factors which influence tissue healing

INFECTION AND FOREIGN TISSUE

Infection can delay healing and in extreme circumstances (Fournier's gangrene or Meleney's synergistic hospital gangrene – necrotizing fasciitis) can cause widespread tissue destruction beyond a wound. Lesser degrees of infection still occur in 5–7% of surgical procedures (depending on contamination at operation) and remain one of the major reasons for a delay in return home postoperatively and for impaired wound healing. Infection directly modulates the immune system and may delay healing by influencing macrophages, PMNs and lymphocytes with a resultant change in cytokine and growth factor sequences. In the metabolic response to trauma there may be delays in healing related to excessive hormonal response to tissue damage. This may become more extreme in systemic inflammatory response syndrome and multiple organ dysfunction syndrome which follow severe trauma, burns, pancreatitis and uncontrolled infection. Healing after surgery in these circumstances is impaired.

NUTRITION

In addition to a requirement for an adequate calorie intake, which may be three to four times greater than normal in severe burns, for example, protein deficiency produces a depressed antibody response, immunodeficiency and an impaired response to infection. Severely ill surgical patients may not respond to hyperalimentation, particularly by the parenteral route. (See also Chapter 2.) Administration of branched chain and sulphur-containing essential amino acids may help reverse the catabolic state. Enteral feeding with alanine, glutamine and polyunsaturated fatty acids (such as ω_3 fatty acids) prevents bacterial gut colonization and translocation which in turn helps control systemic sepsis, organ failure and impaired wound healing. The extra use of vitamins C and A, and trace elements such as zinc, is controversial in promotion of surgical wound healing. In patients on long-term parenteral feeding they should be considered and deficiency corrected if present.

METABOLIC DISEASES

Metabolic diseases such as diabetes mellitus, uraemia and jaundice have all been shown experimentally to impair wound healing. Such work is based on animal studies, cell culture of keratinocytes and fibroblasts and the acquisition of new protein (usually collagen assessed as hydroxyproline) in implanted mesh sponge or tubes. Measuring tensile strength, either on a tensiometer or as anastomotic bursting pressure, has also shown impairment of healing in these metabolic diseases.

ISCHAEMIA

Impaired blood supply to a healing wound may follow systemic shock or local damage to blood supply. Poor tissue perfusion can be measured clinically directly using flowmeters (such as the laser Doppler), or by the use of tonometry (trans- or subcutaneous oxygen meters).[19] Local impairment of blood supply can result from poor surgical technique but the true extent of this is difficult to quantify.

CONCURRENT THERAPY

It is well established in clinical trials that chemotherapy, radiotherapy and immunosuppression following steroid use, AIDS or malignancy can impair healing. Recognition of immunosuppression can easily be measured through tests of immunological function and experimental methods can identify the stage of healing which is affected.

Practical considerations

Incised surgical wounds (or clean fresh incised traumatic wounds which are not associated with contamination or devitalized tissue) can be closed with sutures, staples or tissue adhesives. Careful apposition of tissues allows healing by primary intention. Attention to technical factors and surgical skill gives cosmetically acceptable scars in skin, or functional restoration in tissues such as nerve or tendon. Bowel anastomosis needs simple apposition of bowel ends; many different techniques exist that use a wide range of sutures or staples. The most likely cause of leakage is impaired blood supply to the anastomoses. Vascular arterial anastomosis demands a leak-proof technique using a permanent suture. These variations in approach are considered in the next section.

Contaminated or devitalized traumatic wounds need debridement and should not be sutured primarily. Once clean they can be closed by secondary (or delayed primary) suture. Waiting for clean granulation tissue and control of infection may take several days. Open non-cavity wounds can be grafted with split thickness skin or flaps. Allowing a wound to close by secondary intention takes longer but the cosmetic effect can be more acceptable by allowing wound contraction to occur. Antibiotics are used when there is clear local or systemic evidence of tissue infection. There is good evidence that surgical wounds which are not infected, but are heavily contaminated, can be safely closed by primary suture provided broad-spectrum prophylactic antibiotics are given empirically. This form of treatment remains controversial; after perforated appendicitis wounds are generally treated by secondary closure in North America, but by primary closure (with antibiotic prophylaxis) in the UK. (See also Chapter 5.)

Sutures

Sutures are used for closing wounds in all body tissues and are the most frequently implanted foreign materials.[20] The history of suture development details the use of a variety of naturally occurring materials, but in more recent times technology has allowed for the 'tailor-made' development of suture materials with specific attributes. Despite this, a single ideal suture, suitable for every surgical situation still does not exist and, therefore, it is important that surgeons have an understanding of the different types of suture materials available and when and where to use them.

Evidence of suturing wounds dates back to between 5000 and 3000 BC with the invention of eyed needles made of bone. Early references to suture materials were made in the Caraka Samhita written 3000 years ago and in the Sushruta Samhita 2500 years ago in which the use of plaited horsehair, cotton, leather strips and tree bark fibres was described for closing wounds. Primitive men used cautery and tendon strip ligatures to control bleeding and closed wounds with acacia thorns and the powerful jaws of (decapitated) ants.[21]

The Edwin Smith papyrus details Egyptian wound closure techniques dating back to 1600 BC.[1] The treatment of a gash – 'You should draw together for him his gash with stitching. You should bind it with fresh meat for the first day. If you find that wound open and its stitching loose you should draw together for him the gash with two strips of linen.' Linen strips coated with resin or with an adhesive mixture of honey and flour appeared in Ancient Egyptian medicine, as forerunners of our modern-day skin closure tapes ('steristrips').[22]

Cornelius Celsus suggested that sutures should be soft (wool or linen) and not overtwisted. He also described fibulae, or small metal clips, similar to the Michel clips of today. Galen repaired the severed tendons of gladiators with sutures, giving some hope for recovery of function where previously there had been only paralysis. He used linen, silk and catgut sutures. Avicenna, in about 920 AD, realized that in the presence of gross infection, traditional materials such as linen thread broke down rapidly. He used pigs' bristles as an alternative. Gold wire sutures were introduced by Fabricius in 1550 and silver wire by Marion Sims in 1850. Today, stainless steel wire sutures are used in certain types of surgery,

particularly sternotomy closure after cardiovascular surgery. Silk sutures gained popularity, along with waxed thread, in the eighteenth century, although catgut was still probably the material most often used. In the nineteenth century Joseph Lister stored catgut in a solution of olive oil and carbolic acid, and to improve its handling characteristics he chromicized catgut and found the unexpected additional benefit of delayed suture absorption.

Since the mid-twentieth century, technological advances have produced a range of synthetic absorbable and non-absorbable materials for use as sutures, in braided and monofilament forms. Both synthetic and natural sutures benefited from advances made in the textile industry which allowed for braiding of suture material and coating of sutures with a variety of agents (wax, liquid paraffin, silicone, polytetrafluoroethylene and polybutylate) to improve handling and knotting capabilities and also to reduce the infective potential through the capillarity of suture interstices.

Coupled with the development of suture materials has gone the development of the eyeless atraumatic needle, in routine use since the 1950s. Metal used in needle manufacture has progressed from carbon steel (often chromicized against rust) to modern stainless steel. A variety of needle tips has been fashioned for use in different tissues: triangular-tipped (cutting) needles for easy penetration; round-bodied needles for minimal trauma. Needle sizes and shapes are now available in a wide range, with needles as small as 30 μm in diameter, for microvascular work, being barely visible to the naked eye (Table 3.1).

Table 3.1 Comparative gauges of suture materials

Metric no. (diam. in mm × 10)	Catgut/collagen	Non-absorbables, synthetic absorbables
0.1	–	–
0.2	–	10/0
0.3	–	9/0
0.3	–	8/0
0.4	–	8/0
0.5	8/0	7/0
0.7	7/0	6/0
1.0	6/0	5/0
1.5	5/0	4/0
2.0	4/0	3/0
3.0	3/0	2/0
3.5	2/0	0
4.0	0	1
5.0	1	2
6.0	2	3 & 4
7.0	3	5
8.0	4	5

Wound healing and the choice of suture

The purpose of a suture is to hold tissue in apposition until healing is sufficient for the continued presence of the suture to be unnecessary. An 'ideal' suture, for all applications, does not exist and the choice of suture material is always, therefore, something of a compromise. When choosing a suture, consideration must be given to the strength of the tissue to be sutured, its healing rate and healing capacity. This will largely decide the size of the suture required and whether the material should be absorbable or non-absorbable.

Wounds in the first few days of healing have little intrinsic strength; indeed, tissue strength is lost within 0.5 cm of the wound edges due to the action of collagenases. Adequate support of the wound with sutures placed beyond this area of tissue reaction is essential during this period.[23,24] Gradually, the tensile strength of the healing tissue increases and suture support becomes less important. Different tissues heal at different rates, but even a year or more after wounding most wounds will only have about 70% of tensile strength of the unwounded tissue.[25] In addition, several factors can confound the healing process; in particular, infection, haematoma, steroids and coexisting disease causing immune incompetence, malnourishment and cachexia.

Tissues which heal rapidly and are not under mechanical stress, can be sutured with absorbable sutures (as in gastrointestinal surgery). Tissues which are exposed to disrupting forces during healing, or heal slowly, require prolonged support and generally require suturing with non-absorbable suture material (as in cardiac and vascular surgery and abdominal wall closure). Non-absorbable sutures should be avoided in bile duct and ureteric surgery because they can act as a nidus for stone formation.

Skin sutures need to be left *in situ* for different periods of time depending on the area of the body which has been sutured. The skin of the face and neck heals rapidly and sutures can be removed after 4–6 days. In this short time the 'tram-line' scars will not develop and therefore sutures may be placed in an interrupted fashion and still achieve excellent cosmetic results. Most of the skin elsewhere on the body requires suture support for 8–14 days to achieve adequate wound healing. Sutures left as long as this, may leave 'tram-line' scars unless a subcuticular technique is used (Fig. 3.1). Skin may be sutured with absorbable materials, thereby avoiding the need for suture removal. This can be particularly useful in children, but a subcuticular rather than

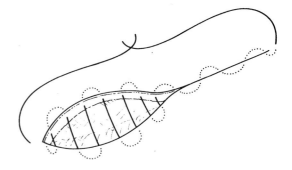

Fig. 3.1 Technique of subcuticular suture (using absorbable or non-absorbable material) which gives cosmetically acceptable scars in skin.

an interrupted technique should be used to minimize scarring. Synthetic, monofilament, non-absorbable sutures are the most popular for skin closure and give the best cosmetic results.

Sutures are foreign bodies and although modern synthetic monofilament sutures are almost completely inert, braided and 'natural' sutures can excite a significant inflammatory response. Bacteria can be difficult, or impossible, to eradicate once colonization of the suture or knot interstices has occurred. This can predispose to wound infection, with abscess and sinus formation, wound dehiscence and incisional hernias. It is known that the number of bacteria required to produce infection can be reduced by 10^4/g tissue in the presence of a silk suture.[26] Sutures should be avoided or used with caution in the presence of established infection or severe contamination, when healing by secondary intention, or delayed primary suture, should be employed.

In practice, much larger sutures are usually used than are strictly necessary, in relation to the breaking strengths of the tissues.[27] Smaller sutures have smaller needles and these may not allow adequate tissue 'bites' to be taken. They are also more difficult to handle and are often more expensive than larger, more popular sutures. In some situations, notably ophthalmology, microvascular surgery and plastic surgery, fine sutures are routinely employed.

Sutures are sterilized by manufacturers using ethylene oxide (Vicryl ®, Dexon ®, PDS ®, linen, Prolene ®) or gamma irradiation (catgut, silk, Nylon, Dacron ®). Steel sutures may be sterilized by autoclave, as can linen, Nylon, Dacron and Prolene sutures as an alternative. (See also Chapter 5.)

Suture classification

1. absorbable or non-absorbable;
2. natural or synthetic;
3. monofilament or multifilament (twisted or braided);
4. dyed or undyed;
5. coated or uncoated.

Ideally, sutures should disappear when their job is done.[28] However, variable and often rapid loss of the tensile strength of absorbable suture materials makes them an unreliable choice when suturing tissues which are subjected to significant mechanical stress (e.g. abdominal wall closure), or in situations in which premature suture failure would have immediate and catastrophic consequences (e.g. vascular surgery). The majority of acute wound failures are due to the 'cutting out' of intact sutures from tissues, rather than suture or knot failure and this can result following the use of any suture type. However, in general, absorbable materials excite a greater tissue reaction than non-absorbable sutures and this augmented inflammatory response may weaken the integrity of the tissue bite. While most cases of 'burst abdomen' are probably due to cutting out of intact sutures,[29] premature suture failure can be responsible for late wound weakness and herniation.[30] There are enthusiasts for abdominal wall mass closure with synthetic absorbable materials, but the risks of suture (and wound) failure, particularly in situations of impaired healing, probably outweigh the disadvantages of using synthetic non-absorbable sutures (persistence of foreign material and irritation from knots).

Monofilament sutures have no interstices in which to lodge bacteria but they are more difficult to handle and require more throws to each knot for security than braided sutures. Monofilament sutures can be absorbable (e.g. polydioxanone – PDS) or non-absorbable (e.g. polypropylene – Prolene).

Multifilament sutures are generally easier to handle, with greater knot security, but do allow capillarity and interstitial bacterial colonization.[26] This can increase the risk of wound infection, particularly with non-absorbable sutures. Multifilament sutures can be absorbable (e.g. polyglactin – Vicryl) or non-absorbable (e.g. silk).

Sutures are dyed in a variety of colours to enhance their visibility during surgery. Dyes do not affect the absorption characteristics of the suture.

Sutures are coated (or treated) with a variety of agents to improve general handling and passage through the tissues (e.g. poloxamer 188 on Dexon), to occlude suture interstices (e.g. wax on silk) and to retard absorption (e.g. chrome tanning of catgut).

Tables 3.2 and 3.3 list the properties and uses of different suture materials.

Needles

Needles (Fig. 3.2) may be curved or straight, and depending on size may be used with needle holders or used as 'hand needles'. Hand needles risk 'needle-stick' injury and their use should be discouraged, particularly when there is a risk of viral transmission. There is a variety of different curvatures available, from 1/4 circle, through 3/8, 1/2 and 5/8 circle to 'J-needles' and compound curved needles. Needles may be 'eyed', requiring the suture to be threaded, or 'autraumatic' with the needle swaged on to the suture. Needle points and cross-section can be variable. They may be 'round-bodied' in cross-section and only sharp at the tip. These are used for suturing bowel, fat, peritoneum and other soft tissues, and separate tissues rather than cutting them. 'Taper-cut' needles also have a round body, but are sharpened on several sides towards the tip allowing the needle to cut through tissues while keeping the needle tract size to a minimum. These are particularly useful in cardiac and vascular procedures. 'Cutting needles' have a variety of point shapes designed for different surgical uses. These may be flattened and 'sword-like', or triangular in cross-section with the apex cutting edge on the inside of the needle curvature (conventional cutting), or on the outside of the needle curvature (reverse cutting). Cutting needles are designed for ease of penetration of tough or dense tissues, including skin. They cut, rather than separate tissues and can, therefore, cause local bleeding by cutting blood vessels. Other needle modifications include 'blunt' needles for suturing friable tissues, e.g. the liver and 'heavy' needles which are particularly strong and bear little resemblance to the size of the suture material.

Use of surgical needles

Needle holders of an appropriate size for the suture concerned should be used; needle holders are easily damaged by needles that are too large. The needle should be grasped on the flattened part of the shank, if present, for the best grip and to prevent slippage and rotation. If the needle does not have a flattened part then it should be grasped at a point about one-third of the needle length from the swaged end. The needle should not be grasped too near its attachment with the suture material and never by its point as this will distort or blunt it.

Table 3.2 Suture materials in common use in surgery – non-absorbable

Suture	Types	Raw material	Tensile strength retention *in vivo*	Absorption rate	Tissue reaction	Contraindications	Frequent uses	How supplied
Silk	Braided or twisted multifilament. Dyed or undyed. Coated or uncoated (with wax or silicone).	Natural protein. Raw silk from silkworm.	Loses 20% when wet; 80–100% lost by 6 months.	Fibrous encapsulation in body at 2–3 weeks. Absorbed slowly over 1–2 years.	Moderate to high.	Not for use with vascular prostheses or in tissues requiring prolonged approximation under stress. Risk of infection and tissue reaction make silk unsuitable for routine skin closure.	Ligation and suturing where long-term tissue support is unnecessary.	10/0–2 with needles. 4/0–1 without needles.
Linen	Twisted.	Long staple flax fibres.	Stronger when wet. Loses 50% at 6 months; 30% remains at 2 years.	Non-absorbable. Remains encapsulated in body tissues.	Moderate.	Not advised for use with vascular prostheses.	Ligation and suturing in gastrointestinal surgery. No longer in common use in most centres.	3/0–1 with needles. 3/0–1 without needles.
Surgical steel	Monofilament. Multifilament.	An alloy of iron, nickel and chromium.	Indefinite.	Non-absorbable. Remains encapsulated in body tissues.	Minimal.	Should not be used in conjunction with prosthesis of different metal.	Closure of sternotomy wounds. Previously found favour for tendon and hernia repairs.	Monofilament: 5/0–5 with needles. Multifilament: 5/0–3/0 with needles.
Nylon® a (Ethilon® a Dermalon® b Nurolon® a)	Monofilament. Braided multifilament. Dyed or undyed.	Polyamide polymer.	Loses 15–20% per year.	Degrades at approx. 15–20% per year.	Low.	None.	General surgical use; e.g. skin closure, abdominal wall mass closure, hernia repair. Plastic surgery, neurosurgery, microsurgery, ophthalmic surgery.	Monofilament: 11/0–2 with needles (including loops in some sizes); 4/0–2 without needles. Multifilament: 6/0–2 with needles; 3/0–1 without needles.

Material	Structure	Composition	Absorption	Tissue reaction		Uses	Sizes
Polyester (Ethibond®[a] Tecron®[b] Mersilene®[a] Dacron®[b])	Monofilament. Braided multifilament. Dyed or undyed. Coated (polybutylate or silicone) or uncoated.	Polyester polyethylene terephthalate.	Indefinite.	Non-absorbable. Remains encapsulated in body tissues.	Low.	None. Cardiovascular, ophthalmic, plastic and general surgery.	Monofilament: (Ophthalmic) 11/10; 10/0 with needles. Multifilament: 5/0–1 with needles. Ethibond®[a] 7/0–5 with needles.
Polybutester (Novafil®[b])	Monofilament. Dyed or undyed.	Polybutylene terephthalate and polytetramethylene ether glycol.	Indefinite.	Non-absorbable. Remains encapsulated in body tissues.	Low.	None. Exhibits a degree of elasticity. Particularly favoured for use in plastic surgery.	7/0–1 with needles.
Polypropylene (Prolene®[a])	Monofilament. Dyed or undyed.	Polymer of propylene.	Indefinite.	Non-absorbable. Remains encapsulated in body tissues.	Low.	None. Cardiovascular surgery, plastic surgery, ophthalmic surgery, general surgical subcuticular skin closure.	10/0–1 with needles.

[a] Ethicon trademark.
[b] Davis and Geck trademark.

Table 3.3 Suture materials in common use in surgery– absorbable

Suture	Types	Raw material	Tensile strength retention *in vivo*	Absorption rate	Tissue reaction	Contraindications	Frequent uses	How supplied
Catgut	Plain	Collagen derived from healthy mammals.	Lost within 7–10 days. Marked patient variability.	Phagocytosis and enzymatic degradation within 70 days.	High.	Not for use in tissues which heal slowly and require prolonged support.	Ligate superficial vessels, suture subcutaneous tissues, stomas and other tissues that heal rapidly. Ophthalmic surgery.	6/0–1 with needles; 4/0–3 without needles.
Catgut	Chromic	Collagen derived from healthy mammals. Tanned with chromium salts to improve handling and to resist degradation in tissue.	Lost within 21–28 days. Marked patient variability.	Phagocytosis and enzymatic degradation within 90 days.	Moderate.	As for plain catgut.	As for plain catgut.	6/0–3 with needles; 5/0–3 without needles.
Polyglactin 910 (Coated Vicryl[a])	Braided multifilament.	Copolymer of lactide and glycolide in a ratio of 90:10, coated with polyglactin 370 and calcium stearate.	Approx. 60% remains at 2 weeks. Approx. 30% remains at 3 weeks.	Hydrolysis. Minimal until 5–6 weeks. Complete absorption 60–90 days.	Mild.	Not advised for use in tissues which require prolonged approximation under stress.	General surgical use where absorbable sutures required, e.g. gut anastomoses, vascular ligatures. Has become the 'workhorse' suture for many applications in most general surgical practices, including undyed for subcuticular wound closures. Ophthalmic surgery.	8/0–2 with needles; 5/0–2 without needles.

Suture	Structure	Composition	Tensile strength	Absorption	Tissue reaction	Contraindications	Uses	Sizes
Poly-glyconate (Maxon®[b])	Monofilament. Dyed or undyed.	Copolymer of glycolic acid and trimethylene carbonate.	Approx. 70% remains at 2 weeks. Approx. 55% remains at 3 weeks.	Hydrolysis. Minimal until 8–9 weeks. Complete absorption by 180 days.	Mild.	Not advised for use in tissues which require prolonged approximation under stress.	Popular in some centres as an alternative to Vicryl and PDS.	7/0–2 with needles.
Polyglycolic acid (Dexon®[b])	Braided multifilament. Dyed or undyed. Coated or uncoated.	Homopolymer. Polyglycolic acid. Available with coating of inert, absorbable surfactant poloxamer 188 to enhance surface smoothness. 97% excreted in urine within 3 days.	Approx. 40% remains at 1 week. Approx. 20% remains at 3 weeks.	Hydrolysis. Minimal at 2 weeks, significant at 4 weeks. Complete absorption 60–90 days.	Minimal.	Not advised for use in tissues which require prolonged approximation under stress.	Uses as for other absorbable sutures.	9/0–2 with needles; 9/0–2 without needles.
Polydioxanone (PDS®[a])	Monofilament. Dyed or undyed.	Polyester polymer.	Approx. 70% remains at 2 weeks. Approx. 50% remains at 4 weeks. Approx. 14% remains at 8 weeks.	Hydrolysis. Minimal at 90 days. Complete absorption at 180 days.	Mild.	Not for use in association with heart valves or synthetic grafts, or in situations in which prolonged tissue approximation under stress is required.	Uses as for other absorbable sutures, in particular where slightly longer wound support is required.	PDS®: 10/0–8/0 with needles. PDS II®: 7/0–2 with needles.

[a] Ethicon trademark.
[b] Davis and Geck trademark.

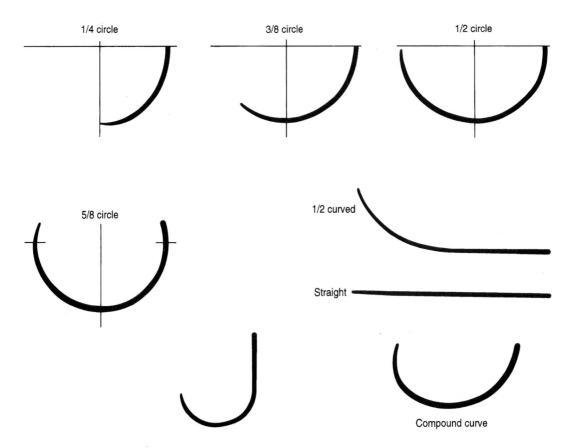

Fig. 3.2 Types of needles used for sutures. All modern needles have the suture swaged on to prevent a 'shoulder' damaging tissue and to allow easy passage.

The needle and suture size appropriate to the required bite size should be chosen; needles that are too small tend to become bent and broken. The passage of the needle through the tissue should follow its direction of curvature.

Principles of suturing

1. Tissues should be handled gently and wound edges protected from contamination, drying, abrasion or crushing.
2. Haemostasis should be meticulous, but overuse of diathermy should be condemned, particularly at the skin edges, as burning of the skin may occur causing a delay in healing and increase in the size of the scar.
3. Contaminated and devitalized tissue should be excised. If severe contamination exists then the wound should *not* be sutured, but treated by delayed primary suture or left open to heal by secondary intention.

4. Choose the correct size and type of suture for the task, bearing in mind the healing characteristics of the tissue in question and the tensile strengths involved. Do not use sutures that are larger than necessary and avoid implanting non-absorbable material where possible. (See also Chapter 5.)
5. Sutures should be tied tightly enough to approximate the wound edges without 'strangling' the tissues. Wound edges become swollen in the early phase of healing. This will exacerbate ischaemic problems caused by overtight sutures and may result in tissue necrosis and 'cutting out' of the sutures with wound breakdown.
6. Surgeons' knots (Fig. 3.3) should always be used with particular regard to 'laying' each throw of the knot in the correct orientation to prevent breakage and slippage of the suture. Synthetic monofilament sutures are more difficult to handle than multifilament and natural sutures and require a greater number of throws to each knot to ensure security. Large knots, if close to the skin, should be 'buried' to prevent irritation.

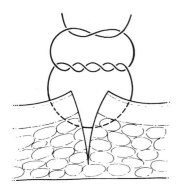

Fig. 3.3 The surgeon's knot – double then single square reef knot. A further double reef knot makes the knot secure.

7. Suture materials should never be gripped with instruments as this weakens them and can lead to suture breakage.
8. Always use appropriate lengths of suture with adequate bites to do the job. Mass closure of the abdominal wall demands sutures bites of no less than 1 cm from the wound edge and about 1 cm apart.[24] This will require a total suture length of at least *four times* the length of the wound.[31]
9. Attention should be directed to appropriate inversion of the sutured tissue edges (e.g. end-to-end anastomoses Figs. 3.4 and 3.5) or eversion (e.g. skin Fig. 3.6a,b,c), to facilitate healing and prevent complications (e.g. anastomotic leakage). Inversion and eversion can be achieved using a variety of different suture techniques.

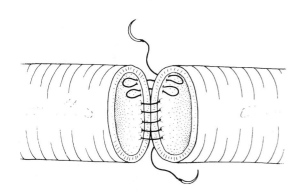

Fig. 3.4 Continuous all layers suture in end-to-end anastomosis of small bowel. The 'loop on the mucosa' Connell stitch is not haemostatic but ensures inversion of the 'corners'.

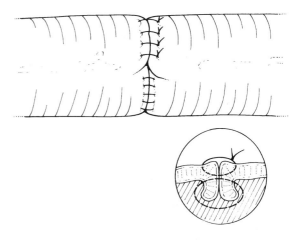

Fig. 3.5 The second interrupted seromuscular layer in end-to-end anastomosis of small bowel. This further ensures mucosal inversion and can be performed as a single layer without the internal all layers suture (Fig. 3.4). The insert shows the effect seen on transverse section.

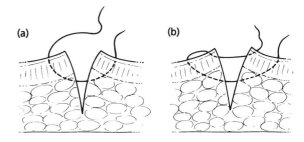

(a)   (b)

(c)

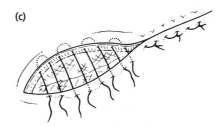

Fig. 3.6 (a) Simple suture of skin. (b) Vertical mattress suture of skin. (c) Horizontal mattress suture of skin.

10. Once the wound has been sutured, it remains at risk of becoming infected and should, in general, be covered with an appropriate dressing and inspected regularly until healing is sufficiently advanced. However, inspection should not disturb the 'seal' of the wound, otherwise infection may be introduced.
11. Make sure adequate instruction is made regarding the timing of suture removal.

Clips and staples

Mechanical stapling devices were first invented by Professor Humer Hultl of Hungary and used successfully in the early part of this century in the operation of distal gastrectomy. Since then a range of staplers has been developed for a wide variety of surgical procedures.

Skin wounds may be closed with staples or clips (classically after thyroid surgery or the long wounds following vascular or orthopaedic surgery). These give a good cosmetic result, are quick and easy to use, but are considerably more expensive than the equivalent length of suture. Proponents would argue that the savings in operating theatre time more than make up for the extra expense.

Stapling devices enable gastrointestinal anastomoses to be fashioned in situations of difficult access where hand-sewn anastomoses are difficult. This allows for lower anterior rectal resections and anastomoses to be achieved, reducing the need for colostomies. Difficult oesophageal anastomoses can be performed using staples, often without the need to open the chest (including oesophageal transection in the emergency treatment of bleeding oesophageal varices). Stapling devices are straightforward and quick to use and the anastomotic leak rate is not significantly different from those created by hand suturing in experienced hands.

There are three basic types of gastrointestinal stapling device available; linear, side-to-side and end-to-end staplers.[32] Side-to-side staplers are available with or without a knife blade for transection of a viscus between staple rows; end-to-end staplers have circular knife blades.

1. *Linear stapler* (Fig. 3.7)
   Linear terminal everting staple line: Used for end closure of a viscus (e.g. duodenal stump closure in Polya gastrectomy).
2. *Side-to-side stapler* (Fig. 3.8)
   a. Linear inverting anastomosis with transection: Used for side-to-side intestinal anastomoses (e.g. gastroenterostomy).
   b. Linear staple line without transection: Used for fashioning enteric reservoirs (e.g. ileal pouch).
   c. Linear staple line with transection: Used for closure of a viscus (e.g. small bowel resection).
3. *End-to-end stapler* (Fig. 3.9)
   Circular inverting anastomosis: Used for end-to-end gastrointestinal anastomoses (e.g. closure of colostomy following Hartmann's procedure).

Laparoscopic surgical advances in recent years owe much to the refinement of clip and stapling devices for use with laparoscopic instruments. Most laparoscopic procedures would be impossible without laparoscopic clip applicators, in particular, as laparoscopic suturing is a difficult technique and one which can add considerably to the operation time.

Other wound considerations

In addition to the range of aspects already considered, which many surgeons would consider to be the most important aspect of wound care in their practice, a number of other considerations need to be taken into account. These include the use of non-surgical methods to assist in healing, the care of patients with chronic wounds and the development of services for patients with wound problems.

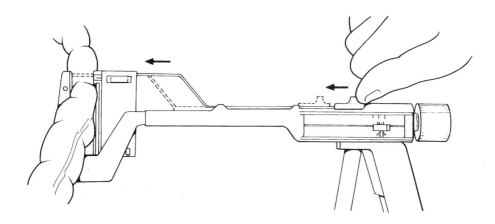

Fig. 3.7 A linear stapling device used to close a bowel end.

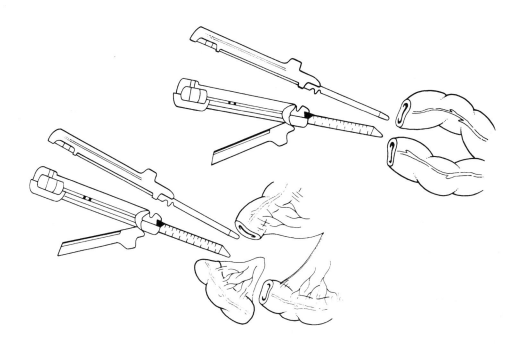

Fig. 3.8 A side-to-side stapling device which can divide and close bowel or allow side-to-side anastomosis.

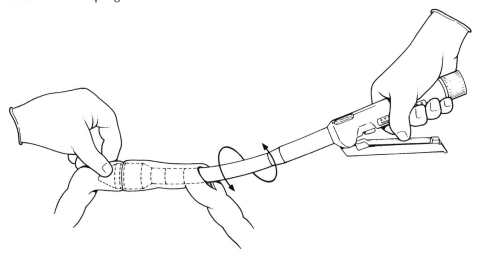

Fig. 3.9 An end-to-end stapling device used to anastomose bowel.

NON-SURGICAL ASPECTS OF HEALING

Since the work of Winter in the 1960s[5] there has been an explosion in the development of dressing technologies that has led to the availability of a bewildering array of materials with differing physical properties and possible modes of action.[33]

The first type of modern wound contact material was the semi-permeable film which was initially developed as an incise drape for theatre use but subsequently was found to be of benefit in treating open wounds. Many clinicians now use this material as a standard dressing to cover primary sutured wounds or for skin graft donor sites and, although there are limitations in its use as a material to manage cavity wounds, it is ideally suited to flat, open surfaces.

Although alginates were first discovered in the 1880s and their current use is diverse, their development as a dressing early in this century was initially as a haemostatic material for intraoperative use. In recent years their development as a dressing for open wounds has improved the management of several types of chronic wounds. Their use as a material with haemostatic properties immediately postoperatively has been described[34] and they may also be used as an alternative to gauze packing. Alginates form a gel in contact with saline or body fluids which allows painless removal, which is not the case when changing a gauze dressing.

Hydrogel materials, which consist of hydrophilic polymers which attract liquids, can be used to either donate or absorb fluid to or from a wound. They are presented either as sheets or amorphous gels which are effective in providing both a moist environment and acting as a non-surgical debriding agent.[35]

Hydrocolloids are a family of compounds which are a combination of gel-forming agents, elastomers and adhesives, developed as wound dressings after their initial use as components of stoma devices. These are available as wafers, powders and gels, and appear to have a beneficial effect on healing,[36] particularly in chronic non-healing wounds.

Foams have existed in various forms for many years and are currently available as sheet, foams and *in situ* forming materials. These materials range in their absorbency and use on both superficial and cavity wounds, depending on their physical structure.[37]

In addition to these major categories of wound management materials, materials with improved absorbency compared with traditional gauze or Gamgee have been developed. Materials which act as deodorising agents have also been developed with effective compression bandages in the management of leg ulceration.

CARE OF PATIENTS WITH CHRONIC WOUNDS

The major developments in this field relate to a more structured system of care for patients with leg ulceration. There are many studies which have addressed the extent of this problem, and the difficulties of obtaining acceptable healing rates.[38] The group at Charing Cross which pioneered the use of a four-layer bandaging system have extended their service to provide a community-based clinic with healing rates at 12 weeks increasing from 22 to 69%.[39]

Progress has also been made in the provision of services to patients with diabetic foot ulcers. The recognition of the need for a multidisciplinary team with physicians, surgeons, nurses, radiologists and paramedical professionals, all providing appropriate skills and expertise for such patients, has led to a significant decrease in amputation rates for patients attending such clinics.[40]

With regard to pressure sores, although surgical intervention is only one component of management, there is an increasing recognition of the importance of both adequate preventative and therapeutic aids and appliances. In many hospitals and nursing homes the number of patients with pressure sores is being used as a measure of the quality of care being offered to patients, and the number of successful legal claims for damages for patients developing sores, which are potentially preventable, is increasing.[41]

DEVELOPMENT OF SERVICES

The setting up of dedicated leg ulcer clinics, either in hospital or in the community, has shown the benefits of dedicating staff and resources in a particular department or area. Similarly, the setting up of diabetic foot clinics has led to a dramatic improvement in outcome for patients with such conditions.

The realization that the numbers of patients who suffer from chronic wounds are likely to increase (with an increased requirement of health care resources)[42] is a cogent reason for recognizing that wound healing and wound care is an important aspect of health care.

The future of wound healing and wound care

It is clear that topical application of growth factors can accelerate healing in chronic wounds. The most commonly studied factors are PDGF, EGF, FGF and TGF-β which promote angiogenesis, collagen synthesis and epithelialization with an increased rate of tensile strength acquisition.[43] It is unlikely that growth factors will be used in uncomplicated healing wounds, as optimal healing cannot be accelerated. They will, however, have a role in compromised healing; in immunosuppressed or malnourished patients, after chemo- or radiotherapy, or in chronic leg ulcers or pressure sores. Attention to the stage of healing and the interaction of applied growth factors may allow a more practical and successful approach as the complexity of the wound healing cascade is recognized.

The understanding of fetal wound healing and its relevance to healing in adults poses another challenge. Modulation of healing by the use of molecular biological techniques may become possible in the not too distant future. Although neonates heal by repair the sequence is accelerated compared with adults, but in the fetus regeneration is associated with rapid healing without acute inflammation, wound contraction or scar formation.[44] The control of inflammation and scar formation may have tremendous impact in the development of new treatments in the near future.

Following the recognition that a moist wound

environment was the most conducive to tissue healing some 30 years ago, there has been an exponential increase in surgical dressings.[45] Simple film dressings have now been complemented by a range of materials that can absorb large amounts of exudate and promote healing by secondary intention. Dressings that interact with the healing wound, or are biologically active in their own right and therefore promote healing, are exciting developments on the horizon.

The increasing knowledge of the biological basis of wound healing requires increasing awareness by all concerned in clinical care. The recognition that appropriate surgical skills are important to reduce the risk of wound complications postoperatively is essential, as is the requirement for the use of appropriate sutures and devices to assist healing. The importance of appropriate dressings and devices to assist healing of chronic wounds that all clinicians will meet cannot be underestimated. The need for better understanding of when and how to offer surgical intervention to complement other aspects of patient care is urgent.

The integration of individuals of different professional backgrounds is important if coordinated care is to be provided for patients with the diversity of wound problems existing in clinical practice.

Acknowledgement

We are grateful to Ethicon Ltd for permission to reproduce Figs 3.2, 3.7, 3.8 and 3.9.

References

1. Majno G. *The Healing Hand: Man and Wound in the Ancient World*. Cambridge, MA: Harvard University Press, 1975.
2. Forrest RD. (i) Early history of wound treatment. (ii) Development of wound therapy from the Dark Ages to the present. *J Roy Soc Med* 1982; **75:** 198–205; 263–73.
3. Metchnikoff E. *Immunity in Infective Diseases* (Trans FG Binnie). Cambridge, UK: Cambridge University Press, 1905.
4. Burke JF. The effective period of preventive antibiotic action in experimental incisions and dermal lesions. *Surgery* 1961; **50:** 161–8.
5. Winter GD. Healing of skin wounds and the influence of dressings on the repair process. In: Harkiss KJ (ed.) *Surgical Dressings and Wound Healing*. London: Crossby Lockwood, 1971: 46–60.
6. Sicard RE. *Vertebrate Limb Regeneration*. New York: Oxford University Press, 1985.
7. Clark RAF, Henson PM. *The Molecular and Cellular Biology of Wound Repair*. New York: Plenum Press, 1988.
8. Wysocki AB. Fibronectin profiles in normal and chronic wound fluid. *Lab Invest* 1990; **6:** 825–31.
9. McKay IA. Epidermal cytokines and their roles in cutaneous wound healing. *Br J Dermatol* 1991; **124:** 513–18.
10. Chen WYJ. Characterisation of biologic properties of wound fluid collected during early stages of wound healing. *J Invest Dermatol* 1992; **99:** 559–63.
11. Balkwill FR (ed.). *Cytokines: A Practical Approach*. Oxford: Oxford University Press, 1991.
12. Clark RAF. Growth factors and wound repair. *J Cell Biochem* 1991; **46:** 1–2.
13. Blitstein-Willinger E. The role of growth factors in wound healing. *Skin Pharmacol* 1991; **4:** 175–82.
14. Deuel TF. Growth factors and wound healing: platelet derived growth factor as a model cytokine. *Ann Rev Med* 1991; **42:** 567–84.
15. Schultz G. EGF and TGF in wound healing and repair. *J Cell Biochem* 1991; **45:** 346–52.
16. Grotendorst GR, Grotendorst CA, Gilman T. Production of growth factor PDGF and TGF-β at the site of tissue repair. In: Hunt TK, Pines E, Barbul A (eds) *Biological and Clinical Aspects of Tissue Repair*. New York: Alan R Liss 1988: 47–54.
17. Matrisian LM. Metalloproteinases and their inhibitors in matrix remodelling. *Trends Genet* 1990; **6:** 121–5.
18. Banda MJ. Proteinase induction by endothelial cells during wound repair. In: Hunt TK, Pines E, Barbul A (eds) *Biological and Clinical Aspects of Tissue Repair*. New York: Alan R Liss, 1988: 117–30.
19. Gottrup F. Measurement and evaluation of tissue perfusion in surgery. In: Leaper DJ, Braniki FJ (eds) *International Surgical Practice*. Oxford: Oxford University Press, 1992.
20. Capperauld I. Suture materials: a review. *Clin Mat* 1989; **4:** 3–12.
21. Artandi C. A revolution in sutures. *Surg Gynecol Obstet* 1980; **150:** 235–6.
22. Vickery CJ, Leaper DJ. Care of surgical wounds. *Postgrad Doctor* 1994; **17:** 297–304.
23. Adamson RJ, Musco F, Enquist IF. The clinical dimensions of a healing incision. *Surg Gynecol Obstet* 1966; **123:** 515.
24. Leaper DJ, Pollock AV, Evans M. Abdominal wound closure: a trial of Nylon, polyglycolic acid and steel sutures. *Br J Surg* 1977; **64:** 603–6.
25. Douglas DM. The healing of aponeurotic incisions. *Br J Surg* 1952; **40:** 79–84.
26. Bucknall TE, Teare L, Ellis H. The choice of a suture to close abdominal incisions *Eur Surg Res* 1983; **15:** 59–66.
27. Howes EL, Harvey SC. The strength of healing wounds in relation to the holding strength of the catgut suture. *N Engl J Med* 1929; **200:** 1285–90.
28. Moynihan BGA. The ritual of a surgical operation. *Br J Surg* 1920; **8:** 27–35.

29. Lythgoe JP. Burst abdomen. *Postgrad Med J* 1960; **36:** 388–91.

30. Bucknall TE, Ellis H. Abdominal wound closure – comparison of monofilament Nylon and polyglycolic acid. *Surgery* 1981; **6:** 672–7.

31. Jenkins TPN. The burst abdominal wound: a mechanical approach. *Br J Surg* 1976; **63:** 873–6.

32. Leaper DJ. Mechanical stapling in surgery. In: Keen G (ed.) *Operative Surgery and Management*, 2nd ed. Bristol: IOP Publishing, 1987.

33. Thomas S. *Wound Management and Dressings*. London: The Pharmaceutical Press, 1990.

34. Gupta R, Foster ME, Miller E. Calcium alginate in the management of acute surgical wounds and abscesses. *J Tissue Viabil* 1991; **1:** 115–16.

35. Thomas S. A new approach to the management of extravasation injury in neonates. *Pharmaceut J* 1987; **239:** 584–5.

36. Alvarez OH, Mertz PM, Eaglstein WH. The effect of occlusive dressings on collagen synthesis and epithelialization in superficial wounds. *J Surg Res* 1983; **35:** 143–8.

37. Turner TD, Schmidt RJ, Harding KG. *Advances in Wound Management*. Chichester: J Wiley, 1985.

38. Nelzen O, Berquist D, Lindhagen L. Leg ulcer aetiology – a cross sectional population study. *J Vasc Surg* 1991; **14:** 557–65.

39. Moffat CJ, Franks PJ, Oldroyd MC *et al.* Community clinics for leg ulcers and impact on healing. *Br Med J* 1992; **305:** 1389–92.

40. Edmunds ME. Experience of a multidisciplinary diabetic foot clinic. In: Connor H, Boulton AJM, Ward (eds) *The Foot in Diabetes*. Chichester: J Wiley, 1987.

41. *Pressure Sores – A Key Quality Indicator*. London: Department of Health, 1994.

42. Harding KG, Jones V, Sinclair AJ. Wound care in an ageing population. *J Wound Care* 1993; **2:** 236–9.

43. Chemoattractants and growth factors. In: Cohen IK, Diegelmann RF, Lindblad WJ (eds) *Wound Healing. Biochemical and Clinical Aspects*. Philadelphia: WB Saunders, 1992: 237–46.

44. Cohen IK, Haynes JH. Overview of fetal wound repair. *Proceedings: Australian International Wound Management Conferences*, 1994: 28–36.

45. Thomas S. *Handbook of Wound Dressings*. London: J Wound Care/Macmillan, 1994.

CHAPTER 4

Molecular genetics for general surgery

ELIZABETH H SMYTH, DANIEL E PORTER

Introduction

Genetic information is encoded in deoxyribonucleic acid (DNA) sequences. Deoxyribonucleic acid is the chemical from which chromosomes are composed and exists as a double helix formed from combinations of only four different bases – adenine, guanine, cytosine and thymine. In the double helix, adenine always pairs with thymine and guanine with cytosine. A gene is a hereditary unit of DNA which can be transcribed into a particular protein. To produce a particular protein, DNA must first be transcribed into messenger ribonucleic acid (mRNA). Within any given gene there are DNA sequences which are required for the production of the final protein (exons) and others which are nonsense sequences (introns) which are removed following transcription by the process of RNA splicing. These steps take place in the nucleus. The mature mRNA is then transported into the cytoplasm where it is translated into protein, each combination of three bases coding for a single specified amino acid.

Only a small percentage of the total DNA is thought to represent structural genes (approximately 20 000 genes are expressed in the adult human). Variations in the DNA base sequences within the

same genes between different individuals are common. These variations are not important in that they still specify the same protein end product. They are, however, scientifically very useful and this concept of genetic polymorphism is widely employed in the analysis of the structure of genes.

Genes are packaged in 23 pairs of chromosomes (22 pairs of autosomes and a pair of sex chromosomes – XX in the female and XY in the male). The members of these pairs (homologues) segregate randomly from each other during cell division by meiosis so that each resultant gamete contains half the genetic material of the parent cell. There is also exchange of genetic material between homologous chromosomes by crossing over during the earliest stages of meiosis.

Alterations to the DNA, which in turn lead to alterations in the protein product, are known as mutations and may take one or more of several forms:

1. Substitution of a single base. In sickle cell disease a thymine is substituted for an adenine which results in a glutamic acid molecule replacing valine in the globin chain. This is sufficient to alter the entire structure and function of the haemoglobin.
2. Deletion of one or more bases. There is a 5 kilobase deletion near the $3'$ end of the LDL

receptor gene in certain types of familial hypercholesterolaemia and in lethal osteogenesis imperfecta there is a deletion within the gene encoding α_1-like collagen.

3. Frame shift. Insertion or loss of one or more bases throws the reading frame out of phase during the transcription of mRNA, e.g. some types of thalassaemia.

A few diseases exhibit simple Mendelian inheritance and are easily understood. These are classified as being:

1. autosomal recessive where two copies of the abnormal allele must be inherited for the disease phenotype to be expressed, e.g. cystic fibrosis (Fig. 4.1a);
2. autosomal dominant in which the disease phenotype is expressed if even a single copy of an abnormal allele is inherited, e.g. adult onset polycystic kidney disease, Huntington's chorea (Fig. 4.1b);
3. sex-linked (or more precisely, X-linked) diseases which are very much more common in males than in females because the genes for these diseases are situated on that part of the X chromosome which has no homology with the Y chromosome, e.g. haemophilia, colour blindness (Fig. 4.1c).

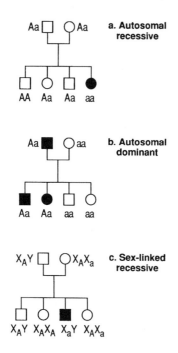

Fig. 4.1 Pedigrees illustrating simple Mendelian inheritance in single gene disorders. A: dominant allele; a: recessive allele.

Most conditions, however, are not nearly so simple as this. Account must be taken of variable expressivity (differing degrees of severity of the disease even when the lesions at the molecular level are identical) and variable penetrance (the probability that an individual who has inherited a particular mutation will express the disease phenotype). The vast majority of human diseases are multifactorial in origin in that they require the interaction of both genetic and environmental influences – the 'nature-nurture' phenomenon – or indeed of several genes (polygenic diseases) with or without additional environmental factors. Examples of conditions where genes and environment interact to cause disease are cleft lip and palate, Dupuytren's contracture, atherosclerosis and many, if not all, forms of cancer.

Evidence for a strong genetic component comes from an association of the disease within families and an earlier age of onset than might generally be expected. For example, in Type II familial hyperlipidaemia there is an unusually high incidence of deaths at very young ages from the complications of atherosclerosis such as myocardial infarction and cerebrovascular accidents.

Within the speciality of genetics as a whole, cancer genetics is emerging as an exciting and rapidly advancing field and is probably the area of most interest to surgeons. Much of the remainder of this chapter will therefore relate to this topic with reference to specific laboratory techniques applicable to unravelling the complexities of the various mutations contributing to the evolution of cancer and examples of some of the more recent advances.

Cancer genetics

Carcinogenesis is a stepwise process. That is, the serial acquisition of specific lesions in the tumour cell DNA correlates with a progressively neoplastic phenotype. The DNA lesions responsible may be classified according to the nature of the molecular event. Alterations in chromosome number (aneuploidy), translocations (such as the Philadelphia chromosome in chronic myeloid leukaemia, where part of chromosome 9 is translocated to chromosome 22), deletions, point mutations and changes in the DNA methylation pattern (see below) have all been observed. These often involve genes which, in one way or another, regulate cell growth or cell death and thus it can be seen how such changes may result in the disordered pattern of cell growth which becomes a cancer. A large percentage of the cytosine residues in human DNA are methylated. This methylation plays a role in the regulation of gene expression and in chromosome condensation. Loss of DNA methylation inhibits chromosome condensation and may lead to mitotic non-disjunction of the chromosomes, resulting in aneuploidy.

There are two broad categories of genes involved in carcinogenesis: oncogenes and tumour suppressor genes.

ONCOGENES

Within the DNA of every cell are sequences known as proto-oncogenes which are involved in regulating the basic essential functions of the cell with regard to control of cell growth and differentiation. Genetic damage (mutation) to a proto-oncogene converts it into an active oncogene. Typically, this results in a gain of function leading to increased cell turnover and more disordered growth. Proto-oncogenes may be activated by amplification, structural alteration or loss of the control mechanism either by insertional mutagenesis or by translocation. Examples of each of these and the tumours in which they are commonly implicated are given in Table 4.1.

Much of the original work on oncogenes came from the study of retroviruses. These RNA viruses are capable of manufacturing DNA and of integrating this into the host cell genome. Certain RNA viruses were noted to induce tumours rapidly in susceptible hosts. It was then observed that the DNA of many tumour cells contained base sequences which were extremely similar to those of the retroviral transforming genes. The main difference between the two is

that the cellular oncogenes contain introns which the viral equivalents do not have. Interestingly, in spite of these exciting scientific discoveries no solid tumour in humans has been convincingly linked with a retrovirus, although various DNA viruses have been implicated in the aetiology of specific tumours (Table 4.2). The human immunodeficiency virus (HIV) is a retrovirus which has been linked with Kaposi's sarcoma but in this case it is the immune suppression associated with the viral infection rather than integration of viral genes into the host cell DNA which is thought to predispose to tumour formation.

Although over 60 separate oncogenes have now been identified, there is evidence that they nearly all exert their biological effect by one of only a few mechanisms. The first of these is the phosphorylation of proteins which in turn act as transforming factors. Second, many proto-oncogenes encode transcription factors which have a role in the control of transcription of DNA to mRNA. The third mechanism is transmission of signals by GTPases which are in turn involved in modulating a chain of cellular activation processes. Others such as *int* and *sis* encode growth factors while yet others, e.g. *bcl2*, confer immortality.

TUMOUR SUPPRESSOR GENES

These are again sequences of DNA present within all normal cells which exert a negative control over cell growth.[1] Alteration of a tumour suppressor gene causes loss of function and thus permits disordered

Table 4.1 Activation of proto-oncogenes and the tumours in which they are commonly implicated

Oncogene	Structure/function	Tumour
sis	Growth factor analogue	Astrocytoma
erb-B	Receptor in plasma membrane	Breast
ras	G-protein	Pancreas, colon, lung, melanoma, Thyroid, others
mos	Cytoplasmic serine/tyrosine kinase	Breast
myc	DNA-binding protein	Breast, colon, Burkitt's lymphoma, Lung, ovary, others
jun/fos	Form DNA-binding heterodimer	Renal, colon, ovary, lung, others

Table 4.2 Various DNA viruses implicated in the aetiology of specific tumours

Cancer	Virus
Liver	Hepatitis B
Burkitt's lymphoma	Epstein–Barr virus
Nasopharyngeal carcinoma	Epstein–Barr virus
Cervix	Human papilloma virus types 16 and 18

cell growth. Much of the evidence for the existence of this family of genes came initially from work on hereditary cancers but is equally applicable to sporadic tumours. The prime example of this is Knudson's work on hereditary retinoblastoma which led him to postulate the two-hit hypothesis. Retinoblastoma is a rare tumour which occurs in both hereditary and sporadic forms. Hereditary retinoblastoma occurs at an earlier age and is more frequently bilateral than the sporadic form. This could be explained if the affected individual inherited a mutation in one copy of the retinoblastoma gene (RB1). As all cells contain two copies of the gene and the mutation is recessive at the cellular level, retinoblastoma does not develop unless there is a further mutation in the normal copy of the

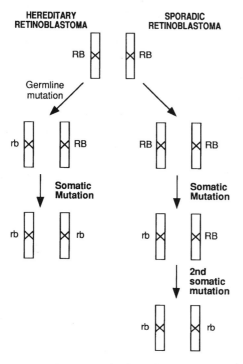

Fig. 4.2 Knudson's two-hit hypothesis. RB: normal retinoblastoma gene; rb: mutated retinoblastoma gene.

gene. The inherited and subsequent mutations are termed germline and somatic respectively. Individuals who have not inherited a germline mutation in the RB1 gene require two somatic events to create a tumourigenic genotype. (Fig. 4.2). The probability of a single somatic event is obviously much greater than that of two, hence the reason why hereditary tumours tend to have a younger age of onset. Although the causative mutation is recessive at the cellular level, such tumours exhibit a dominant pattern of inheritance. Some examples of the locations of probable tumour suppressor genes and the cancers in which they have been implicated are given in Table 4.3.

The p53 tumour suppressor gene deserves special mention as it plays a role in such a diversity of cancers and is also responsible for the rare but fascinating spectrum of hereditary cancers which constitute the Li–Fraumeni syndrome; p53 is located on the short arm of chromosome 17 (denoted 17p in genetic terminology).

Because of its function in acting as a G1 checkpoint control for DNA damage during cell division, p53 has been termed 'guardian of the genome'. Wild-type p53 (i.e. normal p53) binds to double-stranded DNA in a sequence-specific manner. Mutated p53 proteins have lost this sequence-specific binding property. Cells containing normal p53 are arrested in the G1 phase of the cell cycle to allow repair of damaged DNA before proceeding into S phase, or self-destruct if the damage cannot be repaired. Cells with mutated p53 carry straight on into S phase before repair of DNA is complete. If p53 is inactivated, either by mutation or by binding to another protein, cells are rendered genetically less stable and are liable to accumulate further mutations and chromosomal rearrangements at a greater rate, leading to selection of those cells with malignant growth potential (Fig. 4.3). One of the many proteins which can inactivate wild-type p53 is mutant p53 protein itself, this phenomenon being known as the dominant negative effect. Whereas wild-type p53 has tumour suppres-

Table 4.3 Locations of probable tumour suppressor genes and the cancers in which they have been implicated

Tumour suppressor gene	Location	Cancer
BRCA-1	17q	Breast/ovary
DCC	18q	Colon
APC	5q	Colon
WT1	11p	Wilm's tumour
RB1	13q	Retinoblastoma
NF1	17q	Neurofibrosarcoma
VHL	3p	Renal cell carcinoma in Von-Hippel Lindau syndrome

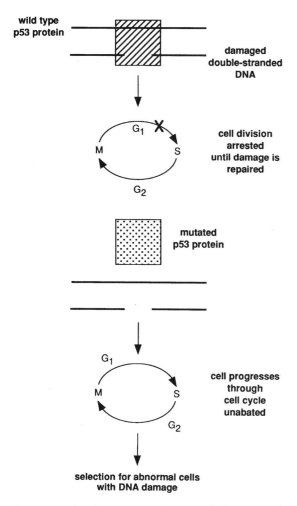

Fig. 4.3 Role of p53 in preventing cell division within DNA-damaged cells.

sing activity, the mutated protein has the properties of an oncogenic product.

HEREDITARY PREDISPOSITION TO CANCER

Some 5–10% of common cancers, or possibly even more, occur as a result of a genetic susceptibility.[2] A given disease may occur in familial clusters due to chance, due to shared environmental influences or because of genetic factors. To determine the likelihood of a genetic component being operational in any given familial cluster, the complex technique of segregation analysis is employed. This involves testing the probability of obtaining the observed distribution of affected and unaffected family members (taking obligate gene carriers into account) under a variety of different genetic models such as autosomal domi-

nant, autosomal recessive, polygenic, etc. A maximum likelihood score is derived which may favour one model so strongly as to virtually exclude all others. All studies of this type are by their very nature subject to ascertainment bias in that the families are selected on the basis of their strong family history of cancer. Nevertheless, segregation analysis remains a useful tool in the search for genes predisposing to common cancers such as breast, ovarian and colon, even if its only contribution is to suggest that such a search by more precise scientific means should prove a fruitful exercise.[3]

Some family cancer syndromes carry such a strong tumour predisposition that they are relatively easy to define and thus to investigate. One such example is familial polyposis (or adenomatous polyposis coli [APC]). Carriers of a mutation in the APC gene develop multiple polyps which literally carpet the colon at an early age, typically in their teens. Many of these individuals will go on to develop invasive carcinoma by the age of 30 unless preventative measures are taken.

The association of germline p53 mutations with the Li–Fraumeni syndrome has already been mentioned. In this rare familial disorder, sarcoma occurs in the proband (index case) before the age of 45 years, at least one first-degree relative develops cancer aged under 45 and sarcoma is diagnosed in a second-degree relative at any age.[4] The spectrum of tumours frequently seen in this syndrome includes soft tissue sarcomas and osteosarcoma, early onset breast cancer, leukaemia, malignant brain tumours and adrenocortical carcinoma. Although the majority of families manifesting this pattern of hereditary cancers have p53 mutations, some families have been documented in whom no such mutation could be found on screening.[5,6]

It is now well recognized that families do exist which exhibit a high incidence of breast cancer or breast and ovarian cancers inherited in autosomal dominant fashion with variable penetrance. A proportion of these show linkage to a locus on the long arm of chromosome 17 (17q) containing the putative tumour suppressor gene BRCA-1. This will be discussed more fully in the section entitled 'Genetic alterations in breast cancer'.

Genetic alterations in colorectal cancer

The evolution of colorectal cancer provides an excellent illustration of stepwise carcinogenesis. The accumulation of several discrete genetic changes correlates well with the phenotypic progression

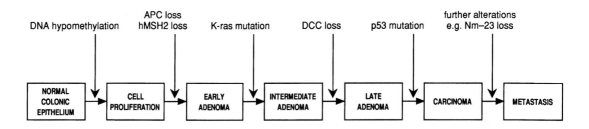

Fig. 4.4 The multistep process of colorectal carcinogenesis. Adapted from ref. 7, with permission.

from benign adenoma to malignant carcinoma.[7] No one mutation is by itself sufficient to cause tumour progression. However, any single mutation may create a state in which further mutations are more likely to occur, known as genetic instability. Although there is some evidence that certain genetic changes tend to occur in a defined order, it is the total number of these alterations rather than their order which is more important in determining malignant potential (Fig. 4.4).

Colorectal carcinogenesis involves both activation of proto-oncogenes and inactivation of tumour suppressor genes. Much heterogeneity exists between different tumours, i.e. no mutation is found in all tumours and indeed a wide variety of changes is seen in many tumours.

Hypomethylation of the DNA is frequently observed in colorectal tumours. As previously discussed, changes in the DNA methylation pattern confer genetic instability. Approximately half of all large bowel tumours and many large adenomas have point mutations in K-*ras*. These are rarely observed in adenomas which are less than 1 cm in diameter. K-*ras* mutation is associated with a more dysplastic appearance of the cell and with clonal expansion.

Several chromosomal regions show frequent allelic loss (see 'Genetic techniques' below) in colorectal cancer cells. These are reported to be the sites of specific tumour suppressor genes. Mutations and losses of the p53 gene on chromosome 17p are found in over three-quarters of colonic carcinomas and represent the most frequent specific genetic alteration in these tumours. The function of p53 was discussed in an earlier section. Its role as a tumour suppressor gene in this situation is confirmed by the fact that transfection of wild-type p53 into colonic cancer cells inhibits colony formation. Cells expressing the normal gene fail to synthesize new DNA and thus fail to progress through the cell cycle.

The second most common site of allelic loss in colonic tumours is on chromosome 18q. The tumour suppressor gene DCC (deleted in colon cancer) has now been localized to this region. The protein product

of this gene bears considerable homology to some neuronal cell adhesion molecules. Diminished expression causes a marked decrease in cell–cell adhesion with reduction in normal growth-inhibiting signals (i.e. loss of contact inhibition).

Two genes lie close together on chromosome 5q. These are MCC (mutated in colon cancer) and the APC gene, mutations of which have been implicated in sporadic cases as well as the familial adenomatous polyposis (FAP) syndrome. Extensive data show that virtually all APC mutations, whether in the germline or somatic in colorectal tumours, are 'nonsense' type, deletion causing frame shift or other inactivating mutations consistent with the simple hypothesis of a tumour suppressor gene. There is also a clear correlation between clinical phenotypes and specific mutations. The APC gene product is thought to be involved in a complex with the cell adhesion molecule, E cadherin. Loss of this protein is thus similar in effect to loss of DCC.

Another condition known as hereditary non-polyposis colorectal cancer (HNPCC) together with FAP accounts for the majority of cases of hereditary colorectal cancer.[8] Hereditary non-polyposis colorectal cancer is defined by the Amsterdam criteria: at least three relatives with colorectal cancer, one of whom must be a first-degree relative of the other two, at least one case diagnosed below the age of 50 years and at least two generations affected. Families which fit this definition have been found to show linkage to at least two separate loci on chromosomes 2p and 3p. The gene on 2p has been identified as a homologue of the DNA mismatch repair gene *mut*S in *Escherichia coli* and is designated hMSH2 (for human *mut*S homologue 2). That on 3p has yet to be fully characterized but these families also manifest signs of a general DNA replication disorder. Even among families with apparently similar patterns of cancer inheritance, it must be realized that considerable genetic heterogeneity may exist.

Genetic alterations in breast cancer

Both oncogene amplification and tumour suppressor gene deletion have been extensively investigated in breast carcinogenesis by means of chromosome studies and electrophoretic analysis of DNA fragments. *Neu*-oncogene amplification is found in up to 30% of primary breast cancers. This is associated with elevated *Neu* mRNA and protein expression and appears to be an independent marker of agressive tumour behaviour. Other oncogenes implicated in breast carcinogenesis include *C-erbB1*, *C-myc* and *int-2*, *hst-1* and *bcl-1* located on the long arm of chromosome 11.

Loss of constitutional heterozygosity studies reveal deletions of tumour suppressor genes including the retinoblastoma gene on chromosome 13 and p53 on chromosome 17. In keeping with Knudson's two-hit hypothesis, the non-deleted copy is frequently inactivated by mutation. Over 20 sites of frequent loss of heterozygosity have been identified throughout the genome, one of which encompasses the gene BRCA-1.

A heritable predisposition has been estimated to contribute at least 20% towards breast cancer in women under the age of 40.[9] Epidemiological studies suggest one or more mutated tumour suppressor genes are carried by at least one in every 250 individuals and inherited in autosomal dominant fashion. Between 60 and 80% of female carriers of such a gene will develop breast cancer in their lifetime compared with a population figure of 10%. Linkage analysis (see 'Genetic techniques' below) in breast cancer families has identified a tumour suppressor gene called BRCA-1 on the long arm of chromosome 17 which is responsible for perhaps 40% of all heritable breast cancer cases.

A second breast cancer susceptibility gene, BRCA-2, has been located on the long arm of chromosome 13. Both genes have now been cloned making predictive testing for mutations a reality for the near future.

Inherited p53 gene mutation has also been demonstrated to predispose to an increased risk of breast cancer both as part of the Li–Fraumeni syndrome and in non Li–Fraumeni breast cancer families, perhaps contributing 0.5% towards the total burden of breast cancer in the general population.[10,11]

Genetic techniques

As understanding of the role of genetics in surgical disease has progressed, so powerful molecular techniques have begun to be applied both in surgical research and in clinical practice. Some of the more important techniques are discussed briefly below.

STRUCTURAL CHROMOSOME ANALYSIS

This is a microscopic technique which requires dividing cell nuclei to be inspected in metaphase when the chromosomes are visible. Staining enables specific chromosome regions to be identified by dividing the chromosome arms into dark- and light-staining bands (Fig. 4.5). Analysis of chromosomes in metaphase can reveal abnormalities which may be associated with surgical disease. Nephroblastoma, for example, is characterized by deletions of the short arm of chromosome 11. Non-lethal constitutional deletions (those which occur in every cell due to an inherited chromosome defect) may encompass a tumour suppressor gene, one copy of which is thereby inactivated predisposing to a cancer syndrome. Identification of individuals with polyposis coli and a deletion of chromosome 5q and of individuals with retinoblastoma and 13q deletion was instrumental in locating the crucial susceptibility genes for these conditions.

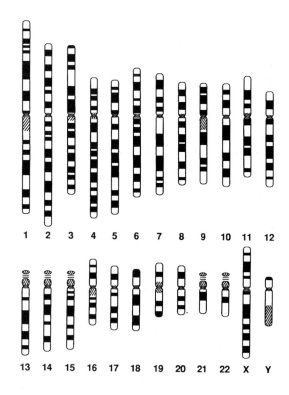

Fig. 4.5 Chromosome bands identified in metaphase of cell division.

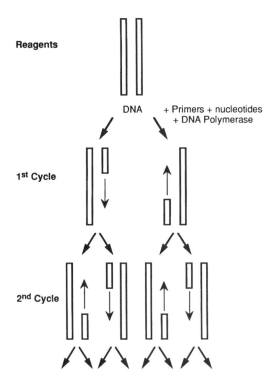

Reagents

DNA   + Primers + nucleotides
       + DNA Polymerase

1st Cycle

2nd Cycle

nth Cycle : up to 10^8 copies of target DNA sequence

Fig. 4.6   Principles of polymerase chain reaction.

FLOW CYTOMETRY

Cells passed through a focused laser beam scatter light according to the amount of DNA within their nuclei. This phenomenon enables the degree of aneuploidy (DNA content of cells differing from diploid) to be assessed. This may be clinically important, for example in discriminating some types of rhabdomyoma which, although histologically identical, behave in a benign manner when diploid and aggressively when aneuploid. Similarly, aneuploidy may be a useful marker of malignant potential in borderline epithelial ovarian tumours.

POLYMORPHIC MARKERS

These are fragments of DNA which exist in more than one form in the population. Since human somatic cells are diploid, each copy of a polymorphic marker in a cell nucleus may exist in two identifiable forms (alleles). Two types of naturally occurring genetic polymorphic markers are commonly utilized in molecular biology.

Restriction fragment length polymorphisms (RFLPs)

These are markers which are produced by means of restriction enzyme cleavage of the DNA strand. A single nucleotide base alteration in the DNA sequence may determine if the enzyme will cleave at that point or not, thereby giving rise to fragments of different lengths. RFLPs are detected through electrophoretic separation of the fragments and subsequent imaging using a technique known as Southern blotting.

Microsatellite repeating elements

These are markers which consist of repeating dinucleotides which vary in length and occur in each chromosome at intervals of every few thousand bases. They can be identified by means of the polymerase chain reaction.

POLYMERASE CHAIN REACTION (PCR)

Polymerase chain reaction is an *in vitro* DNA amplification procedure which, within hours, can amplify a specific segment of DNA, usually 50–10 000 bases in length, by as much as 100 million fold. This enriches the target DNA sample to such a degree that subsequent experimentation such as sequencing of the genetic fragment is greatly simplified.

Basic methodology involves the addition of 'primer' sequences which match the flanking sequences of DNA on either side of the fragment (e.g. microsatellite or gene) to be amplified, together with a pool of building-block DNA nucleotide bases and DNA-polymerase enzyme. Through temperature modulation the target double-stranded DNA is duplicated many times over, first by denaturing to two single strands, and then through synthesis of two new complementary strands from building-block nucleotides using each single strand as a template (Fig. 4.6).

Two important genetic analytical processes utilize polymorphic markers. These are loss of constitutional heterozygosity and linkage analysis.

LOSS OF CONSTITUTIONAL HETEROZYGOSITY

Where two different alleles exist at a known polymorphic marker locus in diploid constitutional DNA, loss of one allele in tumour DNA from the same individual is known as loss of constitutional heterozygosity. This might indicate that one copy of a tumour suppressor gene close to the marker locus

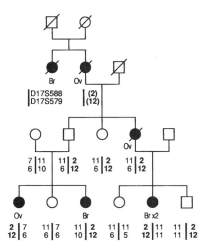

Fig. 4.7 A breast-ovarian cancer family illustrating inheritance of alleles from two adjacent markers mapping to chromosome 17q close to BRCA1. In this family allele 2 of marker D17S588 and allele 12 of marker D17S579 segregate through the pedigree with individuals affected by malignancy. Ov: ovarian cancer, Br: unilateral breast cancer, Brx2: bilateral breast cancer.

has been deleted in the tumour DNA. Although the whole genome exhibits a background rate of loss of heterozygosity in 10–20% of blood–tumour paired samples, higher rates of allele loss occur, for example, close to the APC gene in colorectal cancer tissue.

LINKAGE ANALYSIS

The approach most commonly employed to localize a susceptibility gene for familial disease is known as linkage analysis. Within a given family, individuals will have one allelic form of a polymorphic marker on each of the two chromosome copies on which that marker is located. The individual may be homozygous for the marker, in which case the two alleles will be identical, or heterozygous, in which case two different allelic forms of the marker will be present. These markers are heritable. Thus each parent randomly contributes one or other allele to each of two haploid gametes which, after zygotic fusion, proceed to constitute the alleles of the marker detected in the offspring's genetic make-up. Markers, like genes, are aligned in linear fashion along each chromosome. If the polymorphic marker under analysis is physically close to the disease-causing gene on the chromosome then the chance that a particular allele will segregate with individuals who have the disease (and therefore obviously carry the gene) through several generations of a family is high. This phenomenon, known as *linkage* of susceptibility gene and marker locus, allows mathematical analysis of marker data in blood

DNA from affected and unaffected family members. The probability for or against linkage can thereby be calculated. Thus chromosome bands can be confirmed or excluded as sites of susceptibility genes in familial disease. These loci are then subjected to intensive screening to identify and sequence genes causing heritable traits (Fig. 4.7).

Clinical applications

SCREENING

Examination of a detailed family history may reveal individuals at increased risk of subsequent cancers to whom screening might be offered. This of course assumes that a specific and sensitive mode of screening for the cancer in question is available. The identification of persons carrying a particular gene mutation might allow such screening to be more accurately targeted towards those at highest risk. This is the case with carriers of the APC gene mutation who are advised to undergo colonoscopy from their early teens and, if affected by multiple polyps, to have prophylactic subtotal colectomy with ileorectal anastomosis. Such screening programmes naturally raise many ethical questions to which there are no easy answers. The issues of confidentiality both amongst individual family members and interested third parties such as life insurance companies are of paramount importance but as yet have not been the subject of legislation.

In conditions where the precise mutation in a tumour suppressor gene cannot yet be identified, linkage analysis may be used to calculate the probability that the disease in that family is caused by a given gene and to identify probable carriers of the mutation. Screening and prophylactic measures may then be targeted towards those individuals most likely to benefit.

HUMAN GENOME MAPPING PROJECT (HGMP)

The HGMP was publicly initiated in 1986 at a symposium in Cold Spring Harbor, USA. At present its 5-year goals (October 1990–September 1995) include completion of a fully connected human genetic map with polymorphic markers spaced at approximately 100 000 base pair intervals. A final goal (within a 15-year period) is the physical mapping and sequence description of all human genes together with their controlling regions. Internationally, data are compiled on an annual basis through workshops which review research on individual chromosomes. Initial benefits are anticipated to be in the health care field through the identification and sequencing of genes that confer susceptibility to common disorders such as diabetes, heart disease, cancers and psychiatric conditions; diseases which epidemiological studies suggest have a strong genetic component. Scarce resources may then be targeted at small, defined population groups shown through genetic screening to be at high risk of morbidity or mortality from these conditions.

GENE THERAPY

The rapid advances being made in molecular knowledge have created the potential for using genetic mechanisms to improve detection and treatment, particularly in the field of oncology.[12] Tumour cells may be tagged with a foreign marker gene, the presence of which can then be used to detect minimal residual disease following chemotherapy. Cytokines such as the interleukins and interferons are known to be tumouricidal but are toxic in the doses required for systemic administration. If the genes for these products could be inserted into cells which could then be specifically targeted to cancer cells, the safety of treatment and the potential response would both be greatly enhanced by achieving a high local concentration without systemic toxicity.

Many genes are preferentially expressed in tumour cells. In some cases it has been possible to couple a drug-activating enzyme to the promotor sequence such that a chemotherapeutic agent, delivered to all cells, will only be active in tumour cells. Other avenues currently being explored include the suppression of oncogene expression and replacing defective tumour suppressor genes.

References

1. Macdonald F, Ford CHJ. *Oncogenes and Tumour Suppressor Genes*. Oxford: BIOS Scientific Publishers, 1991.
2. Davies KE, Read AP. *Molecular Basis of Inherited Disease*. Oxford: IRL Press, 1988.
3. Bishop JM. Molecular themes in oncogenesis. *Cell* 1991; **64**: 235–48.
4. Steel CM. Genetic abnormalities in cancer. *Current Opinion in Biotechnology* Vol. 1. Current Biology Ltd, 1990: 188–95.
5. Weinberg RA. Oncogenes, tumor suppressor genes and cell transformation: trying to put it all together. *Origins of Human Cancer: A Comprehensive Review*. Cold Spring Harbor: Cold Spring Harbor Laboratory Press, 1991: 1–16.
6. Malkin D, Friend SH. The role of tumour suppressor genes in familial cancer. In: Hastie ND (ed.) *Seminars in Cancer Biology*, Vol. 3. London: Academic Press, 1992: 121–30.
7. Fearon ER, Vogelstein B. A genetic model for colorectal tumorigenesis. *Cell* 1990; **61**: 759–67.
8. Dunlop MG. Screening for large bowel neoplasms in individuals with a family history of colorectal cancer. *Br J Surg* 1992; **79**: 488–94.
9. Steel CM, Cohen BB, Porter DE. Familial breast cancer. In: Hastie ND (ed.) *Seminars in Cancer Biology*, Vol. 3. London: Academic Press, 1992: 141–50.
10. Steel M, Thompson A, Clayton J. Genetic aspects of breast cancer. *Br Med Bull* 1991; **47**: 504–18.
11. Eccles MR, Phipps RF. Oncogenes and tumour suppressor genes in breast cancer. *Br J Hosp Med* 1993; **50**: 529–36.
12. Sikora K. Genes, dreams and cancer. In: Mead GM (ed.) Current issues in cancer (series) *Br Med J* 1994; **308**: 1217–21.

PART II

Management principles

CHAPTER 5

Prevention of postsurgical infections

STEPHEN J KARRAN

He who tells the truth will be chased out of nine villages.

Old Turkish Proverb

The role of audit and surveillance

Surgical audit and particularly surveillance programmes involving detailed assessment of patients returning into the community,[1,2] confirm that postoperative infections remain the most common and sometimes the most serious cause of *avoidable* complications ensuing from surgery.

Few centres in the United Kingdom have, as yet, achieved the thoroughness and sensitivity of surveillance systems which have been firmly established for many years in North America. Notable examples, among many such surveillance programmes, are the systems established by Peter Cruse in Calgary,[3] David Birnbaum[4] in Victoria, British Columbia and Lee in Mineapolis.[5] Time and again the merits of such programmes have been demonstrated, first, by accurately identifying existing problems, reducing them by targeted action, and finally maintaining the improvement achieved by continuing surveillance. Such programmes have been shown to be highly cost effective. For surgery to proceed into the new millennium without absorbing and applying these lessons will be nothing less than an abdication of responsibility by both the profession and by administration, who so far have failed to provide the genuine support that is vital to success. Criteria for such programmes are given in Table 5.1.

Studies carried out in Southampton over the last two decades have confirmed the truth of the lessons that Cruse and others have long taught. For example, the *genuine* complication rate, detected only by community surveillance or similar recall follow-up, gives the clearest and the most accurate indication of the excellence (or otherwise) of an individual surgeon's performance. It is also a clear marker of the effectiveness of a surgical unit and the hospital in which surgery is performed.[2] These lessons have sadly not as yet been learnt by our profession at large and therefore hardly suprisingly by those in charge of our destinies as clinicians.[6]

Among the lessons taught by the likes of Cruse and Birnbaum is that once an accurate, complete and

Table 5.1 Recommendations for surgical audit meetings

Must be:

Regular (at least once every 2 weeks)
Structured, e.g. informal 'leader' – optimally a rotating privilege
Compulsory for all surgical staff
Welcoming to nursing, anaesthetic and other relevant staff
Recorded fully and accurately
Protected in law
Timely, i.e. providing surveillance
Ongoing, i.e. also to provide surveillance
Active and proactive to effect change
Complete, i.e. to discuss *successes* (especially unexpected and also *'near misses'*)
Enthusiastically supported by management

Ethos must be:

Confidential
Consultant led
Never a 'witch hunt'
Honest
All (*especially seniors*) must accept constructive criticism
Educational – otherwise a waste of time

Based on *Recommendations of the Wessex Working Party on Surgical Audit*, 1988; and *Recommendations of Royal Colleges of Surgeons, 1989.*

relevant surveillance system is put in place the genuine complication rate can fall automatically by up to 50% as a direct result of the surveillance programme itself ('the Hawthorn effect'). There is no incentive to clinicians as effective as the knowledge that their performance is being monitored. Examples of dramatic improvements in surgical performance include the reduction in postoperative surgical catheter-related urinary tract infections, postoperative wound haematomas and the consequent wound infections following 'clean' surgery such as hernia repair[7] and breast surgery.[8]

One day, perhaps, both surgeons and managers and (particularly accountants) will acknowledge that there is, quite simply, no more effective way of providing the quality service which all patients deserve than by getting it right first time.

Prevention of contamination

The key to the avoidance of postoperative infections is strict adherence to all the well-known principles of aseptic technique, allied to relevant sterilization of equipment and all surgical materials and the judicious use of antiseptics (Table 5.2). By these methods tissues 'at risk' are protected against possible contamination.

Although there is active debate about the effective-ness of some traditional surgical rituals, such as the value of face masks, there is no debate about the principle of striving ceaselessly to prevent exposed susceptible tissues, such as the wound, from inoculation with potential pathogens. This principle applies with equal validity to contamination from outside the patient (and this includes his or her own skin and nares etc., i.e. exogenous contamination), as to contamination from infected material such as bile or faeces from within (endogenous contamination).

Clearly, major differences exist between the flora responsible for exogenous and endogenous routes of contamination. There are also major differences in the stablility of such flora. The flora of the colon has, for example, in all probability, been consistent for thousands of years. By contrast, the pattern of exogenous pathogens, has, for largely unknown reasons, altered significantly over the last century. Streptococci posed the major threat during the Crimean War and up to the turn of the century. Gradually their pathological pre-eminence gave way to staphylococci, though even today streptococci can cause havoc, particularly among immunosuppressed patents.[9] Few will forget the recent furore over 'flesh-eating bugs'!

A further critical factor in the ever changing threat posed by bacterial pathogens, especially of the exogenous variety, has been the use, and particularly the abuse, of antibiotics during the last three decades. The emergence of multiply resistant organisms, sometimes of quite 'exotic' varieties, the ever present

Table 5.2 Methods of sterilization and disinfection

NB all equipment must be scrupulously cleaned prior to sterilization

Heat

An autoclave (preferably porous load) should be used for sterilization of surgical instruments.

1.	Autoclave	Steam under pressure e.g. 132° for 3 min at 2.2 bar.	Destroys all microorganisms including spores
	a) Porous load (in CSSD)	Vacuum removed.	Wrapped instruments which can be stored. Quality assured.
	b) Simple	No vacuum.	Unwrapped instruments (use immediately or up to 3 h if covered).
2.	Boiling	5 min from time water boils.	Does not destroy spores, for medium risk instruments only.
3.	Pasteurization	80°C 1 min.	Disinfects only, e.g. bedpan washers.
4.	Hot air ovens	160°C 3 h. high temperature may destroy instruments.	Destroys spores, mainly used for glassware.
5.	Ethylene oxide	Gas at a low temperature. Flammable. Found in very few centres. Instruments have to be aired for 7 days.	Destroys spores, etc. Used for very expensive sensitive equipment.
6.	Ionization radiation	Commercial use.	Plastics.

Chemicals

Mainly used for disinfection, as most not active against spores.

Many corrosive   :   damages instruments
      irritant   :   Health and Safety issues

must be made up and stored correctly.

1.	Glutaraldehyde e.g. Cidex®, Gigasept®	Kills bacteria, fungi, viruses rapidly. Tubercle bacilli. Spores. Sterilization.	60 min 3–10 h min. 3 h, preferably longer; *Autoclave Method Better.*
		Disinfection e.g. endoscopes Use when no other alternative.	4–60 min according to type of instrument, site of use and whether patient compromised.
2.	Hydrogen peroxide e.g peracetic acid, Steris®	Wide activity against bacteria, fungi, viruses. Peracetic acid also destroys spores and mycobacteria. New–for endoscopes, less irritant than glutaraldeyhde, more corrosive.	
3.	Hypochlorites e.g. Milton®, Presept® Sodium dichloroisocyanurate (NaDCC)	Active against most organisms. Corrosive: damages instruments. Mainly used for surface cleaning.	
4.	Phenol e.g. Cidex®, Stericol®	Destroys most bacteria (not spores or viruses). Used as surface agent only.	
5.	Alcohol e.g. 70% industrial methylated spirits, ethanol	Rapidly destroys bacteria and fungi. Less active viruses, no effect on spores. Mainly used for thermometers. Very useful for hand cleansing combined with chlorhexidine or povidone iodine.	
6.	Chlorhexidine (Hibiscrub®)	Kills bacteria, more effective gram positive than gram negative. Skin disinfectant. Not suitable for equipment.	
7.	Povidine iodine e.g. Betadine®, often contains 1% alcohol	Active against bacteria. Some activity against viruses and fungi. Less prolonged activity than chlorhexidine. Used as a skin disinfectant.	

Table courtesy of Dr Ann Pallett.

Table 5.3   Attributes of the 'ideal' surgeon[a]

1.   Careful patient selection
2.   Gentle tissue handling → minimize devitalization
3.   Immaculate haemostasis
4.   Avoidance of unnecessary foreign material
5.   Wise suture choice
6.   Immaculate anastomotic technique
7.   Avoidance of spillage of bile, faeces, etc.
8.   Careful use of appropriate prophylaxis, e.g. antibiotic, antithrombogenic
9.   Avoidance of time wasting
10. Willingness to learn (i.e. humility)
11. Dedication to meaningful audit and many others

[a] after Lord Moynihan:
   'the heart of a lion,
   the eyes of a hawk,
   the hands of a woman,
   and also 'her intelligence' (Linda Graham, personal communication)

threat of methicillin-resistant staphylococci (MRSA), and also highly destructive fungi and yeasts, all pay tribute to the supreme carelessness of the medical profession and the pharmaceutical industry. The sins of our predecessors, and indeed of our own youth, are currently being visited upon us in no uncertain manner.

The importance of surgical technique

Poston and Winstanley in Chapter 6 have stressed the importance of surgical technique in the management of the cancer patient. This message is at least as important in the prevention of postoperative infections. Enormous individual surgeon variations can be seen in many studies. The large study by McArdle from Glasgow provides convincing proof of this. In one of our own studies,[10] in which the complication rate after re-anastomosis following Hartmann's procedure was studied, a more than ten-fold difference was seen between individual consultant surgeons.

The reasons for discrepancies in postoperative infection rates are multiple, with leakage from anastomoses being but one major contributor (Table 5.3). Within the responsibility of the surgeon lie a multiplicity of critical decisions. These include the suitability of the patient for surgery, the necessity for, and appropriateness of, the planned surgical procedure, and the choice of sutures or other foreign materials such as meshes, as all of these carry individual risks of trapping or encouraging infection.

Our own audit studies over the last 20 years have indeed confirmed that the price of freedom (i.e. from infection – and also litigation) is eternal vigilance.

Fitness of the patient

Over the centuries certain high risk categories of patients have become manifest. The malnourished, the immunosuppressed, the jaundiced are but a few such patients (Table 5.4). Despite the caveats regarding the infective risk in diabetes (see Chapter 9), when even a suspected high risk patient presents to the surgeon, it is imperative that the question be asked 'is it necessary to do anything more than the routine (e.g. consider the addition of antibiotic prophylaxis) for such a patient ?'. The surgeon must then decide on an *individual* patient basis what the relevant risks are when such extra precautions are instituted and weigh these against the risks of failing to provide such added protection. It is thus imperative that surgeons familiarize themselves with all currently available antimicrobial agents. In particular, it is essential that they understand not only the *in vitro* sensitivities (i.e. the spectrum of activity), but also the relevant pharmacokinetics of the compound, with particular reference to such matters as its absorption, distribution, half life (t/2), tissue penetration, metabolism and excretion. Failure to take these elementary educational steps can imperil their patients. More than one commercially driven antibiotic study is rejected for publication when submitted to peer review because of misleading, and even dangerous, protocols, even though these may have deceived unsuspecting local ethics committees. Finally, of course, the risk of all possible adverse reactions that can occur with such antibiotics must be fully appreciated.

Such considerations naturally apply to all patients warranting surgical phrophylaxis (e.g. elective colorectal procedures) but even more important in high

Table 5.4   High risk factors

Emergency surgery

Immunosuppression

  (a) Malnutrition
  (b) Co-morbidity, e.g.
      Liver disease
      Renal failure
      Diabetes (see also Chapter 2)
      Myopathies
      Neurological disease
      Other endocrine/metabolic disease
  (c) Drugs
      Steroids
      Antineoplastic drugs
  (d) Post-radiotherapy
  (e) Malignancy

Localized factors

e.g. Exploration of common bile duct
Crohn's disease
Malignancy
Central venous access

risk patients for several reasons. Not only is the 'physiological safety margin' usually reduced in such patients (e.g. because of depressed renal or hepatic function) but also the pharmacokinetics and tissue distribution can be grossly altered by suboptimal physiological conditions.

It should go without saying, that following the identification of any high risk factor, wherever possible, an attempt should be made to modify any such factors which might thereby reduce the risk. Otherwise, even a minor degree of contamination can result in disastrous clinical sequelae.

Unfortunately, however, in many instances, and particularly in emergency situations, there is very little if anything that can actually be done to reduce these risks significantly.

Antimicrobial prophylaxis

In the last three decades dramatic reductions in the infective risks of surgery have been achieved by rational approaches to prophylaxis. The scientific basis of such therapy was initially clearly defined by the pioneering work of Sir Ashley Miles and Professor John Burke working in the former's laboratory. In essence, the guiding principle of prophylaxis may be stated thus: the relevant antibiotic (i.e. one which is active against the organisms likely to be responsible for any contamination of previously clean tissues, whether that be from exogenous or endogenous sources) must adequately penetrate the tissues at risk (e.g. the wound) *immediately prior* to any inoculation by contaminating organisms. Tissue levels of *at least* 4 × the MICs (i.e. the *in vitro* minimal inhibitory concentrations) of these organisms must be achieved and maintained throughout the period of risk. However, as soon as that period of risk has passed, the antibiotics are no longer required – indeed they present an unnecessary hazard and should be withdrawn forthwith. Likewise, inappropriately prolonged antibiotic administration prior to the risk of contamination can only lead to an increased likelihood of production of resistant organisms – and this risk applies not only to the individual patient but to others as well. The same hazard applies to the environment itself. The unnecessary prolongation of administration after the end of this 'risk period' will similarly foster such dangers. In addition, the risk of unwanted effects of a wide variety, including hypersensitivity reactions, renal and hepatic impairment, CNS toxicity (and particularly ototoxicity with the aminoglycosides) will be increased. Diarrhoea, and even potentially fatal pseudomembranous colitis, are everyday risks in this form of management that must always be remembered. Finally, no health care system can afford the inevitable wastage of valuable resources that inappropriate, unconsidered prophylaxis inevitably produces. (See Antibiotic policies, p. 59.)

Period of risk

This is clearly the period during which exposed tissues such as the wound or the peritoneum might become contaminated. This applies equally to either external (exogenous) sources of infection or to infective sources already within the body (endogenous).

The period of risk for exogenous sources is usually extremely easy to assess. Invariably it is the same as the 'skin-to-skin' time, providing, of course, that there is no interference with the wound or occlusive dressings after the return of the patient to the ward. Thus an 'umbrella' time of an hour or two should be more than adequate to cover many procedures such as an 'open' cholecystectomy. More prolonged procedures will, however, require a more extensive period of cover. Depending on the pharmacokinetic properties (such as the half-life) of the antibiotic used, it may well be necessary to provide an additional dose, over and above the original prophylactic dose, which is given most commonly nowadays intravenously at the induction of anaesthesia. Other routes and methods of administration must be modified accordingly (see below).

More contentious, however, is the judgement of what constitutes the actual period of risk against endogenous contamination.

When, in an open cholecystectomy, for example, the infected gall bladder has been safely removed and the cystic duct stump securely ligated, providing there is no bile leak present such as from accessory biliary radicals within the gall bladder fossa, the period of risk comes to a definitive end. This is usually immediately prior to the closure of the wound.

In many studies conducted in the 1970s and 1980s it was clearly shown that a single dose of a suitable broad-spectrum antibiotic (without anti-anaerobic activity as anaerobes are seldom a hazard in this situation[11,12]) given intravenously at induction of anaesthesia[13–15] was as effective as three doses of the same antibiotic given over a 24-hour perioperative period. (The most commonly chosen antibiotic was a second- or even third- generation cephalosporin such as cephazolin or cefuroxime.) These studies confirmed conclusively that the period of risk for such elective procedures was indeed relatively short, i.e. less than an hour or so.

More recently it has been shown that similar protection can be given to these patients with a single oral tablet of the 4-quinolone, ciprofloxacin, *providing* it is given at least 30 minutes prior to any premedicant drugs. Several of these drugs, principally opiates and anticholinergic drugs, either, delay and/or reduce the absorption of this and similar antibiotics. If this occurs the fundamental principles of prophylaxis are negated. Any benefits that such antibiotics might produce must, therefore, rely on the principle of early treatment rather than prophylaxis. Confusion in this area is rife, so much so that many so-called prophylactic regimen should more accurately be labelled as being 'prophyltreatment'.[11]

Regardless of which method of prophylaxis is chosen, usually a 4-to-6 hour period of cover is provided. As stated above, this has been repeatedly proven to be more than adequate and is usually achieved with a single dose of the suitable antibiotic depending on its pharmacokinetic properties.

An additional benefit of single-dose prophylaxis, which has been less often documented, however, has been an up to three-fold reduction in postoperative respiratory infective complications and undiagnosed (and undiagnosable), postoperative fevers. These would often, otherwise, be treated with a short therapeutic course of antibiotics[16] on most surgical units.

Colorectal surgery

When we regard optimal prophylaxis for these common procedures, however, the situation is not so clear as it is with elective biliary surgery. Failure to provide prophylaxis in colorectal surgery has been associated with a <50% serious infective complication rate.

In this situation it is, of course, necessary to provide additional cover against *anaerobic* bacteria, particularly the bacteriodes. Failure to do so can produce extremely unpleasant complications, and these may well be delayed, producing late wound infections or deep abscesses. Certainly, such complications generally present later than postoperative infections caused by both Gram-negative rods and Gram-positive cocci.

The major contentious issue with colorectal surgery relates to the possible ongoing endogenous infective risk following colonic anastomosis.

On theoretical grounds a straightforward right hemicolectomy, undertaken as an elective procedure by the same surgeon, should have a much lower leak rate and thus a lower infective risk than a difficult low anastomosis undertaken within a narrow pelvis.

In the former case there should generally be virtually no problems of exposure, lighting, blood supply or general viability of the bowel except, of course, in Crohn's disease. By contrast, the difficulties that can only too often occur in performing an anastomosis deep in a dimly lit, narrow pelvis, with possibly a less than perfect blood supply to the bowel ends, are only too well known. Even in the best of hands leaks can occur. The incidence of radiologically detected leaks, in such cases, far outnumbers the incidence of clinically obvious leaks. It is not far fetched, therefore, to assume that the number of 'microbiological leaks' is even higher.

Furthermore, the contents of the gut which might escape into the peritoneum and beyond are usually totally different in these contrasting situations in terms of both inoculum size and flora. Small gut content, flowing past the anastomosis of a right hemicolectomy, whilst not sterile, is invariably far less hazardous to the peritoneum should it escape than the contents of the proximal colon flowing past a low risk pelvic anastomosis. Keighley and his colleagues[17] demonstrated many years ago the almost undiminished microbiological hazard of such colonic effluent, even after apparently successful colonic evacuation.

This observation, incidentally, lends credence to the philosophy embraced in many North American centres, of a 'dual' approach to prophylaxis in colorectal surgery, i.e. the combination of systemic prophylaxis with orally administered, non-absorbable, antibiotics. This approach is gaining favour – even in the United Kingdom despite a theoretical increased risk of producing resistant organisms, superinfections (e.g. fungal) or ever inducing pseudomembranous colitis.

However, the theoretical differences in risk between right-sided and low left-sided anastomoses mentioned above have not generally been borne out in clinical studies. One of the problems in this particular failure to show a difference is the fact that many elective right hemicolectomies are given to less experienced surgeons to perform because they are less difficult. In addition, when hemicolectomies are undertaken as emergencies, they are also often performed in less than ideal circumstances, such as in the middle of the night and again often by less experienced surgeons. Such practices have rightly been vigorously denounced by the recent Confidential Enquiry into Peri-Operative Deaths (CEPOD).[18]

Recommendations

Despite the apparent success of shorter courses of prophylactic cover in colorectal surgery in recent years,[19,20] a full 24-hour cover against both aerobes and anaerobes remains generally advisable. This is conveniently provided by a three-dose regimen of a suitable cephalosporin such as cefuroxime 750 mg, together with metronidazole 500 mg. The initial dosage of cefuroxime (i.e. at the time of induction) may be doubled to 1.5 g to provide a suitable 'loading dose'.

This recommendation applies providing there are no major worries about the intraoperative procedure, particularly the integrity of the anastomosis. If any such worries should exist it is wise to convert the prophylactic regimen into a short-course therapeutic regimen. This is conveniently achieved by continuing the same antibiotics until the patient has remained apyrexial for at least 24 hours.

There is, of course, a plethora of different and effective antibiotic regimen available and some of these involve single agents (i.e. effective against both aerobes and anaerobes) e.g. a carbapenem such as Imipenem, or antibiotics containing β-lactamase inhibitors such as Sulbactam and Augmentin. None of these alternatives, however, has proven itself superior to the standard regimen mentioned above. Single agents may have the advantage of convenience, but this is often more than offset by greatly increased costs, and also by the danger of destroying the value of these more potent antibiotics for the treatment of serious, or even life-threatening, infections by encouragement of the emergence of resistant organisms.

Other procedures

Space excludes discussion of other clinical problem areas such as urological surgery, orthopaedics and neurosurgery. The same underlying principles enunciated by Miles and Burke, however, pertain just as much as with the gastrointestinal examples discussed here, i.e. discover the microbiological risk and cover the period through which it applies. Of considerable interest in recent years, however, has been the realization that some 'clean' surgical procedures, particularly in high risk patients, might justify the use of antibiotic prophylaxis.[7,8]

Antibiotic policies

One of the major advances in the United Kingdom in recent years has been the widespread adoption of antibiotic policies in nearly all hospitals. The importance of such clearly defined policies is that they should ensure:

1. That patients receive only *appropriate* antibiotics for their condition, and that the details of their administration in terms of dosage, distribution, etc. should be optimal.
2. That the risks of encouragement of *resistant* organisms, with all the attendant hazards not only for individual patients but also for the general hospital and even the community itself should minimized.
3. That best *value for money* can be obtained for the hospital. There are several ways in which this can be achieved. For example, whenever possible generic formulations of drugs rather than brand names can be used. Bulk purchasing of commonly used antibiotics can also save vast amounts of limited resources. Implicit in such arrangements is the prevention of commercial interests or personal inducements.

Cost

Avoidable complications such as wound infections waste vast amounts of precious resources.[21]

Summary

In this brief review some of the major determinants of prevention of infection arising in surgical patients have been outlined. The major problems with this 'oldest of surgeons' adversaries' (personal communication, Sir James Fraser) is its multifactorial nature. This review can hope to do no more than stimulate interest, arouse awareness and thus encourage all responsible for minimizing the risks to which every patient undergoing surgery is exposed, to leave no stone unturned in their efforts. No longer should effective audit of infections be regarded as 'an insult to the surgeon's virility' (J. Alexander Williams, personal communication), or the truth be subjected to 'selective forgetfulness' (Hiram Polk, personal communication). An excellent start to essential further reading is *Infection in Surgical Practice* edited by Eric Taylor.[15] Topics discussed in detail range from classification of operations and audit of infection by Peter Cruse, to a wide range of clinical problems including antibiotic resistance.

References

1. Bailey IS, Karran SE, Toyn K *et al.* Community surveillance of complications after hernia surgery. *Br Med J* 1992; **304**: 469–71.
2. Karran SJ, Brough P. Surveillance of day-case surgery. *Proceeding Annual Scientific Meeting Royal College Surgeons, Edinburgh, 1994.*
3. Cruse PJE, Foord R. The epidemiology of wound infection. A 10–year prospective study of 62 939 wounds. *Surg Clin N Am* 1980; **60**: 27–40.
4. Birnbaum D. Risk management vs infection control committees. *Dimensions* 1981; **58**(12): 16–21.
5. Olsen MM, Lee JT. Continuous 10-year wound infection surveillance. Results advantages and unanswered questions. *Arch Surg* 1990, **125**: 794–803.
6. Karran SJ, Ranaboldo CJ, Karran AJ. Review of the perceptions of general surgical staff within the Wessex region of the status of quality assurance and surgical audit. *Ann Roy Coll Surg Engl* 1993; **75** (Suppl): 104–7.
7. Ranaboldo CJ, Karran SE, Bailey IS, Karran SJ. Antimicrobial prophylaxis in 'clean' surgery: hernia repair, *J Antimicrobial Chemother* 1993 (Supple B): 35–41.
8. Platt R, Zucker JR, Zalaznik DF *et al.* Perioperative antibiotic prophylaxis and wound infection following breast surgery. *J Antimicrob Chemother* 1993; **31** (Suppl. B): 43–8.
9. Scott SD, Dawes RFH. Tate JJT *et al.* The practical management of Fournier's gangrene. *Ann Roy Coll Surg Engl* 1988; **70**(1): 16–20.
10. Pearce NW, Scott SD, Karran SJ. Timing and method of reversal of Hartmann's procedure. *Br J Surg* 1992; **79**: 839–41.
11. Keighley MRB, Flinn R. Alexander-Williams J. Multivariate analysis of clinical and operative findings associated with biliary sepsis. *Br J Surg* 1978; **63**: 528–31.
12. Chetlin SH, Elliott DW. Pre-operative antibiotics in biliary surgery. *Arch Surg* 1973; **107**: 319–23.
13. Karran SJ, Moore PL, Goh H, Papachristodoulou AJ. Three-year experience with single dose cephalosporin prophylaxis in biliary surgery. In: Karran SJ (ed.) *Controversies in Surgical Sepsis.* New York: Prager, 1980; 293–302.
14. Strachan CJ, Black J, Powis SJA *et al.* Prophylactic use of cephazolin against wound sepsis after cholecystectomy. *Br Med J* 1977; **i**: 1254–6.
15. Karran SJ, Allen S, Lewington V *et al. Cefuroxime Propylaxis in Biliary Surgery.* Royal Society of Medicine International and Congress Series 1980; no. 38: 27–34. London: Royal Society of Medicine.
16. Karran SJ, de la Hunt M, Townend I *et al.* Prevention of infection in high risk biliary operations. *Antibiotic Chemother* 1985; **33**: 59–72.
17. Keighley MRB, Arabi Y, Alexander-Williams J. Comparison between systemic and oral antimicrobial proplyaxis in colorectal surgery. *Lancet* 1979; **i**: 894–7.
18. Buck N, Devlin HB, Lunn JN. *Confidential Enquiry into Perioperative Deaths (CEPOD).* Nuffield Provincial Hospitals Trusts and Kings Fund, 1987.
19. Rowe-Jones DC, Peel ALG, Kingston RD *et al.* Single-dose cefotaxime plus metronidazole as prophylaxis against wound infection in colorectal surgery: multicentre prospective randomised study. *Br Med J* 1990; **300**: 18–22.
20. Karran SJ, Sutton G, Gartell P *et al.* Imipenem prophylaxis in elective colorectal surgery. *Br J Surg* 1993; **80**: 1196–8.
21. de la Hunt MN, Chan AY, Karran SJ. Postoperative complications: how much do they cost? *Ann Roy Coll Surg Engl* 1986; **68**: 199–202.
22. Taylor E. *Infection in Surgical Practice.* Oxford: Oxford Medical Publications, 1992.

CHAPTER 6

Principles of surgery in malignant disease

GRAEME J POSTON, JOHN H R WINSTANLEY

Does surgical oncology exist?

For centuries, surgery has been the principal mode of treatment for patients suffering from cancer. Surgical efforts were aimed either at tumour destruction or removal. The first curative excision of an ovarian tumour was by McDowell in 1809 and in 1885 Billroth performed the first gastrectomy. Shortly afterwards, Volkmann performed the first protectomy for a rectal tumour, and at the turn of the century Halstead was advocating radical mastectomy. In 1896 the Glasgow surgeon Beatson reported a clinical improvement following oophorectomy in a patient with advanced breast cancer.

During the first decade of the twentieth century, radical prostatectomy (Young), radical hysterectomy (Wertheim) and abdominoperineal rectal excision (Miles) were all described, and in 1913 Torek performed the first oesophagectomy. In 1927 Divis was the first to resect a lung metastasis and in 1933 Graham performed the first successful pneumonectomy for lung cancer. Whipple described the first pancreatoduodenectomy for ampullary carcinoma in 1935. In 1945, Huggins followed up on Beatson's hormone manipulation hypothesis, advocating orchidectomy

and adrenalectomy for prostate cancer, for which he deservedly won the Nobel Prize for Medicine.

There is a tendancy today to regard the treatment of patients suffering from cancer as the remit of medical oncologists (chemotherapists) and clinical oncologists (the rather bizarre title now given to radiotherapists). This concept is based on the observation that they see only patients suffering from one disease process, namely cancer – *ergo* all patients with cancer should be treated by these particular clinicians. Such a remit cannot be absolute, since neither of these modalities offer any hope of cure to the vast majority of patients suffering from the common lethal (predominantly solid) forms of cancer. The use of chemotherapy and radiotherapy for the common solid tumours can only be recommended outside of clinical trials either as an adjunct to surgical resection or for palliation of surgically incurable disease.

The majority of common solid tumours (lung, breast, colon and rectum, stomach, pancreas, etc.) present clinically to surgeons and remain the major cancer killers. For patients with these common solid tumours, successful surgical excision offers the only chance of cure. Radiotherapy can cure the common skin cancers (basal cell carcinoma and squamous carcinoma) as effectively as surgical excision and chemotherapeutic regimen now offer hope to patients with rare cancers such as leukaemia and testicular teratoma, In addition, radiotherapy and chemotherapy can reduce the bulk of some advanced solid tumours. For patients with advanced disease, appropriately timed surgery, in combination with planned chemotherapy and radiotherapy, remains an important option for good palliation of symptoms.

Failure to produce higher cure rates in patients with these tumours is due to one of four factors: (1) the lesion has already disseminated beyond the operative field by the time of detection; (2) the cancer is multifocal in a vital organ; (3) the surgeon is unable to detect distant disease (overt or microscopic); (4) inadequate excision of the tumour and/or its local/regional spread.

In many areas of surgery for common tumours, there appears to have been a minimal advance over the past 50 or so years. If one looks at 5-year survival for patients following excision of a Dukes' Stage C rectal cancer in 1994 compared with 1932,[1] there appears, at face value, to be little improvement in outcome. However, this observation belies the fact that in 1932, many fewer patients could be offered safe surgery for a rectal cancer than today. Advances in surgical technique and prevention of blood loss, general anaesthesia and blood product replacement, antisepsis and antibiotic therapy, better preoperative imaging, use of adjuvant therapies and better understanding of tumour biology mean that many more patients receive timely, appropriate and potentially curative treatment than ever before. One example of these developments is the introduction of the American Society of Anaesthesiologists' (ASA) classification of patients' physical status, correlating this with operative/anaesthetic mortality. Class 1 patients have no physiological or organic disturbances, while Class 5 includes patients with little chance of survival but who require surgery as a potential life-saving procedure. Most cancer patients admitted for elective surgery fall within Classes 2–3. When these factors are combined with far greater patient education, awareness and expectation, then overall outcomes start to improve. Furthermore, on the back of these advances, radical and potentially curative surgery becomes possible for advanced cancers previously regarded as incurable. One obvious example is liver resection for primary and secondary hepatic tumours.

General principles of surgical oncology

Whereas medical and clinical oncologists previously maintained a general cancer practice, the surgical treatment of the common solid tumours was historically the brief of the general surgeon. General surgeons would treat cancer patients within a case mix that included patients with relatively minor ailments like varicose veins and herniae, along with non-malignant, but life-threatening, disorders such as aneurysms and peptic ulceration. The development of vascular and urological surgery as distinct entities allowed the residual rump of general surgery to concentrate on two site-specific areas of cancer; breast and gastroenterology. These two areas between them account for nearly 50% of cancer death certifications in the UK. In the cases of breast and colon and rectum, surgical excision of the primary tumour may cure nearly half of all patients at the time of initial presentation. Significantly, the greatest proportion of postoperative deaths in general surgery occur after colorectal surgery, particularly undertaken for cancer in the emergency setting.[2]

SPECIALIZATION

All physicians who regularly treat cancer patients recognize that specialization produces better outcomes. Clinical and medical oncologists now specialize in disease-specific areas; improving outcomes both by rapidly enhancing the individual clinician's experience and also by regular participation in clinical trials. Similarly, when surgeons specialize in specific complex cancer surgery there is both a reduction in operative morbidity and mortality, and also an improvement in overall survival.[3] In specialist tertiary centres, operative 30-day mortality for procedures such as oesophagectomy, pancreatoduodenectomy and partial hepatectomy does not exceed 2%, and in most is under 1%. In the present climate of health purchasers and providers, it will probably soon become the accepted norm that, unless a surgeon can demonstrate a personal audit that equals the outcome of the best centres in the literature, then specific operations will not be purchased from their unit.

We would therefore argue that successful surgical oncologists concentrate on site-specific practices, which may include one or two common tumours, and perform a repertoire of procedures which will benefit all patients who suffer from these particular cancers, and at different stages in their disease process.

COMBINED CLINICS

Since modern solid cancer treatment is a combination of all three treatment modalities, surgery, radiotherapy and cytotoxic chemotherapy/hormone therapy, then the appropriate management strategy should be determined jointly by the surgical, clinical and medical oncologists.[5] Although strategically ideal, for many surgeons with busy (and burgeoning) practices, regular joint clinics are seen as a luxury. In such a situation, shared care of the patient with a clinical or medical oncologist is the norm, alternating follow-up with all parties following a previously agreed management protocol. The successful surgical oncologist is one who resists influences that attempt to reduce him or her to the role of (albeit competent) technician in removing the 'lump', but having little or no say in pre- and postoperative patient management.

Cancer surgeons must keep abreast of oncological developments outside surgery. This is relevant not only to the implications of adjuvant and neoadjuvant chemotherapy and radiotherapy, but also to the rapidly expanding understanding of the oncological process at the molecular level.

THE CANCER PATIENT

Whilst cure remains the ideal goal, for most cancer patients the practical objective is good quality of life. When selecting surgical options for a patient with cancer, the surgeon must have a clear understanding of the natural history of the disease, in particular the patterns of metastasis. In addition, both the surgeon and the patient should understand the aims for surgical intervention and the risks of such interventions to the individual patient.

A major factor in poor outcome is poor or inappropriate patient selection. There may be little point in resecting a tumour in a patient with unstable angina, nor is there any place for radical surgery of a local lesion in a patient with disseminated malignancy. If a patient undergoes a general surgical operation within 3 months of a major myocardial infarction, the risk of perioperative cardiac death is 30%. If the operation is deferred until 6 months after the infarct, the risk falls to 15%. Even 12 months out, the risk of perioperative cardiac death is 5%. One in five patients with congestive cardiac failure do not survive major surgical intervention.

On the other hand, patients with widespread malignancy may have a poor quality of life because of local disease (e.g. the woman with a fungating breast cancer), and so might benefit from surgery to achieve local control. There are also patients with advanced and incurable local disease who benefit from timely surgical palliation which might improve both the quality and the length of life (e.g. the patient with gastric outflow obstruction and jaundice due to pancreatic cancer). Just as in the administration of chemotherapy and radiotherapy, the cancer surgeon must avoid 'overdoing' and 'underdoing' surgical intervention. Certainly, in palliative surgical intervention, it is in the patient's interest that the procedure is performed as safely and effectively as possible by the most experienced surgeon available. This should allow the patient to recover with the minimum of morbidity, and thus leave hospital quickly to gain the greatest possible quality of life for whatever time they have left. Classic examples of bad practice include leaving the senior house officer at the end of the list to perform or close a defunctioning colostomy, or taking the junior surgical trainee through a triple bypass for pancreatic cancer to practise anastomotic technique. *Primum non nocere* (above all, do no harm) is paramount in the decision-making process in palliative cancer surgery. The surgeon should only ever intervene in cases where patients have incurable malignancy if there is a realistic opportunity to achieve symptomatic relief, thereby prolonging life of reasonable quality.

Cancer patients are usually malnourished and this may lead to poor wound healing, greater risk of concurrent infection and delayed convalescence. Some cancers may precipitate coagulopathies, such as vitamin K depletion in obstructive jaundice and thrombophlebitis migrans in visceral malignancy. Furthermore, cancer patients are at greater risk of developing deep vein thrombosis during surgery, with subsequent risk of pulmonary embolism.[4]

Any experienced surgeon with a large cancer practice recognizes that cancer patients (and their families) need far more time than those patients with other conditions such as hernia or gallstones. One complicated patient can throw a busy outpatient clinic into chaos. Therefore surgeons with a major oncological interest should separate out their cancer clinic from any general practice that they undertake. The cancer clinics should be run by experienced medical and nursing staff and, ideally, jointly with other disciplines relevant to the patient. These include not only the medical and clinical oncologists, but ready access to cytopathology and specialist imaging. These last two areas become especially important to the management of tertiary referral patients who may have travelled long distances to attend the clinic, and in whose interests it is important to keep hospital attendance to a minimum. Furthermore, in addition to the regular clinic nursing staff (whose familiarity brings comfort to cancer patients who regularly attend), involvement at an early stage of colleagues specializing in palliative care (physicians and nurses) in the management of patients whose disease is inevitably incurable, pays immense dividends in the longer term.

THE SURGICAL ONCOLOGIST

Dr Glenn Steele Jr of Harvard Medical School has stated that 'the surgical oncologist is essentially a function of his or her training'.[5] Surgical training is undergoing a major overhaul in virtually every major Western country. This is partly in response to the changes in practice (particularly specialization) within the profession and also in response to political pressure regarding hours worked and health care reforms. In addition to the basic pathological principles of adequate tumour resection, training a cancer surgeon requires a broad-based background involving exposure to a whole range of surgical techniques including vascular and reconstructive surgery. As alluded to earlier, the cancer surgeon must be conversant with the techniques of medical oncology and radiotherapy colleagues. Perhaps equally important, cancer surgeons must have a thorough grounding in laboratory-based research techniques, since they will need to grasp developments in molecular, clinical and psychosocial oncology if they are to lead in the practice of their chosen oncological speciality.

SCREENING FOR CANCER

It is now apparent that screening to detect common cancers at an early stage in their development may improve overall outcome for the general population of cancer sufferers. Screening programmes vary widely in their cost, sophistication and overall accuracy. Although the benefit may be very great to the individual patient who is found to have an early cancer, the cost to the providers of health care (usually the rest of society) may also be considerable, and these precious resources might otherwise be deployed to greater overall social benefit. There are several prerequisites for a successful cancer screening programme. First, the cancer is common in the population under study. Second, the test itself has a high specificity and sensitivity. Third, the test is relatively cheap and cost effective. Fourth, the test has a high patient acceptance rate. Last, and perhaps must important, the test detects the cancer at a time when therapeutic intervention has a high probability of cure and is not simply bringing forward the time of diagnosis before inevitable death (lead time bias). Against these factors, one has to measure the psychological morbidity of the anxiety generated by false positive results, and subsequent negative impact of this on further acceptance of the screening programme.

Surgery may be required in the detection and treatment of several precancerous lesions. Familial polyposis is inherited as an autosomal dominant gene on chromosome 5 and left untreated will result in extensive large bowel adenomatosis with inevitable cancer development by the mid-twenties.[6] Prophylactic proctocolectomy before the age of 25 significantly reduces the prevalence of colon cancers and prolongs the life in these patients. Other precancerous lesions amenable to surgical excision include buccal leukoplakia, cervical carcinoma *in situ*, chronic ulcerative colitis and ductal carcinoma *in situ* of the breast.[7] In addition, colon and breast cancer may exhibit familial predispositions, thereby self-selecting kindreds for closer screening of individuals at risk.[8] The major decision for the surgical oncologist in this process is the timing of surgical intervention.

THE SURGICAL PRACTICE

The last general factor in the practice of surgical oncology is determined by the setting in which the surgeons find themselves. In the urban setting of a large general hospital or university medical centre, there may be a large staff of surgeons, each with their own (or several with the same) specialist interests. As such, the surgical oncologist can subspecialize and develop a tertiary practice in either the more complex aspects of surgery or the rarer diseases. Such a practice offers opportunities for both clinical and laboratory research, and also training facilities that may not be easily available elsewhere. In the smaller general hospital, particularly in a more rural setting, the surgeons have also to take part in the general emergency workload and must keep abreast of clinical developments in a much wider field of practice. They may be further hampered by the lack of intensive care facilities, and supported by junior staff much less experienced than those available in larger centres. In this setting, cancer surgeons should adjust their practice to one which is safe and successful for their patients. It is no less satisfying to cure a patient of cancer by safely removing a small primary tumour than it is to resect a giant metastasis.

Biological principles of surgery in malignant disease

THE SPREAD OF CANCER

Successful cancer surgery involves an understanding of the place of surgical expertise within the overall biology of the cancer being treated. Examples include the surgical management of basal cell carcinoma of the skin which essentially involves local excision and adequate skin cover, and the strategic principles of lymphatic resection in breast and colorectal cancer. A cancer is a tumour which has the capacity to invade and metastasize. Classically, spread is by one or more of four routes; direct invasion; lymphatic; blood-borne emboli; and transcoelomic deposits. Death is usually determined by the extent of tumour burden, but less frequently may be due to interference with a vital structure such as the urinary outflow tract, bile duct or airway. In some cases, death is due to destruction of a vital organ (e.g. brain or liver).

Staging for Breast Carcinoma

DEFINITIONS:

PRIMARY TUMOUR (T)

TX   Primary tumour cannot be assessed
T0   No evidence of primary tumour
Tis   Carcinoma *in situ:* Intraductal carcinoma, lobular carcinoma *in situ:* or Paget's disease of the nipple with no tumour
T1   Tumour 2 cm or less in greatest dimension
     T1a   0.5 cm or less in greatest dimension
     T1b   More than 0.5 cm, but not more than 1 cm in greatest dimension
     T1c   More than 1 cm, but not more than 2 cm in greatest dimension
T2   Tumour more than 2 cm, but not more than 5 cm in greatest dimension
T3   Tumour more than 5 cm in greatest dimension
T4   Tumour of any size with direct extension to chest wall or skin
     T4a   Extension to chest wall
     T4b   Oedema *(*including *peau d'orange)* or ulceration of the skin of breast or satellite skin nodules confined to same breast
     T4c   Both T4a and T4b
     T4d   Inflammatory carcinoma

REGIONAL LYMPH NODES (N)

NX   Regional lymph nodes cannot be assessed (e.g., previously removed or not removed for pathologic study)
N0   No regional lymph node metastasis
N1   Metastasis to movable ipsilateral axillary lymph node(s)
     N1a   Only micrometastasis (none larger than 0.2 cm)
     N1b   Metastasis to lymph node(s), any larger than 0.2 cm
         N1bi   Metastasis in 1 to 3 lymph nodes, any more than 0.2 cm and all less than 2 cm in greatest dimension
         N1bii   Metastasis to 4 or more lymph nodes, any more than 0.2 cm and all less than 2 cm in greatest dimension
         N1biii   Extension of tumour beyond the capsule of a lymph node metastasis less than 2 cm in greatest dimension
         N1biv   Metastasis to a lymph node 2 cm or more in greatest dimension
N2   Metastasis to ipsilateral axillary lymph nodes that are fixed to one another or to other structures
N3   Metastasis to ipsilateral internal mammary lymph node(s)

DISTANT METASTASIS (M)

MX   Presence of distant metastasis cannot be assessed
M0   No distant metastasis
M1   Distant metastasis (includes metastasis to ipsilateral supraclavicular lymph node(s))

AJCC/UICC STAGE GROUPING

Stage 0	Tis	N0	M0		Stage IIIA	T0	N2	M0
						T1	N2	M0
Stage I	T1	N0	M0			T2	N2	M0
						T3	N1	M0
Stage IIA	T0	N1	M0			T3	N2	M0
	T1	N1	M0					
	T2	N0	M0		**Stage IIIB**	T4	Any N	M0
						Any T	N3	M0
Stage IIB	T2	N1	M0					
	T3	N0	M0		**Stage IV**	Any T	Any N	M1

89-15M-Rev. 8/91-No. 3485.05

10/91

Fig. 6.1   The staging of cancer : breast carcinoma

Staging for Stomach Carcinoma

DEFINITIONS:

PRIMARY TUMOUR (T)

TX   Primary tumour cannot be assessed

T0   No evidence of primary tumour

Tis   Carcinoma *in situ;* intraepithelial tumour without invasion of lamina propria

T1   Tumour invades lamina propria or submucosa

T2*   Tumour invades muscularis propria or subserosa

T3** Tumour penetrates serosa (visceral peritoneum) without invasion of adjacent structures

T4** Tumour invades adjacent structures

* Note: A tumour may penetrate the muscularis propria with extension into the gastrocolic or gastrohepatic ligaments or the greater or lesser omentum without perforation of the visceral peritomeum covering these structures. In this case, the tumour is classified T2. If there is perforation of the visceral peritoneum covering the gastric ligaments or omenta, the tumour is classified T3.

** Note: The adjacent structures of the stomach are the spleen, transverse colon, liver, diaphragm, pancreas, abdominal wall, adrenal gland, kidney, small intestine, and retroperitoneum. Intramural extension to the duodenum or oesophagus is classified by the depth of greatest invasion in any of these sites including stomach.

REGIONAL LYMPH NODES (N)

NX   Regional lymph node(s) cannot be assessed

N0   No regional lymph node metastasis

N1   Metastasis in perigastric lymph node(s) within 3 cm from edge of primary tumour

N2   Metastasis in perigastric lymph node(s) more than 3 cm from edge of primary tumour , or in lymph nodes along left gastric, common hepatic, splenic, or coeliac arteries.

DISTANT METASTASIS (M)

MX   Presence of distant metastasis cannot be assessed

M0   No distant metastasis

M1   Distant metastasis

AJCC/UICC STAGE GROUPING

Stage 0	Tis	N0	M0
Stage IA	T1	N0	M0
Stage IB	T1	N1	M0
	T2	N0	M0
Stage II	T1	N2	M0
	T2	N1	M0
	T3	N0	M0
Stage IIIA	T2	N2	M0
	T3	N1	M0
	T4	N0	M0
Stage IIIB	T3	N2	M0
	T4	N1	M0
	T4	N2	M0
Stage IV	Any T	Any N	M1

91-15M-No. 3485.12
10/91

Fig. 6.2   The staging of cancer : stomach carcinoma

TUMOUR DOUBLING TIME

From a patient's perspective, the major factor that influences survival time from diagnosis to death in incurable cancer is tumour volume doubling time. The doubling time is influenced by several factors.[9] First, and most obvious, is the rate of mitosis and this is often an inverse factor of the degree of differentiation of the tumour. Well-differentiated tumours usually grow slowly, whilst poorly differentiated cancers tend to grow quickly. The second important factor is the rate of cell death. Cancer cells are very fragile when compared with most healthy tissues. They are usually more susceptible to hypoxia and to sudden environmental changes. Cells which are not diploid will fail to undergo mitosis successfully and will die. In most solid tumours at any given moment, 90% of the cells are either non-viable, dying or already dead. However, a factor that distinguishes cancer cells from normal cells is a loss of ability to undergo apoptosis, or programmed cell death. Restoration of apoptosis will tip the balance of outcome in favour of the patient. Tumour volume reduction by surgical extirpation, radiotherapy, chemotherapy or biological therapy may influence outcome by returning the tumour volume to a lower position on the growth curve. Unfortunately, the patient may still die earlier because of untreated local complications. Finally, growth rate may be modified by cytotoxic or biological intervention.

SUCCESSFUL METASTASIS

Solid tumours tend to follow a growth curve that is not linear, but sigmoid. This is particularly true for metastases in liver, lung and brain which may have been present for 1–2 years before detection. After a tumour embolus has lodged in the venous microcirculation of a target organ it must gain an arterial blood supply to grow beyond a small morulus of cells. The factors driving tumour angiogenesis remain poorly understood, but are the subject of considerable research since, if they could be manipulated, we would have a powerful tool to prevent metastasis. During the phase in which a metastasis is developing its arterial supply, growth is slow. However, as the vasculature is established, growth accelerates.

All experienced oncologists have anecdotal cases of patients whose prognosis appeared hopeless, but who subsequently survived for unexpectedly long periods of time, there are 'good' cancers as well as 'bad' cancers. Traditionally, the degree of differentiation of the primary tumour plays an important role. Well-differentiated metastases do not develop from a poorly differentiated primary. Similarly, a tumour whose conventional spread is by several routes renders it more aggressive than one with the capability of limited direct invasion. An example is the outcome following hepatic metastasectomy in colorectal cancer. Five-year survival is poorer in patients whose primary was Dukes' Stage C than those with Dukes' Stage B.[10] There are no data to prove that the Dukes' stage correlates with the age of a tumour. A colon cancer that has the biological ability to spread via lymphatics is generally more aggressive than one whose spread at the time of presentation was entirely local. The same is true of breast cancer where nodal status is one of the most powerful prognostic tools.[11,12] In colon cancer, it remains obscure what factors distinguish the patient with multiple bilateral liver and lung metastases from the fortunate few (<25%) with solitary or limited (up to 3) liver or lung metastases who might benefit from potentially curative metastasectomy.[10]

ONCOGENESIS

It is probable that many cancers have a long natural history from premalignant lesion to clinical cancer. One obvious citable example is the colorectal cancer of familial adenomatous polyposis (FAP). Clearly, the patient is born with the genetic 'time-bomb' already ticking, and develops mascroscopic malignancies some two decades later. Similarly, patients in breast cancer families and colon cancer (Lynch) families,[8] although not inheriting an autosomal dominant cancer gene, are born with several mutations already present and therefore prone to accelerated carcinogenesis. Fearon and Vogelstein have carefully dissected out the genetic pathway of colorectal oncogenesis.[13–15] The BRCA-1 gene[16] has been identified in breast cancer, and recently the BRCA-2 gene also by workers from the Imperial Cancer Research Institute.[41]

Allelic loss on chromosome 5 (FAP locus) and other nuclear events such as DNA hypomethylation result in a hyperproliferative state, 'initiating' the colonic mucosa. Subsequent events, including point mutations on the *ras* gene may result in adenoma formation. *Ras* point mutations have been identified in over 50% of colorectal adenomas and carcinomas, and are prevalent in most other common gastrointestinal (GI) malignancies.[17] The *ras* genes code for membrane receptor G-proteins which may respond to growth factors; therefore mutations may result in abnormal and accelerated growth responses by the cell to their surrounding environment.

Following mutation of one or more of these dominant oncogenes, development of the malignant phenotype may be accelerated by inactivation of tumour suppressor genes. One such suppressor gene is p53 which lies on chromosome 17; p53 codes for a peptide of molecular weight of 53 kD, which acts as a brake on DNA replication. Any point mutation of the wild-type p53 gene results in an inefficient mutant protein product with accelerated DNA synthesis. There is a second tumour suppressor gene (DCC or deleted in colon cancer gene) on the long arm of chromosome 18 (18q), mutation of which is associated with colon cancer progression in 70% of cases.[15] The DCC gene encodes for a cell adhesion molecule, and may prove to be the key that unlocks our understanding of the enzymatic process involved in disruption of the basement membrane and the start of direct invasion. Certainly, it is now possible to correlate the aggressiveness of a given cancer to its genetic mutations and this holds great promise for future screening programmes. Not only could it be possible to identify individuals at risk of developing a particular cancer, especially those who might develop the disease early in life, but also enable us to channel scarce resources to screen an at risk population. (See also Chapter 4.)

TUMOUR STAGING

At the macroscopic level, every undergraduate medical student learns by rote the routes of spread and staging classifications of the common cancers. For those of us in oncological surgical practice, these have practical implications which dictate our day-to-day activity. Every common solid cancer can now be staged prognostically according to the TNM (tumour, node, metastasis) system developed jointly by the American Joint Committee on Cancer (AJCC)

and the Union Internationale Contre le Cancer (UICC) (Figs 6.1 and 6.2). Such staging systems determine the appropriateness of surgical and non-surgical treatment strategies; allow comparative audit of outcome between different cancer centres; and form the basis of comparative trials of differing treatment modalities (Table 6.1).

In addition to his or her role in diagnosis and treatment of cancer, the surgeon may also be asked to assist in the staging process. Prior to widespread availability of computerized tomography (CT), staging laparotomy played an important role in the management of lymphoma. Careful laparotomy in patients with ovarian cancer will determine the necessity of subsequent chemotherapy. Finally, at the completion of a surgical resection, the placement of radio-opaque surgical clips determines the field for postoperative adjuvant radiotherapy. These staging systems may subsequently be modified by molecular changes observed in these tumours.

BIOPSY

The diagnosis of cancer is based on histological or cytological examination of tissue removed by either surgical, endoscopic or radiological methods. Sampling error remains a problem; positive biopsies of malignancy have high specificity, but negative biopsies have low sensitivity. In surgical practice, excisional biopsies, rather than incisional biopsies are

Table 6.1 Staging of colorectal Cancer (Astler–Coller modification of Dukes', AJCC/UICC)

Dukes' Stage	AJCC/UICC	Definition	5-Year survival (%)
Initial extension			
A	I	Mucosa only	95
B1		Within wall	85–90
B2(M)		Microscopically through wall	75–80
B2(G)	II	Grossly through wall	60–70
B3		Involves adjacent structures	30
Lymph nodes +ve			
C1		Within wall	50–60
C2(M)		Microscopically thorough wall	50
C2(G)	III	Grossly through wall	40–50
C3		Involves adjacent structures	20–30
(D)	IV	Distant metastases	5% without intervention

always to be preferred. Excision should ensure an adequate amount of tissue for a diagnosis and allows examination of the interface between tumour and normal tissue to assess invasion. Excisional biopsy also reduces the risk of cancer cell dissemination and abolishes problems of sampling error.

RESECTION MARGINS

The importance of resection margins varies according to tumour type. Common principles exist in most cases, the most fundamental of which is that the lesion should not be transgressed by the resection margin. Other principles include giving the pathologist enough normal material to exclude multifocal or confluent disease, classic examples being multifocal ductal carcinoma *in situ* (DCIS) in breast cancer or polyps in colon cancer. In some areas the requirements of the resection margin have reduced over the years. Traditionally, malignant melanomata required a margin of 5 cm, but careful studies have demonstrated that a 3 cm margin, and probably only a 1 cm margin are more than adequate, depending on tumour stage.[18, 19]

When a potentially curable solid cancer is not cured because of inadequate removal, the surgeon must accept responsibility. This argument is based on the premise that a cancer starts in one place, and its growth and spread is predictable. Therefore for some time in its early growth it is possible to completely excise the cancer and any adjacent metastatic spread. This hypothesis holds sway in colorectal cancer particularly with regard to lateral margins during proctectomy,[20] but, despite the teachings of Halstead, is all too often not the case in breast cancer. In several cancers, most notably head and neck

tumours and oesophageal neoplasms, multiple frozen section examinations are necessary at the resection margin to ensure adequacy of the excision.

LYMPHATIC CLEARANCE

The management of lymph nodes in cancer surgery serves two functions. Traditionally, lymphatic clearance may 'cure' the cancer, reducing the incidence of local recurrence. More contemporary thought suggests that nodal status may indicate the need for adjuvant therapy. The importance of lymph node dissection remains tumour specific.

It is quite clear that adequate lymph node clearance affects outcome in breast, colorectal and gastric cancer surgery. Contemporary debate rests on the level of surgical resection: axillary sampling plus radiotherapy versus axillary clearance in breast surgery,[11,12] Level 2 (R2) versus Level 3 (R3) resection in gastrectomy (see Table 6.2).[21] Similarly, in surgery for papillary carcinoma of the thyroid, should the lymphatic resection include all the draining lymphatics *en bloc* or be confined to only those lymph nodes obviously involved?[22] By contrast, most surgical oncologists accept that the benefit to be gained from prophylactic lymphadenectomy of regional lymph nodes in the treatment of malignant melanoma is debatable, particularly in the treatment of trunk melanomata which could spread equally to both axillae and both groins.[12]

ANASTOMOTIC TECHNIQUE

In colorectal surgery, several other operative factors influence outcome: the experience of the operating

Table 6.2 1906 Gastric cancer cases 1966–86, Yongata, Japan: 367 (19%) curative resections of patients with serosal involvement (2.2% overall operative mortality)[21]

	5-Year survival	
	R2 dissection	R3 dissection
	188 cases	165 cases
Operative mortality	3 (1.6%)	5 (3.0%)
Survival:		
Overall	49%	50% NS
N0	49%	84% NS
N1	71%	56% NS
N2	42%	35% NS
N3	31%	26% NS
Hepatoduodenal N3	0%	31%

R2 operations predominantly during earlier years, R3 operations in later years
R3 + R2 + hepatoduodenal, retropancreatic, colonic and mesenteric nodes

surgeon and the intensity of their practice.[3] Anastomotic technique is also important, both with regard to anastomotic failure and also the rate of local recurrence.[23,24]

ADJUVANT THERAPY

A better understanding of the biology of cancer spread allows us to channel scarce resources in adjuvant therapy to more appropriate and 'deserving' patients. Since, as already stated, neither chemotherapy nor radiotherapy (either external beam or local/topical) can cure breast or GI cancers, and are not without significant and sometimes fatal toxicity, their random and general use in the adjuvant setting cannot be supported. Adjuvant therapy is aimed at reducing any as yet undetected residual microscopic tumour burden after resection of all macroscopically evident tumour burden. By identification of patients at risk of late recurrence, particularly by their tumour stage at presentation, clear adjuvant therapy policies are emerging in breast and colorectal cancer. In breast cancer, all women who opt for wide local excision of invasive tumours should be offered radiotherapy to the site of excision (Table 6.3).[27]

In addition, if axillary lymph node sampling is preferred to axillary clearance, then positive sampling should be followed by adjuvant radiotherapy to that axilla. Pre- or postoperative radiotherapy to the rectal bed for Dukes' B and C lesions reduces the risk of local recurrence after excision of rectal cancers.[28,29] This does not lead to prolongation of survival, but does reduce the sequaelae of sometimes intolerable symptoms that may follow cancer recurrence in the sacral plexus.

Most postmenopausal women with breast cancer are now offered the anti-oestrogen drug tamoxifen for between 2 and 5 years after excision of their primary lesion with intent to cure. Its continued use after 5 years is the subject of the current ATOMS trial. Initial policies on adjuvant tamoxifen were based on the findings from the Nolvadex Adjuvant Trial Organization (NATO) and Scottish trials, which showed an improved survival and reduction in contralateral tumours.[30,31] The evidence that this response is dependent on oestrogen-receptor status or nodal status is conflicting, so in practice neither of these are used as selection criteria. Premenopausal patients are much less clear cut. The Peto overview has shown a clear survival advantage for node positive patients who receive adjuvant chemotherapy.[32] It must be remembered that this is a survival advantage (living longer) but not an increase in absolute cure rates.

In colorectal cancer, a consensus is now emerging around patients with Dukes' Stage C lesions, in whom adjuvant chemotherapy with 5-fluorouracil (5-FU) (the only cytotoxic to show consistently an effect on colorectal cancer in the clinical setting) offers a small but real survival benefit of about 8%. This benefit is there whether or not the treatment is given systematically or regionally (by portal vein infusion) to the liver.[33,34] Similar results are now being shown in the Dukes' Stage B lesions.[34] Less certain is the role of adjuvant therapy in gastric, pancreatic and oesophageal cancer. All three cancer sites are the subject of ongoing clinical trials of adjuvant therapy, and clinicians who profess an interest in these areas should be attempting to place their patients in such studies. Ultimately, understanding of cancer biology forms the basis of the balance between the radicality of surgery (attempting to improve outcome) and the conservation of normal tissues and structures (excision of which may have absolutely no impact on

Table 6.3 Ten-year follow-up results of adjuvant chemotherapy following surgery for breast cancer

Study	Regimen	Group	Disease-free survival(%)			Overall survival(%)		
			Treatment	Control	p	Treatment	Control	p
NSABP[25]	L-PAM	All patients	38	29	0.06	48	41	0.3
		Pre-menopause	46	29	0.02	61	37	0.02
		Post-menopause	34	28	0.49	41	43	NS
Milan[26]	CMF	All	43	31	0.01	5	47	0.1
		Pre-menopause	48	31	0.01	59	45	0.01
		Post-menopause	38	32	0.32	52	50	NS

NSABP: National Surgical Adjuvant Breast Project; L-PAM:L-phenylalanine mustard:CMF: cyclophosphomide, methotrexate and 5-fluorouracil, NS: not significant.

long-term survival). In addition, the experienced cancer surgeon is continually weighing up the benefits of aggressive surgery against the risks of morbidity and mortality of each procedure for each and every patient.

It is now apparent that locally advanced GI and breast cancers will respond to radiotherapy and chemotherapy and such *neoadjuvant* treatment often downstages large tumours, rendering them more amenable to surgical control. In the case of breast cancer, a tumour that earlier required a mastectomy might now only need wide excision. However, there is no evidence that survival is improved by such manoeuvres.

REGIONAL THERAPY

There has been considerable recent interest in the safety and efficacy of anti-neoplastic agents delivered directly into the region of the body affected by malignant disease. The rationale for this is first, drug delivery may increase both the peak drug levels as well as the total target exposure (or 'area under the curve' [AUC] time) compared with that achieved by systemic drug administration. Second, if the cytotoxicity of a particular agent for a specific tumour type is concentration dependent, then greater response rates may result from regional delivery of the drug. Third, along with the increased exposure of the region perfused with the drug, there may be a significant decrease in systemic exposure (and therefore side-effects) to the agent. This is particularly important for agents that are rapidly metabolized in the liver during their first passage through the organ (first pass effect). Established roles of regional therapy in standard clinical practice include intrathecal/intravesical therapy for selected patients with bladder cancers.

More controversial is the use of hepatic arterial perfusion for colorectal liver metastases. There is a major pharmacokinetic advantage of hepatic parenchymal exposure to several agents (most notably 5-FU and FUDR). Response rates of measurable metastases following intrahepatic FUDR range from 30 to 88%. Unfortunately, because of the crossover nature of trials comparing regional and systemic drug delivery in these patients, as yet no survival benefit has been demonstrated for regional delivery. In addition, there is measurable toxicity associated with this technique, including gastritis, chemical cholecystitis, chemical hepatitis and occasionally irreversible biliary sclerosis. This technique is significantly more expensive to deliver (including the cost of a laparotomy) compared with systemic treatment.

BLOOD TRANSFUSION

Over the last decade, a number of studies (mostly retrospective) have attempted to assess the impact of perioperative blood transfusion on outcome in cancer patients.[37] Unfortunately, the current conclusions drawn from these reports fail to give a clear message. The basic hypothesis is that transfusion of allogeneic blood at the time of surgery encourages the growth of residual local disease and disseminated micrometastases. It may also encourage successful tumour implantation during surgery. This effect is mediated by depression of the host immune system, and the degree of this depression may be specific to a given tumour. The effect seems to be greater when whole blood is transfused, compared with packed red cells.[38] Plasma factors implicated in this effect include proteinase-antiproteinase complexes, fibronectin, histocompatibility antigens and anti-idiotypic antibodies.[39] Furthermore, the ability of splenocytes to produce interleukin-2 is reduced by blood transfusion.[40] Although the jury remains out on the problem of blood transfusion and cancer surgery, we should question the necessity of blood transfusion and examine the use of possible alternatives (such as predonated autologous transfusion). In addition, better

Table 6.4 Comparison of results of NSABP protocols C-01 and C-03 following resection of Dukes' Stage C colorectal cancers[35,36]

Patient group	Disease-free at 3 years(%)	Survival at 3 years(%)
C-01 untreated control	60	72
C-01 methyl-CCNU/5-FU/vin	65	75
C-03 methyl-CCNU/5-FU/vin	64	77
C-03 5-FU + leucovorin	73	84

vin: vincristine: NSABP: National Surgical Adjuvant Breast Project.

surgical technique and the use of haemostatic techniques such as organ isolation, argon beam coagulation and fibrin glues may reduce blood loss sufficiently to render transfusion unnecessary.

Practical implications of surgical principles in malignancy

We have already stated the importance of recognizing those patients who will not benefit from radical surgical intervention, as well as those that will. It is also essential for the successful surgical oncologist not only to lead in his or her field but to keep abreast of developments in other areas. Obvious examples of these principles in surgical oncology include the steady shift away from radical breast surgery towards breast conservation, and the move towards rectal conservation in locally treatable rectal cancer. Both of these have been aided by advances in the safe delivery of radiotherapy and chemotherapy. On the other hand, we have witnessed the move towards more radical surgery in the treatment of metastases, particularly in the case of colorectal cancer which has spread to liver, lung and even, occasionally, brain.

PRINCIPLES OF FOLLOW-UP

Once a patient has undergone an apparently curative surgical intervention (with or without adjuvant therapy), it is the responsibility of the cancer surgeon to ensure adequate follow-up. The aims and objectives of follow-up are to detect early recurrence with intention to cure, and identify incurable progression so as not to defer successful palliation of symptoms. Unfor-

tunately, follow-up protocols are rarely followed rigorously in asymptomatic patients, and so diagnosis of recurrence is delayed until patients have large tumour burdens, disabling symptoms and poor performance status.

The follow-up note 'no sign of recurrence, see $\frac{6}{12}$' is obsolete. Follow-up demands specific timed protocols including screening scans and serum markers to detect recurrence and progression. These protocols should also indicate management algorithms to be followed in the event of tumour progression.

PROTOCOLS FOR FOLLOW-UP

In the case of the (decreasing) number of cancers treated by surgery alone, this follow-up is the sole responsibility of the surgeon. Cancer surgeons must have clear guidelines and protocols of follow-up for each tumour seen in their practice, and these protocols must be clearly understood and adhered to by all members of the surgical team. In these increasingly litigious times, these protocols must be robust and defensible against critical peer review. In the case of shared or joint outpatient management, all clinicians should have a clear understanding of both the objectives and methods of follow-up. Although self-evident, endpoints such as disease-free interval and overall survival must be explicitly laid out. Clearly, if the disease recurs or progresses and there is no other treatment option available, is there any benefit in bringing forward the time of detection? In following this line, clinicians must be absolutely certain they are totally abreast of the literature on the subject and the local availability of other forms of treatment.

COLORECTAL CANCER

One such area that has seen a major shift of emphasis on follow-up policy is colorectal cancer. First, it is

Table 6.5 Follow-up schedule for disease-free patients under 75 years after resection for colorectal cancer

Schedule (months)	Physical exam.	CEA	Liver US Scan	Chest X-ray	Colonoscopy
3	X	X			
6	X	X	X	X	
9	X	X			
12	X	X	X	X	
18	X	X	X	X	
24	X	X		X	X and every 3 years
Annually	X	X		X	

CEA: Carcinoembryonic antigen; US: Ultrasound.

now clear that the probability of success (particularly in reducing local recurrence rates) is dependent on the skill and experience of the operating surgeon.[3, 23, 24] Second, patients with up to three unilateral liver metastases which can be resected with an adequate (1 cm) margin have a 33% probability of being alive 5 years later and a 25% chance of being disease free at this time *and therefore cured*.[10] On the basis of these findings we have developed our own follow-up protocol for colorectal cancer (which needs to be tested against the outcome of accepted best practice) and management strategy for patients with recurrent disease (Table 6.5).

The situation with breast cancer is less clear. While mammography is frequently used in follow-up, other methods, including isotope bone scans, chest X-rays and serum markers, are not universally adopted. The mainstays of breast follow-up are clinical examination to detect local and nodal recurrence every 3 months in the first year, 6 monthly for the next 4 years and annually thereafter. Mammograpy is often carried out annually, although some centres undertake this every 2 years. Generally, there is little point in continuing mammography beyond the age of 70. There is no clear evidence that treatment of asymptomatic distant breast metastases alters survival.

FOLLOW-UP SETTING

Other factors that influence follow-up include the practice venue (including the availability of laboratory and imaging facilities) and the inclusion of patients in clinical trials. Since the entry criteria of clinical trials are more rigorous, the follow-up protocol more rigid and the endpoints usually more clearly defined, many clinicians accept that patients in clinical trials get a better 'deal' when it comes to follow-up. If resources are limited then they should be concentrated on the detection of new primary disease and potentially curable recurrence. Furthermore, resources should be directed locally towards the detection and palliation of incurable recurrence. In the setting of tertiary care, a major objective of follow-up should be the development and introduction of effective new treatments for recurrent disease.

QUALITY OF LIFE

One factor that has recently been largely ignored by surgeons, but is paramount in the palliation of symptoms, is measurement of quality of life. Karnofsky introduced his crude but effective scoring system over a generation ago, and there are many variants (ECOG, WHO, HAD Rotterdam, etc.) in use today. Surgeons must be familiar with these systems and introduce them into their clinical practice. They are a useful adjunct to their armamentarium in the justification of surgical procedures in malignant disease when comparing outcomes between centres and also when discussing their repertoire with potential purchasers of health care. Cancer is no different from any other chronic disease; the aim should be to keep the patient independent, active and symptom free until they die.

The skills of a surgical oncologist

In addition to an extensive training and research base in oncology, the surgical oncologist must be a leader in the field of the practice to which he or she devotes their skills. On no account should surgical oncologists allow themselves to be lead by the medical or clinical oncologists because of their failure to keep abreast of developments in a particular area. The surgical oncologist should be a skilled technical surgeon who pursues excellence in the practice of his or her own clinical art. It is debatable whether every surgical oncologist should be equally skilled in such procedures as partial hepatectomy, hindquarter amputation, major plastic/reconstructive surgery or major retroperitoneal dissection. Such procedures should only be undertaken in tertiary centres which concentrate experience and expertise. Where a patient's disease process extends geographically beyond the ability of one surgical oncologist, as with medical and clinical oncology, it behoves the surgical oncologist to seek the guidance and support of other dedicated cancer surgeons. The cancer surgeon's operative skills should be measured by comparative audit of outcome.

Other surgical skills, in addition to cancer resection, include techniques of systemic and regional vascular access for cytotoxic chemotherapy. Successful collaboration with radiotherapy colleagues includes providing access for brachytherapy (slow delivery of local radiation treatment) and the possible introduction of intraoperative radiotherapy in the not too distant future. If not part of the surgical oncologists skills, then it is necessary to collaborate with colleagues in reconstructive and vascular surgery in such areas as breast reconstruction, free tissue transfer for pharyngo-oesophageal replacement, and vascular reconstruction in major liver and groin resections.

Finally, surgical oncologists must master interpersonal skills. This is not only self-evident in dealings with other oncologists, but with other surgeons on whose skills they may rely. A successful tertiary practice is dependent on keeping the referring physician well informed of progress and outcome of each and every individual patient referred. These attributes are also necessary in the development of good relationships with palliative care physicians and nurses who will be vital to the long-term benefit of patients whose disease is beyond the skills of the cancer surgeon. These skills are called for day in and day out when the cancer surgeon is dealing with the most important person in the practice, the cancer patient.

References

1. Dukes CE. The classification of cancer of the rectum. *J Pathol Bateriol* 1932; **35**: 323–6

2. *Glasgow Audit of Surgical Deaths: Anual Report 1993*. Glasgow: Greater Glasgow Health Board, 1994.

3. McArdle CS, Hole D. Impact of variability among surgeons on postoperative morbidity and mortality and ultimate survival. *Br Med J* 1991; **303**: 1501–5.

4. Thromboembolism Risk Factors (THRIFT) Consensus Group. Risk of and prophylaxis for venous thromboembolism in hospital practice *Br Med J* 1992; **305**; 567–74.

5. Steele G Jr. Surgical oncology–definition/training. In: Steele G Jr., Cady B (eds.) *General Surgical Oncology*. Philadelphia: WB Saunders, 1992; 1–9.

6. Bodmer WF, Bailey CJ, Bodmer J *et al* Localisation of the gene for familial adenomatous polyposis on chromosome 5. *Nature* 1987; **328**: 614–6.

7. Collins RHJ, Feldman M, Fordtran JS. Colon cancer, dysplasia and surveillance in patients with ulcerative colitis. *N Eng J Med* 1987; **316**: 1654–8.

8. Lynch HT, Albano WA, Lynch JF *et al*. Recognition of the cancer family syndrome *Gastroenterology* 1983; **84**: 672–3.

9. Cohen AW, Wood WC, Gunderson LL, Shinna M. Pathological studies on rectal cancer. *Cancer* 1980, **45**: 2965–8.

10. Hughes KS, Simon R, Songhorabodi S *et al*. Resection of the liver for colorectal carcinoma metastases: multi-institutional study of patterns of recurrence. *Surgery* 1986; **106**: 278–84.

11. Veronesi U. Rationale and indications for limited surgery in breast cancer: current data *World J Surg* 1987; **11**: 493–8.

12. Cady B. Lymph node metastases: indicators, but not governors, of survival. *Arch Surg* 1984; **199**: 1067–72.

13. Vogelstein B, Fearon Er, Hamilton SR *et al*. Genetic alterations during colorectal tumour development. *N Engl J Med* 1988; **319**: 525–32.

14. Vogelstein B. Fearon ER. Kern SE *et al*. Allotype of colorectal carcinoma. *Science* 1989; **244**: 207–11.

15. Fearon ER, Vogelstein B. A genetic model for colorectal tumorogenesis. *Cel* 1990; **61**: 759–67.

16. Porter DE, Cohen BB, Walace MR *et al*. Linkage mapping in familial breast and ovarian cancer; improved localisation of a susceptible locus on chromosome 17q 12–21. *Int J Cancer* 1993; **93**: 188–98.

17. Bos JL, Fearon ER, Hamilton SR *et al*. Prevalence of *ras* gene mutations in human colorectal cancer. *Nature* 1987; **327**: 293–7.

18. Handley WS. The pathology of melanotic growths in relationship to their operative treatment. *Lancet* 1907; **1**: 927–33, 996–1003.

19. Breslaw A, Macht SD. Optional size of resection margins for thin cutaneous melanomata. *Surg Gynecol Obstet* 1977; **145**: 691–2.

20. Macfarland JK, Ryall RDH, Heald RJ. Mesorectal excision for rectal cancer. *Lancet* 1993; **341**: 457–60.

21. Kaibara N, Sumi K, Yonakawa M *et al*. Does extensive dissection of lymph nodes improve the results of surgical treatment of gastric cancer? *Am J Surg* 1990; **159**: 218–21.

22. Hay ID, Grant CS, Taylor WF, McConalay WM. Ipsilateral lobectomy versus bilateral lobar resection in papillary thyroid carcinoma: a retrospective analysis of surgical outcome using a novel prognostic scoring system. *Surgery* 1987; **102**: 1088–94.

23. Sugarbaker PH, Corlew S. Influence of surgical techniques on survival in patients with colorectal cancer: a review. *Dis Colon Rectum* 1982; **25**: 545–57.

24. Docherty JG, Aykol AM, McGregor JR, Galloway DJ. Anastomotic technique has an influence on outcome following colorectal cancer surgery. In: Steichen FM, Walter R (eds), *Minimially Invasive Surgery and New Technology*. St Louis: Quality Medical Publishing; 1994 414–20.

25. Fisher B, Fisher ER, Redmond C. Ten year results from the NSABP clinical trial evaluating the use of L-phenylalanine mustard (L-PAM) in the treatment of primary breast cancer. *J Clin Oncol* 1986 **4**: 929–41.

26. Bonnadonna G, Valagussa P, Rossi A *et al*. Ten year experience with CMF based adjuvant chemotherapy in resectable breast cancer. *Breast Canc Res Treat* 1985; **5**: 95–115.

27. Recht A, Connolly JL, Schnitt J *et al*. Conservative surgery and radiation therapy for early breast cancer: results, controversies and unsolved problems. *Semin Oncol* 1986; **13**: 434–9.

28. Marks G. Mohiuddin M, Goldstein SD. Sphincter preservation for cancer of the distal rectum using high dose prepoperative radiation. *Int J Radiat Oncol Biol Phys* 1988; **15**: 1065–8.

29. Thomas PR, Lindblad AS. Adjuvant postoperative radiotherapy and chemotherapy in rectal carcinoma: a review of the Gastrointestinal Tumour Study Group experience. *Radiother Oncol* 1988; **13**: 245–52.

30. Controlled trial of tamoxifen as single adjuvant agent in the management of early breast cancer: analysis at six years by Nolvadex Adjuvant Trial Organisation (NATO). *Lancet* 1985; **1**: 836–40.

31. Controlled trial of tamoxifen as single adjuvant agent in the management of early breast cancer.

Analysis at 8 years by Nolvadex Adjuvant Trial Organisation. *Br J Cancer* 1988; **57**: 608–11.

32. Peto R *et al*. Early Breast Cancer Trialists Collaborative Group. Systemic treatment of early breast cancer by hormonal, cytotoxic or immune therapy: 133 randomised trials involving 31,000 recurrences and 24,000 deaths amoung 75,000 women. *Lancet* 1992; **339**: 1–15, 71–84.

33. Taylor I, Machin D, Mullee M *et al*. A randomised controlled trial of adjuvant portal vein cytotoxic perfusion in colorectal cancer. *Br J Surg* 1985; **72**: 359–62.

34. Moertel CG, Fleming TR, MacDonald JS *et al*. Levamisole and fluorouracil for adjuvant therapy of resected colon carcinoma. *N Engl J Med* 1990; **322**: 352–8.

35. Wolmark N, Fisher B, Rockette E *et al*. Postoperative adjuvant chemotherapy or BCG for colon cancer: results from NSABP protocl CO–1, *J Natl Canc Inst* 1988; **80**: 30–36.

36. Wolmark N, Rockette E, Wickerhorn DL *et al*. Adjuvant therapy of Dukes A, B and C adenocarcinomas of the colon, with portal vein fluorouracil hepatic infusion: preliminary results of National. Surgical Adjuvant Breast and Bowel Project Protocol C 2. *J Clin Oncol* 1990; **8**: 1466–75.

37. Weiden PL. Do perioperative blood transfusions increase the risk of cancer recurrence? *Eur J Cancer* 1990; **26**: 987–9.

38. Blumberg N, Heal JM, Murphy P *et al*. Association between transfusion of whole blood and recurrence of cancer. *Br Med J* 1986; **293**: 530–3.

39. Kerman RH, Van Buren CT, Payne W. Influence of blood transfusion on immune responsiveness. *Transp Proc* 1982; **14**: 335–7.

40. Stephan RN, Kisola JM, Dean RE *et al*. Effect of blood transfusion on antigen presentation function and on interleukin–2 generation. *Arch Surg* 1988; **123**: 235–40.

41. Wooster R, Neuhausen SL, Mangion J *et al*. Localisation of a breast cancer susceptibility gene BRCA2 to chromosome 13q 12–13. *Science* 1994; **265**: 2088–90.

CHAPTER 7

Principles of adjuvant therapy in malignant disease

JW DAWSON, I TAYLOR

The term 'malignant disease' describes a wide spectrum of conditions, characterized by the loss of normal control of growth and replication of cells. Many early cancers can be cured by local treatment such as the removal of the tumour or the organ in which it originates. More advanced tumours may not be cured by surgery alone because of the metastatic potential of the tumour. The results of primary surgical treatment may be impoved by additional treatment using another modality. The use of such an additional modality to improve the results of primary treatment is known as adjuvant therapy. Cytotoxic drug therapy, radiotherapy and hormone therapy are the main adjuvant therapies currently available and each may be used independently or combined as part of a coordinated approach to treatment by the surgeon and oncologist.

Adjuvant therapy in early malignant disease

If a tumour is diagnosed and removed at an early clinical stage, i.e. before local invasion or distant dissemination have occurred, cure will result. The failure of surgery alone to eradicate malignant disease is due either to local invasion of structures adjacent to the tumour or to distant dissemination via blood or lymphatics. Unfortunately, metastasis to both local and distant tissues is not always possible to diagnose, despite the use of the most sensitive investigations to identify it. This is because metastases may be microscopic and may remain subclinical for some time after their deposition in distant tissues. Micrometastases have been shown to have a more rapid cell turnover than large bulky tumours and thus should be more amenable to cytotoxic agents.[1,2]

In many cases of cancer with no obvious local or distant spread, metastases appear later, often many years after the primary resection. It is generally assumed that these arise from micrometastases disseminated around the time of surgery though the mechanism of metastasis remains open to further investigation. There is evidence to suggest that dormant micrometastases develop into macroscopic tumours although the stimulus for this is unknown. However, the presence of occult liver metastases in, for example, colorectal cancer, is associated with a poor prognosis.[3,4]

The pathophysiology giving rise to varying patterns of metastatic disease remains incompletely understood. Identifiable patterns are found in different diseases and are important in understanding the rational basis for their adjuvant therapy. For example, gastrointestinal cancers spread via the portal venous system to give rise to liver metastases whereas malignant melanoma spreads via the lymphatics. Factors such as cellular adhesion and the ability to produce enzymes that facilitate the invasion into target organs determine whether the metastases will become viable.[5,6] In colorectal cancers, about half of patients thought to have undergone curative surgery subsequently develop metastasis,[7,8] whilst in breast disease the subsequent development of metastasis is related to the stage of the primary.

It is presumed that failure of primary treatment in patients who suffer recurrent disease are those in whom micrometastases have regrown. In such cases systemic chemotherapy is rarely curative. This is thought in part to be due to the development of tumour-resistant cell-lines or the limiting toxicity of the therapy. Systemic chemotherapy, which might be of palliative value only in patients with advanced disease, might have been curative if applied at an earlier stage in the disease. Patients who are at high risk of recurrent disease (those with advanced stage or high histological grade of tumour) may benefit from systemic chemotherapy earlier in the course of their disease. This view is supported by various animal model studies that have demonstrated that carcinomas of lung, breast and colon and melanomas which are incurable by primary treament alone, can be treated effectively by the use of adjuvant chemotherapy.[9–11] In these animal models the efficacy of adjuvant treatment is diminished by: (1) advanced stage of tumour, (2) increased interval from surgery to adjuvant therapy, (3) increased intervals between doses of chemotherapy and (4) reduced dose of cytotoxic chemotherapy. In animal models, drugs that are marginally effective for advanced tumours may be curative when the tumour burden is very small.

Thus, adjuvant therapy may be given to eradicate presumed but not demonstrable tumour cells present either in structures adjacent to the original tumour, or in regional drainage sites. Treatment is designed to reduce the chance of local recurrence and of distant metastasis arising from dissemination which might have occurred around the time of surgery and is likely to be of greatest benefit in those patients at highest risk.

Adjuvant radiotherapy is given to reduce locoregional recurrence in adjacent structures or regional lymph nodes. Chemotherapy is directed towards the eradication of metastatic tumour cells in distant sites of metastasis such as liver, lungs or bone marrow.

Adjuvant therapy in advanced malignant disease

Adjuvant therapy may also be used to improve the results of primary treatment in advanced malignancies. Resection of the primary tumour may be apropriate despite macroscopic metastatic disease being apparent at operation. Conditions such as an obstructing carcinoma of the colon require surgical treatment and in such circumstances it is rational to supplement this with postoperative chemotherapy in an attempt to modify the course of the disease. Similarly, advanced ovarian cancers are treated by 'debulking' surgery to reduce the tumour mass which improves the benefit of subsequent cytotoxic chemotherapy. Experimental data suggest that surgical debulking recruits remaining cancer cells into phases of growth more susceptible to chemotherapy.[12] In addition, the term adjuvant treatment has been applied to chemotherapy given after resection of localized colorectal liver metastases. This is delivered on the assumption that although all macroscopic tumour has been removed, micrometastatic (occult) disease is likely to be present which would influence overall survival.

Germ cell tumours such as malignant teratomas and seminomas of the testis are treated with a combined approach by surgeon and oncologist. There has been a dramatic improvement in the prognosis of teratoma over the last 15 years, even in advanced disease. Initial orchidectomy is followed by adjuvant cytotoxic chemotherapy and even patients with advanced disease can expect a 75% remission rate and 50% cure rate. Seminoma is treated by orchidectomy followed by radiotherapy to regional lymph nodes and achieves cure rates of up 90%.

Neoadjuvant therapy

The difficulties of treating some advanced malignancies with surgery alone has led to the development of 'neoadjuvant' therapy. Extensive local spread may mean that primary resection of the tumour alone offers little hope of complete eradication of the disease. In addition, such surgery might be associated with an unacceptably high morbidity. For example, locally advanced breast cancer may only be resectable by radical mastectomy and possible skin grafting, yet still have an unacceptably high local recurrence rate. Similarly, advanced rectal cancers may require a technically hazardous procedure to be excised adequately because of their proximity to vital structures or involvement with other organs. In addition involved excision margins would result in an unacceptable rate of local recurrence. Preoperative adjuvant therapy may render a tumour more amenable to resection, for example preoperative radiotherapy of advanced rectal cancers has been shown to 'downstage' advanced growths and facilitate organ sparing.[13,14] Similarly, in advanced (T_3–T_4) breast cancer, neoadjuvant chemotherapy has been shown to downstage advanced tumours, making 'unresectable' cancers amenable to surgery or to lower doses and smaller fields of radiation.[15,16] In addition, the incidence of axillary node involvement is reduced in patients with breast cancer treated by neoadjuvant chemotherapy.[17]

Thus, the ideal of neoadjuvant therapy is to reduce the tumour burden at the primary site, increase local control and improve the long-term outcome.

In practical terms there are two main advantages of neoadjuvant therapy:

1. improved local and distant control in certain tumours;
2. preservation of organs which would otherwise have to be completely removed – neoadjuvant therapy, for example, enables breast conservation to be performed rather than mastectomy.

In addition, a precise response to the particular cytotoxic therapeutic regimen may be monitored and adapted accordingly

EXAMPLES OF NEOADJUVANT THERAPY

The use of neoadjuvant therapy is now established as the standard treatment in certain malignant tumours. Squamous cell carcinoma of the anus was previously treated by abdominoperineal excision of the anorectum but had a high local recurrence rate and poor long-term survival. Combined neoadjuvant chemoradiotherapy is now so successful that abdominoperineal resection is reserved for those cases in which persistent disease remains after initial treatment. In nearly 90% of cases a complete response is achieved, while preserving normal anorectal function.[18, 19]

Osteogenic sarcoma is now treated by neoadjuvant cytotoxic chemotherapy followed by limb salvage surgery. Provided there is a good response to intial treatment, amputation may be avoided and a less radical resection of the tumour-bearing bone performed. Especially designed prostheses are used to preserve limb function. Histology of the resected specimen is evaluated to determine the degree of response to chemotherapy. Current regimen achieve a response in 70–80% of patients. Patients with a good histological response to neoadjuvant therapy have an improved outcome compared with those with a poor response (92 vs 54% 5-year disease-free survival).[20,21]

Radical surgery is effective in controlling local disease in the early stages and sometimes even in quite advanced cancers. Patients with advanced, resectable head and neck tumours have a survival rate of 40%.[22] However, surgery is often mutilating and may involve major reconstructive procedures. In patients with advanced laryngeal carcinoma, neoadjuvant chemotherapy followed by definitive radiotherapy achieved a 49% complete response rate and allowed preservation of the larynx in 64% without compromising overall survival.[23] Randomized trials of advanced squamous cell carcinomas of the pharynx, larynx and oral cavity have shown improved 3-year survival for patients treated with neoadjuvant chemotherapy compared with those treated with radiation or surgery alone (41 vs 23%).[24–26]

The increasing acceptability of neoadjuvant therapy reflects a shift in the concept of how adjuvant therapy may be most effectively directed against malignant disease. The success of neoadjuvant therapy may be because the tumour remains *in situ*, rather than with postoperative therapy which is directed against a residual population of micrometastases left behind after surgery. Cytotoxic chemotherapy and radiotherapy is often successful in reducing the size and extent of the primary tumour – perhaps as a result of good vascular access, especially at the growing edge of the cancer. In theory, by reducing the number of cancer cells before surgery, the chance of resistant clones developing, which will subsequently grow into metastases, could be reduced. There is evidence from experimental animal models that the primary tumour itself has an inhibitory effect on metastases.[27] By giving chemotherapy before the primary tumour (and its metastatic inhibitory effect) has been removed, neoadjuvant therapy may offer an improved chance of control of distant spread. These considerations remain theoretical and illustrate that our understanding of mechanisms of tumour growth and metastatic spread is still evolving.

DISADVANTAGES OF NEOADJUVANT THERAPY

Neoadjuvant therapy is not without hazard and potential disadvantages include the cost and inconvenience of treatment. If ineffective it may compromise local control by delaying surgery and allow potentially aggressive tumours to metastasize. The scarring and fibrosis resulting from neoadjuvant therapy, particularly radiotherapy, may make subsequent surgery more difficult and should be performed within 6 weeks of neoadjuvant therapy to minimize these problems. Pathological staging of the resected specimen may be difficult to interpret following chemoradiotherapy. Surgery prior to this is made difficult by post-irradiation acute inflammation which can cause abnormal bleeding.

Hormonal treatment

The growth of some malignancies is affected by a change in their hormonal environment. The precise mechanism of hormonal dependence is imperfectly understood but is related to the presence of hormone receptors on the malignant cell surface. Hormonal drugs are rarely curative by themselves but may significantly influence the course of the disease when used in conjunction with other treatments. They are relatively non-toxic compared with cytotoxic agents and this makes them attractive options for those patients with tumours known to respond to endocrine manipulation.

Carcinoma of the prostate has long been treated by hormonal therapy. Growth of the tumour is related to endogenous androgens and if these are reduced clinical improvement is seen in about 75% of patients. This is largely symptomatic, however, and the exact survival benefit of hormonal manipulation in prostatic cancer remains unclear. Bilateral orchidectomy is the standard by which other treatments are judged. Other endocrine manipulation includes oestrogen administration (1–3 mg stilboestrol daily). This has a similar efficacy to orchidectomy but more side-effects, the most serious of which is thromboembolism. The use of luteinizing hormone releasing hormone (LHRH) agonists effect a 'medical castration' by causing a block in luteinizing hormone production and subsequent decrease in testosterone production. Treatment with LHRH is attractive because the risk of cardiovascular effects is lower than with oestrogens. Other drugs include the anti-androgens cyproterone and flutemide and are usually second-line drugs when previous attempts at hormonal manipulation have failed.

The effect of hormonal manipulation is most dramatically demonstrated in breast cancer. It has been recognized for many years that marked responses may be achieved by changing the hormonal environment, either by diminishing endogenous hormones in premenopausal women or by adding them in postmenopausal women. The discovery of the oestrogen-receptor (ER) in breast cancer has led to a better understanding of the differences in response by tumours to hormonal manipulation.[28] Oestrogen-receptor positive (ER+) tumours tend to respond better to tamoxifen therapy than do ER negative

(ER−) tumours and are associated with a lower relapse rate and improved overall survival.[29] However, as far as adjuvant treatment is concerned both ER+ and ER− tumours are associated with survival improvement, particularly in postmenopausal women. Oestrogen is the most important factor in the development and control of breast cancer. It affects the differentiation and proliferation of target cells by binding to oestrogen-receptors on the cell surface. At an intracellular level the effect of oestrogen is to stimulate the transcription of various mRNAs, and the production of a number of growth factors which may act in an autocrine or paracrine fashion to stimulate breast cancer proliferation. About 65% of breast cancers are ER+. Breast cancer cells may also express other hormonal receptors including those for progesterone, prolactin, androgen and glucocorticoid. These act as gene regulators and are themselves regulated by oestrogens. They have some use as a predictor of response to endocrine therapy and may explain the efficacy of progestins such as megestrol acetate in advanced disease.[30,31]

Further evidence of the hormonal dependence of some tumours is demonstrated by studies in premenopausal women who have different survival, depending on when in their menstrual cycle the primary tumour is treated.[32] This is likely to relate to a complex relationship between primary and metastatic tumours and is imperfectly understood at present.

The most marked success has been achieved with tamoxifen, which blocks oestrogen-receptors on malignant cells. The use of tamoxifen has minimal side-effects and has demonstrated an increase in disease-free survival and a small effect on actual survival in postmenopausal women. It is the most widely used adjuvant therapy of breast cancer and is routinely given to all postmenopausal women with breast cancer.

Progestogen treatment is used in various other malignancies, namely advanced uterine carcinomas where it generates a 40% response rate overall and ovarian and renal cancers where about 10% of patients may show some objective response.

The adjuvant hormonal treatment of thyroid cancers is standard treatment for well-differentiated papillary and follicular carcinomas. Well-differentiated tumours retain the ability to be regulated by normal endocrine control and are responsive to endogenous thyroid stimulating hormone (TSH). Following thyroid lobectomy to remove the tumour, thyroxine (T_4) is administered to suppress endogenous TSH levels to below the normal range, without causing thyrotoxicosis. This may, by itself, induce tumour regression if surgery is not possible and should be continued for life to minimize the chance of regrowth of the original tumour or the development of multifocal malignancies in the remaining thyroid.

Immunotherapy

Immunotherapy has been advocated as an adjuvant to surgery, particularly in those where the host is known to exhibit some immunological response (e.g. melanoma, Kaposi's sarcoma and renal cell tumours). In animal models very small tumour masses may be eliminated by an immune mechanism though they are totally ineffective against substantive tumour masses. The immunological approach is attractive because of low general toxicity and the theoretical advantage that the patient's own immune system might be harnessed to eradicate disease at a cellular level. Immune techniques may be either general, non-specific enhancement of the patient's immunological state or some active mechanism directed specifically against the tumour.

Passive immunotherapy was first used at the end of the nineteenth century by inoculating animals with cancers and using their antisera. Since these early unsuccessful attemps to modulate the host's response against cancers, interest has continued with the use of monoclonal antibodies (MAbs), targeted against various tumour markers or tumour-associated antigens found on the cell surface, such as carcinoembryonic antigen (CEA) and epithelial membrane antigen (EMA). Monoclonal antibodies may form conjugates with toxins such as ricin which destroy tumour but are limited by the selectivity of the MAb for tumour compared with the normal tissues and by the small amount of toxin that can actually be delivered to the tumour.

Non-specific techniques of enhancing an immune response to tumour include the inoculation of the patient with immunostimulants such as bacillus Calmette–Guérin (BCG) vaccine and *Corynebacterium parvum* toxin. Interferons have also been used to induce a non-specific enhancement of immune response. Unfortunately none of the above techniques has demonstrated objective improvement in outcome. Over the last decade the anti-helminthic levamisole has been used in the USA in trials of adjuvant therapy of colorectal cancer. Levamisole is known to be an immune stimulant which reduces the period of postoperative immunosuppression following surgery. None of the above techniques has shown conclusive benefit and they remain experimental.

Examples of adjuvant therapy in specific cancers

ADJUVANT THERAPY OF BREAST CANCER

Adjuvant therapy is particularly important in breast cancer. The positive impact of adjuvant systemic therapy on disease-free survival and overall survival has been studied over the last three decades and the place of adjuvant therapy in breast cancer is now established beyond doubt.

Local radiotherapy

For many years the approach to the treatment of breast cancer was radical surgery – *en bloc* excision of the breast with wide clearance of associated structures including pectoralis major and minor muscles as well as total clearance of axillary lymph nodes. The basis for such treatment was the hypothesis that the breast cancer spread via local extension and lymphatic drainage to regional lymph nodes. However, radical surgery had little effect on survival compared with conservative surgery and subsequent experience with modified radical mastectomy showed equivalent success rates but a significantly lower morbidity. Breast conservation is now advocated wherever possible. Two-thirds of women have T1 or T2 tumours on presentation and are suitable for conservative surgery. This consists of excision of the primary tumour with at least a 1 cm margin of normal breast tissue, axillary node dissection followed by adjuvant irradiation of the breast. This approach allows the nipple and much of the breast to be conserved.[33, 34]

The aim of local treatment is to achieve local control, i.e. to avoid local recurrence. Breast conservation surgery as an alternative to mastectomy is only made possible by the use of adjuvant radiotherapy to reduce the risk of local recurrence. Recent studies have demonstrated the benefit of radiation to the breast in decreasing local recurrence following conservative surgery. Local recurrence rates following wide local excision alone, without adjuvant radiotherapy are about 30%, whereas with radiotherapy they are reduced to 10–14%. A dose of 4500–5000 cGy to the whole breast, fractionated over 6 weeks is recommended, starting 2–3 weeks after surgery. Additional doses of 100 cGy may be required if the tumour extends to the excision margin.

The prognosis for locoregional recurrence compares favourably with modified radical mastectomy. Prospective randomized trials demonstrate that recurrence developing within 2 years of mastectomy usually implies distant metastases, carrying only a

Table 7.1 Local recurrence for breast cancer patients following local excision with and without irradiation in three studies[36]

No. of patients	Size/stage	Endpoint	LR with radiotherapy (%)	LR without radiotherapy (%)
1504	T_1–T_4	Act LR 10 y	14	29
1450	4 cm	Act LR 8 y	10	39
237	T_1–T_3	Crude LR	10	30

Act: actuarial; LR: local recurrence.

15% 5-year survival rate.[34] Recurrence following breast conservation surgery, however, is usually at the site of the primary and, with further surgery, results in a 5-year survival rate of 60–70%.[34]

Some patients are at particular risk from locoregional recurrence. Risk factors include: large tumours (>3 cm), high histological grade, minimal excision margins and large number of axillary nodes involved. In these circumstances radiotherapy may be required as a 'boost' to the breast if breast conservation has been employed or to the chest wall if the patient has undergone mastectomy.[35] Irradiation to the axilla is avoided unless there is known residual disease after surgery or very large numbers of involved nodes with gross extranodal disease. In these circumstances adjuvant chemotherapy will also have an important role in preventing local recurrence as well as distant.

Risks of irradiation include oedema and thickening of the skin of the breast or chest wall, deformation of the residual breast and, rarely, sarcoma of the chest wall. High voltage machines currently in use now minimize these problems to an acceptable level.

Adjuvant drug treatment

Endocrine therapy

Following surgery, clinicians must decide whether a patient should receive additional endocrine and/or cytotoxic chemotherapy. This is determined by pathological examination of the specimen, the axillary nodal status, the menopausal status and to a lesser extent hormone receptor assays. The most important drug therapy in breast cancer is the use of the anti-oestrogen drug tamoxifen. This appears to act by competing with endogenous oestrogens for receptors on the surface of the malignant cell. Tamoxifen appears to exert an antiproliferative effect and the extent to which this occurs is directly related to the degree to which tamoxifen binds oestrogen receptors. Other studies have also shown that tamoxifen has other effects on growth stimulatory factors.

The definitive study on the value of tamoxifen as an adjuvant therapy was published by the Early Breast Cancer Trialists Collaborative Group (EBCTCG). An overview of 75 000 women entered into various randomized trials showed that both local recurrence rate and death rates were reduced in both node-negative and node-positive patients (recurrence: 25%, mortality: 17%). The reduction in overall survival and in recurrence-free survival was slightly higher in the node-positive group compared with node-negative patients. Recurrence-free survival, a reduction of mortality, and a reduction in the risk of contralateral breast cancer by 39%, were seen in women who were ER$^-$.

Other trials such as the National Surgical Adjuvant Breast Project (NSABP) comparison of ER$^+$ patients receiving tamoxifen vs no tamoxifen found a highly significant disease-free survival. In addition, the tamoxifen group had fewer locoregional recurrences and fewer distant metastases, a reduction in ipsilateral recurrence in patients who had undergone conservation breast surgery and a reduction in contralateral tumours.[37] Although the recommended duration of treatment with tamoxifen is 3 years, many researchers feel that 5 years or longer is more appropriate in maintaining disease-free survival.[38]

Cytotoxic chemotherapy

In addition to adjuvant tamoxifen, systemic cytotoxic chemotherapy should be considered in patients with axillary node involvement. This rationale is based on the assumption that axillary node involvement represents systemic disease and the presence of micrometastases. Carcinoma of the breast is sensitive to various cytotoxic regimen and many patients with advanced disease show a marked response to initial chemotherapy, even though this is not necessarily maintained. In addition, many women die of their metastases when local control is maintained. These observations led to the rationale that chemotherapy given early in the disease (i.e. as adjuvant therapy) may improve the results of primary treatment. There have been many trials of adjuvant chemotherapy in breast cancer and interpretation of results has been difficult. This is, in part, due to the heterogeneous nature of the disease, different drug regimen and the need for a very long follow-up. As a result of large, multicentre trials conducted in Europe and the USA over recent decades more precise indications for adjuvant treatment are now emerging.

Axillary node-positive breast cancer

The situation is most clear in premenopausal women with axillary node involvement. Adjuvant chemotherapy is now considered standard treatment. Bonnadonna has reported a 15-year analysis of a trial using cyclophosphamide, methotrexate and 5-fluorouracil (CMF) in premenopausal node-positive women. In this study a clear advantage in disease-free survival and overall survival was demonstrated in women receiving CMF, specifically during the first 3 years following surgery – this advantage continued over the next 12 years. The regimen achieved a 25–35% reduction in death rates at 10 years.The EBCTCG demonstrated the advantage of using combination chemotherapy such as CMF compared with a single drug regimen. The standard regimen currently used by many oncologists is CMF delivered in six, monthly cycles. Because of its efficacy in treating advanced breast cancer, doxorubicin has been investigated to see if there is an advantage over CMF. The initial use of high dose doxorubicin may so reduce the tumour burden that there are fewer cells to mutate into drug-resistant lines:[34, 39] Other groups have failed to confirm this advantage, however, perhaps because an initial course of treatment with CMF selects cell-lines that are resistant to doxorubicin.

Two other important trials have confirmed the advantage of chemotherapy in node-positive postmenopausal patients. The NSABP trial compared doxorubicin + cyclophosphamide + tamoxifen with tamoxifen alone and found a significantly improved disease-free survivial and overall survival at 3 years in the chemotherapy + tamoxifen group.[30] Similarly, the EBCTCG overview has shown that chemotherapy + tamoxifen is superior to tamoxifen alone in preventing recurrence.[40]

Axillary node-negative breast cancer

The situation in axillary node-negative women is less clear. Follow-up data from various trials indicate that patients within this group may have recurrence rates of 5–14% at 20 years. Women who are node negative but have tumours > 3 cm have a 20-year recurrence rate of > 50%.[34] The NSABP trial found that node-negative women overall had a 25% treatment failure rate at 5 years with > 20% suffering distant disease and > 20% having died at 5 years.[37] The greatest uncertainty for adjuvant cytotoxic chemotherapy has been in the early breast cancers (node-negative patients with tumours < 1 cm). Clinicians have ques-

tioned the benefit of chemotherapy over the morbidity of treatment. Various trials, however, have now demonstrated an advantage for adjuvant cytotoxic chemotherapy in groups of early cancers. The NSABP study demonstrated a significant advantage in disease-free survival and overall survival for both premenopausal and postmenopausal patients at 7 years.[41] A study by the Milan group demonstrated a significant advantage in disease-free survival in both pre- and postmenopausal women with high risk, node-negative cancers. At 8 years disease-free survival was 82 vs 40% for the premenopausal group and 76 vs 36% for postmenopausal women.[39] Nonetheless, the precise role of chemotherapy in these tumours continues to be debated, particularly whether it offers an advantage over tamoxifen for ER$^+$ tumours in postmenopausal women.

High dose adjuvant chemotherapy

Recently, it has been suggested that treatment failures following adjuvant therapy may be due to insufficient doses. Higher doses of CMF and treatment regimen incorporating adriamicin have both demonstrated a possible advantage in node-positive women.[38, 39] High dose adjuvant chemotherapy is now the subject of debate and various trials in Europe and the USA have recently been set up to evaluate any potential benefit.

Neoadjuvant therapy for breast cancer

During the 1980s the value of neoadjuvant chemotherapy was established in the treatment of advanced breast cancer, inducing a complete response in 50% and partial response in 40%.[37] These patients then went on to have mastectomy. Since then, two trials have reported the use of neoadjuvant therapy. The Milan group prospectively studied women with large tumours (> 3 cm) with the aim of reducing their size to enable conservation breast surgery and also to reduce subsequent local relapse. This was successful in 201 of 220 patients (91%) and 8 patients (4%) had complete disappearance of their tumour on histological examination. Disease-free survival and relapse rates were favourable and were related to initial response to neoadjuvant therapy. A French group has reported an early study of neoadjuvant chemotherapy for all stages of breast cancer, again with favourable disease-free survival at 5 years. Comparative Phase III trials are now planned to determine whether neoadjuvant therapy prolongs disease-free survival and overall survival compared with primary surgery followed by adjuvant therapy.

In summary, improvement in disease-free and overall survival is seen in premenopausal patients who undergo cytotoxic chemotherapy. Improvement in disease-free and overall survival is seen in post-menopausal patients who receive tamoxifen. Adjuvant chemotherapy is debatable for node-negative cancers but patients who are at high risk of recurrence (tumour > 3 cm, high histological grade, ER$^-$) are advised to have cytotoxic chemotherapy. The use of high dose and neoadjuvant cytotoxic chemotherapy is currently being investigated, though neoadjuvant therapy for advanced breast cancers has been shown to offer an early advantage over surgery alone. The main problem in defining optimum treatment is determining those patients most likely to benefit. It is hoped the results of ongoing studies will clarify further methods of better treatment.

Adjuvant treatment of colon and rectal cancer

Adjuvant therapy of colon and rectal cancers has been practised increasingly over the last decade in the USA and parts of Europe and is now becoming established in the UK. The positive impact of adjuvant systemic therapy on disease-free survival and overall survival is much less clear than in breast cancer.

Potentially curative surgery is possible in about 75% of patients who present with colorectal cancers. Unfortunately about 50% of all 'curative' patients will develop recurrent disease to which they will ultimately succumb.[42] Determining the need for adjuvant therapy requires the identification of high risk factors. Pathological stage remains the most important prognostic indicator, particularly the degree of regional lymph node involvement and also the histological grade of the tumour.

There is a clear difference in patterns of failure of primary treatment between rectal cancers (those arising below the peritoneal reflection) and colonic (those occuring in the peritoneal cavity). Rectal cancers have a local recurrence rate of 5–20%[3,43] overall but those of Dukes' Stage B$_2$ and Dukes' Stage C have a local recurrence rate of 25–30% and 40–80% respectively. By contrast, colonic lesion have a recurrence rate of only 3–12%. Local recurrence is a particular problem in the pelvis owing to the technical difficulty in obtaining wide excision margins, particularly for low rectal tumours. Local recurrence is thought to relate to the presence of micrometastases in the pararectal pelvic tissues. The complete excision of the mesorectum and lateral pararectal tissues is therefore important to obtain optimum results,[4,44] but may be technically difficult. There is also evidence that other mechanisms may cause local recurrence including implantation from tumour cells shed into the lumen of the bowel and the peritoneum at surgery.[45–47]

Despite a low local recurrence rate, colonic cancers develop distant recurrence, predominantly in the liver, in about 33% of cases.[6] Liver metastases are a major determinant of outcome.[4] Furthermore, about 30% of patients considered to have a disease-free liver at laparotomy will develop overt hepatic metastases within 2 years,[4,48] from micrometastases that are likely to have been present at the time of surgery. About 50% of all colon and rectal cancer patients develop recurrence overall and the majority die of hepatic metastases.[7]

Hepatic metastases are likely to develop from cancer cells shed by the tumour into the portal circulation.[49,50] Unfortunately, by the time of surgery, high ligation of the inferior mesenteric vessels is too late to alter outcome.[51]

The rationale for delivering adjuvant cytotoxic chemotherapy is therefore based on the belief that spread to regional lymph-nodes represents distant spread of the disease. There may already be hepatic seeding of micrometastases at the time of surgery and an improved response rate is likely when the metastatic tumour burden is low. Most cells entering the liver are destroyed but some survive to form micrometastases, eventually developing into hepatic deposits of tumour (Fig. 7.1). Initially the micrometastases derive their blood supply from the portal vein and later develop their own vasculature from the hepatic arteries. The stress of surgery and anaesthesia, hypercoagulability and immune suppression occurring around the time of surgery are all reasons why it is rational to commence adjuvant therapy in the perioperative period.

Trials of postoperative adjuvant cytotoxic chemotherapy have been performed since the mid-1950s but results have been limited by poor trial

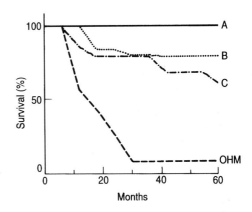

Fig 7.1 Survival curves for colorectal cancer patients without hepatic secondaries (by Dukes' Stage A, B, C) and with occult hepatic metastases (OHM).[4]

designs and suboptimal chemotherapy regimen and it is only since 1990 that a consensus has begun to emerge. Previous trials have been of two types: (1) systemic therapy, either single agent or in combination with other agents and (2) portal vein infusion, either with 5-fluorouracil (5-FU) alone or in combination. The most widely used agent is 5-FU. Despite its limitations, meta-analysis of published data suggests a reduction in mortality by 10–15%.[52]

The first trial to show positive benefit was by Taylor *et al.* in 1985, who used portal vein infusion of 5-FU for 7 days postoperatively as a single cytotoxic agent.[53] A 5-year survival benefit in the treated group of 25% was achieved (70% treated group vs 45% surgery only). Subsequent trials of similar design have confirmed these findings with improvement in survival and reduction in the number of liver metastases, especially in patients with locoregional lymph node spread.[54–57] The Swiss Group for Clinical Research (SAKK) found that perioperative adjuvant intraportal combination chemotherapy reduced the recurrence rate by 21% overall and mortality by 26% in all groups with the greatest improvement in patients with locoregional lymph node involvement (33%).

Various trials of systemic chemotherapy have used 5-FU either alone or in combination with other cytotoxic agents such as *semustine* or vincristine. Recently, 5-FU has been combined with the immunomodulator levamisole and with biomodulators such as folinic acid (leucovorin).

The results of trials using levamisole with 5-FU have aroused considerable interest and controversy. Patients receiving this combination had a significant reduction in recurrence (41%) and mortality (33%); however, this was only seen in those patients with locoregional lymph node involvement. Why levamisole should confer such an apparent advantage is unknown other than by a general effect on the immune system. The metabolites of levamisole are also possibly synergistic with 5-FU and may act in the same way as other biomodulators such as folinic acid (leucovorin).

Current trials in progress include the QUASAR (Quick and Simple Reference) project which will compare the benefit of folinic acid with 5-FU ± levamisole and the SAKK Study which is currently comparing results of systemic chemotherapy with portal vein infusion.

ADJUVANT RADIOTHERAPY IN RECTAL CANCER

Radiotherapy has little place in the primary treatment of gastrointestinal cancers. These tumours are resistant to therapy and therapeutic doses required are poorly tolerated by patients giving rise to unacceptable morbidity from small bowel side-effects, namely radiation enteritis and small bowel adhesions. However, many trials have demonstrated that pre-and postoperative radiotherapy is associated with statistically significant reductions in local recurrence of rectal cancer.[58,59] Unfortunately this is not translated into a benefit in survival. Presumably this is due to the presence of distant metastases, particularly in the liver, which are unaffected by local radiotherapy. Other studies have combined radiotherapy with chemotherapy[58] and demonstrated benefits. The UK AXIS study (Adjuvant X-Ray and Infusion Study) combines radiotherapy (as adjuvant treatment to reduce local recurrence) with portal vein cytotoxic infusion to reduce distant metastases in patients with rectal cancer.

Conclusions

Adjuvant therapy encompasses a range of treatment options and emphasizes the importance of a joint approach to the management of cancer between surgeon and oncologist. It is now an established part of the treatment of many cancers but more precise criteria for adjuvant treatment are still being defined. New cytotoxic agents and regimen continue to be evaluated and it is hoped that a clearer understanding of the mechanisms of metastasis will facilitate the development of effective agents. Over the last two decades, improvements in the treatment of cancer have been incremental; randomized trials of new regimen need to be carefully planned to ensure potential benefits are not obscured nor the hazards of adjuvant therapy suffered unnecesarily by patients.

References

1. Rew DA, Wilson GD, Taylor I. Weaver PC. Proliferation characteristics of human colorectal carcinomas measured *in vivo*. *Br J Surg* 1991; **78**: 60–6.
2. Hunt TM, Flowerdew AD, Birch SJ *et al.* Prospective randomized controlled trial of hepatic arterial embolization or infusion chemotherapy with 5-fluorouracil and degradable starch microspheres for colorectal liver metastases. *Br J Surg* 1990; **77**: 779–82.
3. Heald RJ, Husband EM, Ryall RDH. The mesorectum in rectal cancer surgery – the clue to pelvic recurrence? *Br J Surg* 1982 **69**: 613–16.
4. Finlay IG, McArdle CS. Occult hepatic metastases in colorectal carcinoma. *Br J Surg* 1986; **73**: 732–5.

5. Folkman J. Tumour angiogenesis *Adv Cancer Res* 1985; **43**: 175–83.

6. Lafrenie RM, Buchanan MR, Orr FW. Adhesion molecules and their role in cancer metastasis. *Cell Biophys,* 1993; **23 (1–3)**: 3–89.

7. Cedermark J. Autopsy studies for metastases from primary colorectal tumours *Surg Gynecol Obstet* 1977; **144**: 745–8.

8. Stower JM, Hardcastle JD. The results of 1115 patients with colorectal cancer treated over an 8 year period in a single hospital. *Euro J Surg Oncol* 1985; **11** : 119–23.

9. Martin DS. The scientific basis for adjuvant chemotherapy. *Cancer Treat Rev* 1981; **8**: 169–89.

10. Goldie JH, Coldman AJ. A mathematical model for relating the drug sensitivity of tumour to their spontaneous mutation rate. *Cancer Res.* 1979; **63**: 1727–33.

11. Salmon SE. Kinetics of minimal residual disease. Recent results. *Cancer Res.* 1979; **67**: 5–15.

12. Braly PS, Klevecz RR. Flow cytometry evaluation of ovarian cancer. *Cancer* 1993; **71**;: 1621–8.

13. MRC working party (2nd report). The evaluation of low dose pre-operative X-ray therapy in the management of operable rectal cancer: results of a randomly controlled trail. *Br J Surg* 1984; **71**: 21–5.

14. Mohuddin M, Marks G. High dose preoperative radiation therapy for adenocarcinoma of the rectum, 1976–1988. *Int J Radiol Oncol Biol Phys* 1991; **20**: 37–45.

15. Bonnadonna G. Conceptual and practical advances in the management of breast cancer. *J Clin Oncol* 1989; **10**: 1380–97.

16 Bonnadonna G. From adjuvant to neoadjuvant chemotherapy in high risk cancer: the experience of the Milan Cancer Institute. *Int J Cancer* 1993; **55**: 1–4.

17. Crown J, Vahdat L, Fennelly D *et al.* High intensity chemotherapy with haemopoietic support in breast cancer. *Ann NY Acad Sci* 1993; **29**: 111–6.

18. Nigro ND, Vaitkeviceus VK, Herskovic AM. Preservation of function in the treatment of cancer of the anus. In: Devita VT, Hellman S, Rosenberg SA, (eds) *Important Advances in Oncology.* Philadelphia; JB Lippincott, 1989: 161–77.

19. Cummings BJ, Keane TJ, O'Sullivan B *et al.* Epidermoid anal cancer: treatment by radiation alone or by radiation and 5-fluorouracil with and without mitomycin C. *Int J Radiol Oncol Biol Phys* 1991; **21**: 115–25.

20. Rosen G. Caparros B, Huvos AG *et al.* Preoperative chemotherapy for osteogenic sarcoma: selection of postoperative adjuvant chemotherapy based on the response of the primary tumour to preoperative chemotherapy. *Cancer* 1982; **49**: 1221–30.

21. Glasser DB, Lane JM, Huvos AG *et al.* Survival, prognosis and therapeutic response in osteogenic sarcoma: the Memorial Hospital experience. *Cancer* 1992; **69**: 6948–90.

22. Dimery IW, Hong WK. Overview of combined modality treatment for head and neck cancer. *J Natl Canc Inst* 1993; **8**: 95–111.

23. Department of Veterans Affairs Laryngeal Cancer Study Group. Induction chemotherapy plus radiation in patients with advanced laryngeal cancer. *N Engl J Med* 1991; **324**: 1685–90.

24. Merlano M, Vitale V, Rosso R *et al.* Treatment of advanced squamous cell carcinoma of the head and neck with alternating chemotherapy and radiotherapy. *N Engl J Med* 1992; **327**: 115–21.

25. Urba S. Wolf GT. Organ preservation in multimodality therapy of head and neck cancer. *Hematol Oncol Clin N Am* 1991; **5**: 713–24.

26. Vokes EE, Weichelsbaum RR, Lippman Sm, Hong WK. Head and neck cancer. *N Engl J Med* 1993; **328**: 84–93.

27. Fisher B, Gundux N, Saffer SA. Influence of the interval between primary tumour removal and chemotherapy of kinetics and growth of metastases. *Cancer Res.* 1983; **43**: 1488–92.

28. Lønning PE. Use of endocrine therapy to study the biology of breast cancer. *Cancer Treat Rev* 1993; **19** (Suppl B): 65–77.

29. Fuqua SAW, Chamness GC, McGuire WL. Estrogen receptor mutations in breast cancer. *J Cell Biochem* 1993; **51**: 135–9.

30. Falkson CI, Falkson G, Falkson HC. Postmenopausal breast cancer: drug therapy in the 1990s. *Drugs Aging* 1993; **3**: 106–21.

31. Tripathy D, Henderson IC. Systemic adjuvant therapy for breast cancer. *Curr Opin Oncol* 1992; **4**: 1041–9.

32. Saad Z, Bramwell V, Duff J *et al.* Timing of surgery in relation to the menstrual cycle in premenopausal women with operable breast cancer. *Br J Sug* 1994; **81**: 217–20.

33. Kinne DW. Controversies in primary breast cancer management. *Am J Surg* 1993; **166**: 502–08.

34. Balch CM, Singletary SE, Bland KI. Clinical decision making in early breast cancer. *Ann Surg* 1993; **217**: 217–25.

35. NIH Consensus Development Conference: 18–21 June 1990. Early stage breast cancer: consensus statement. In: Henderson IC (ed) *Adjuvant Therapy of Breast Cancer.* Amsterdam: Kluwer, 1992: 383–93.

36. Wagner H Jr, Smith T. Locoregional management of early breast cancer. *Cancer Detect Prev* 1993; **17**: 207–25.

37. Fisher B, Wickerham DL, Redmond C. Recent developments in the use of systemic adjuvant therapy for the treatment for breast cancer. *Semin Oncol* 1992; **19** 263–77.

38. Harris JR, Morrow M, Bonadonna G. Cancer of the breast. In: Devita VT, Hellman S Rosenberg SA (eds) *Cancer: Principles and Practice of Oncology* 4th edn. Philadelphia: JB Lippincot, 1993: 1264–332.

39. Bonnadonna G. Evolving concepts in the systemic adjuvant treatment of breast cancer. *Cancer Res.* 1992; **52**: 2127–37.

40. Early Breast Cancer Trialists Collaborative Group. Systemic treatment of early breast cancer by hormonal, cytotoxic or immune therapy: 133 randomised trials involving 31,000 recurrences and 24,000 deaths among 75,000 women. *Lancet* 1992; **339**: 1–15.

41. Glick JH, Gelber RD, Goldhirsch A *et al.* Adjuvant therapy of primary breast cancer. *Ann Oncol.* 1992; **3**: 801–7.

42. NIH Consensus Conference. Adjuvant therapy for patients with colon or rectal cancer. *JAMA* 1990; **264**: 1444–50.

43. Philips RS, Hittinger R, Blsovsky L, Fielding LP. Large bowel cancer: Surgical pathology and its relationship to survival. *Br J Surg* 1984; **71**: 604–10.

44. Quirke P, Dixon MF, Durdey P, Williams NS. Local recurrence of rectal adenocarcinoma due to inadequate surgical resection *Lancet* 1986; **ii**: 996–9.

45. Skipper D, Cooper AJ, Marston JE, Taylor I. Exfoliated cells and *in vitro* growth in colorectal cancer *Br J Surg* 1987; **74**: 1049–52.

46. Umpleby HC, Williamson RCN. The efficacy of agents employed to prevent anastomotic recurrence in colorectal carcinoma. *Ann Roy Coll Surg Engl* 1984; **66**: 192–4.

47. O'Dwyer PJ, Martin EW. Viable intraluminal tumour cells and local/regional tumour growth in experimental colon cancer *Ann Roy Coll Surg Engl* 1987; **71** : 54–6.

48. Finlay IG, Meek D, Brunton F, McArdle CS. Growth rate of hepatic metastases in colorectal carcinoma. *Br J Surg* 1988; **75**: 641–4.

49. Fisher ER. Tumor cells in mesenteric venous blood. *Surg Gynecol Obstet* 1995: Jan: 102–8.

50. Leather AJ, Kocjan G, Savage F *et al.* Detection of free malignant cells in the peritoneal cavity before and after resection of colorectal cancer. *Dis Colon Rectum* 1994; **37**(8): 814–19.

51. Pezim ME, Nicholls RJ. Survival after high or low ligation of the inferior mesenteric artery during curative surgery for rectal cancer. *Ann Surg* 1984; **200** (6): 729–33.

52. Gray R, James R, Mossman J, Stenning S. AXIS a suitable case for treatment. *Br J Cancer* 1991; **63**: 841–5.

53. Taylor I, Machin D, Mullee M *et al.* A randomised controlled trial of adjuvant portal vein cytotoxic perfusion in colorectal cancer. *Br J Surg* 1985; **72**: 359–63.

54. Swiss Group for Clinical Research (SAKK). Long term results of single course of adjuvant intraportal chemotherapy for colorectal cancer. *Lancet* 1995 **345**: 349–53.

55. Fielding LP, Hittinger R, Grace RH, Fry JS. Randomised controlled trial for adjuvant chemotherapy by portal vein infusion after curative resection for colorectal adeanocarcinoma. *Lancet* 1992; **340**: 502–6.

56. Wereldsma JC, Bruggink ED, Meijer WS *et al.* Adjuvant portal liver infusion for colorectal cancer with 5-fluorouracil/heparin versus urokinsase versus control: results of a prospective randomised clinical trial (colorectal adenocarcinoma trial I). *Cancer* 1990; **65**: 425–32.

57. Wolmark N, Rockette H, Wickerman DL. *et al.* Adjuvant therapy of Dukes A, B, C adenorcarcinomas of the colon with portal vein 5–FU hepatic infusion; preliminary results of National Surgical Adjuvant Breast and Bowel Project protocol C–02. *J Clin Oncol* 1990; **8**: 1466–75.

58. Krook JE, Moertel CG, Gunderson LL *et al.* Effective surgical adjuvant therapy for high risk rectal cancer. *N Engl J Med* 1991; **315**: 1294–5.

59. Pahlman L, Glimelius B. Pre- or postoperative radiotherapy for rectal and rectosigmoid carcinoma. *Ann Surg* 1989; **211**: 187–95.

Renal failure in general surgery

M SLAPAK

When renal function and hence the concentrating power of the kidney is excellent, a minimum of 300–400 ml of urine must be voided every 24 hours in order to clear the nitrogenous waste resulting from body metabolism. If less urine than this quantity is passed, by definition, oliguria and renal failure exist. In normal circumstances of intake and temperature, failure to pass the 'magic' 1 litre of urine over 24 hours should be grounds for suspicion. Anuria is the state when no urine at all is passed over a 12-hour period. The cause of anuria in surgical cases is either obstruction in the urinary tract, or, rarely, bilateral renal artery thrombosis. In most instances of acute renal failure, oliguria rather than anuria is present.

The consequences are grave if renal failure requiring dialysis occurs after general surgery. Of 95 patients with acute renal failure admitted to the Wessex Regional Renal and Transplant Unit, St Mary's Hospital, Portsmouth, between 1 April 1989 and March 1990, 28 died (29.5%). When ventilatory support was also required the mortality rose to 80%. Other reports testify to the high mortality of this complication.[1–5]

Multiorgan failure,[1] as well as factors such as sepsis,[2] haemorrhage[3] and hypoxia are a major cause of the high mortality associated with the onset of acute renal failure in patients after surgery. Never-theless, in a suprisingly large proportion of patients, unwarranted delay in the diagnosis of the renal failure component and its inappropriate treatment adversely affects the outcome.

Pathophysiology

Although they constitute less than 3% of the body mass, in keeping with their function as a filter, the kidneys receive 20% of the total cardiac output. Over 95% of this flows through the cortex, the site of glomerular function. In situations of physiological stress such as 'fight or flight', temporary cessation of this glomerular flow occurs,[6] with diversion of blood flow to muscle and other tissue more crucial to survival. A similar but more accentuated adaptation occurs in acute pathological conditions such as sepsis, haemorrhage or hypoxia. The consequent cortical ischaemia is often of great severity and duration and thus cortical damage results which may or may not be reversible. The tubules are the main target for this potentially reversible damage brought about by diminished perfusion consequent to peritubular capillary damage. Vacuolation of tubules and red staining protein material in the tubular lumen is seen histolo-

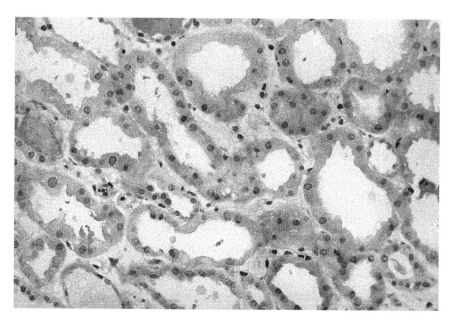

Fig 8.1 Recovering acute tubular necrosis. The vacuolation of the tubules, together with proteinaceous material within the lumen, are seen in this micrograph. There is very sparse celluar infiltrate consequent to the tubular damage. The arrow shows mitotic figures in some of the tubular cells which indicates that regeneration of tubules is now occurring and a degree of recovery can be expected.

gically – the classical appearances of acute tubular necrosis (Fig. 8.1)

Functionally, the decreased flow into the glomeruli, together with the effects of tubular dysfunction on potassium and sodium control, lead to the 'big three' of renal failure from a surgical point of view, namely:

1. fall in urine output;
2. tissue oedema;
3. raised serum potassium.

Autoregulation of glomerular blood flow and thus of urine formation is exerted by control mechanisms situated at the juxtaglomerular junction. These regulate the intraglomerular perfusion pressures. At pressures below 60 mmHg, urine production ceases.

Simplistically, sodium retention is synonymous with oedema, whereas sodium excretion is accompanied by diuresis. Drugs such as the frusemide class of loop diuretics act on the tubules by inhibiting their sodium reabsorbing function, thus allowing greater sodium (with its concomitant water) loss to take place. Osmotic diuretics such as mannitol act by increasing blood volume and – providing blood reaches the glomerulus – increasing the plasma filtrate. Both these diuretics increase cortical blood flow and are thus protective in instances when renal ischaemia may ensue by providing a greater reservoir

of available oxygenated blood for tissue consumption. Dopamine in 'renal' doses (below 10 μg/kg/min) dilates the renal vascular bed via dopaminergic receptors causing an increase in renal blood flow, glomerular filtration rate (GFR), and sodium excretion.

Neither a decrease in urine output, nor a rise in serum creatinine or blood urea occurs after unilateral nephrectomy in a healthy adult. Such is the 'spare capacity' inherent in normal renal function. Compensatory hypertrophy of the remaining kidney takes 10–20 days to make up the deficit in these circumstances. The GFR measures the functional capacity of the kidneys using a strangely contrived unit (creatinine clearance) in which it is hypothesized that the amount of a substance, such as creatinine, passed into the urine per minute is related to the volume of plasma in millilitres per minute which *would* have been entirely cleared of its creatinine content. Since, for practical purposes, creatinine is neither absorbed nor excreted by the tubules, its presence in the urine accurately measures the GFR. Of course, only a fraction of the creatinine in each millilitre of plasma is actually filtered but that fraction is filtered from the total blood volume which passes through the kidneys per minute – well in excess of 1000 ml. The GFR in an adult male is approximately 120 ml/per min. Immediately after unilateral nephrectomy it is halved to 60 ml/per min. Despite this 50% drop in function, enough serum creatinine and urea are filtered to keep the blood levels of these two substances normal. By the same token, a rise in the creatinine above the normal value, for what ever reason, signifies a decrease in the functional capacity of the kidneys of greater than 50%. Thus, a normal urine output in association with a normal serum creatinine a few days postoperatively does not guarantee that one of the ureters has not been accidentally ligated, whilst a normal creatinine clearance does.

Historically, prior to the advent of effective haemodialysis, pioneered by Kolff in 1946,[7] acute renal failure resulted in uraemic death, usually within 7–10 days due to hyperkalaemic cardiac arrest. With effective dialysis, tubular regeneration may take as long as 6 weeks before full return to normal renal function. The observable practical sequelae of the pathophysiological changes of failing renal function are those related to a falling urine output, increasing signs of water retention and the effects of acidosis, with rising potassium, creatinine and blood urea levels.

The above pathophysiological abnormalities can result from pathological processes situated at three main anatomical locations classically described as:

1. Prerenal – abnormal factors extrinsic to the kidneys as in circulatory collapse due to shock, haemorrhage, vomiting and dehydration;
2. Renal – intrinsic renal damange is usually caused by prerenal mechanisms, but also more specifically by ischaemic damage to peritubular vessels, as well as by known nephrotoxic substances such as gentamicin or free haemoglobin;
3. Postrenal – due to obstruction to the passage of urine as a result of stone or tumour, or iatrogenically by ligation of ureters.

The above classification, whilst helpful clinically, must be seen in the context of intrinsic renal damage taking place at a variable rate in both the pre- and postrenal situations. Thus, obstructive symptoms certainly cause intrinsic renal damage but do so far more slowly than severe systemic sepsis. [This delay is similar to that seen in biliary obstruction and liver damage. – Ed.]

Symptoms and signs

The symptoms of uraemia are insidious and therefore easily missed. Fatiguability, nausea and vomiting caused by anaemia and failure to excrete the products of protein breakdown respectively are present in varying degree. Muscle twitching, pruritus and anorexia are common. All or any of these may, however, have alternative and acceptable explanations in patients with complex postoperative pathologies. The main clue is water retention. This may cause dys-

pnoea, swollen ankles and, more rarely, reduced urine output. The telltale signs are mainly those of fluid retention. There is oliguria progressing to anuria. Pitting oedema of the ankles, a sacral pad (i.e. dependent oedema of the sacrum and back), basal crepitations in the chest, a visibly raised jugular pulse, together with a gross disparity between the fluid intake and output, are usually present. Hypertension is often a feature resulting from the increased circulatory volume. Bradycardia due to hyperkalaemia is a late feature as are convulsions and coma. Muscle twitching and a 'flap' may occur early and are thus useful alerting signs.

Biochemical analysis confirms renal failure. Serum creatinine and blood urea are elevated above normal and as failure progresses serum potassium levels rise. Serum creatinine is the single most useful index of renal function, being far less influenced than is the blood urea by extraneous factors such as bleeding into the alimentary tract or elsewhere or by severe tissue catabolism. Sodium levels are often low due to dilution from fluid retention as well from failing tubular function. Characteristically, there is also marked acidosis with CO_2 levels below 30 mmol/l. Urinary chemistry is usually of little diagnostic help. However, a urine sodium of less than 10 mmol/l in the presence of oliguria would strongly mitigate against an intrinsic renal cause for the low urine output. Positive bacteriology may indicate a primary causative septic factor, but far more commonly points to a concomitant urinary tract infection caused by an indwelling Foley catheter.

Causes of acute renal failure in general surgery

A literature review of acute renal failure (ARF) following general surgery is complicated by the variety of definitions for ARF. Oliguria, as defined by volumes varying from 300 to 600 ml/day, serum creatinine levels from 400 to 800 mmol/l, and the need, or otherwise, for dialysis make comparison difficult.

Of 147 patients admitted to the Wessex Renal and Transplant Unit between March 1989 and March 1993, 62 (49%) had preceding general surgical procedures. The six leading causes were:

*   sepsis 40%;
*   postlaparotomy for neoplasm 24%;
*   aortic aneurysm 21%;
*   pancreatitis 5%;
*   multiple trauma 5%;
*   perforated peptic ulcer 5%.

In a series of 1347 patients with ARF admitted between 1980 and 1988[4] who either required dialysis or had a serum creatinine > 600 mmol/l at diagnosis, the mean age was 60 years. When surgery preceded the renal failure, the mortality in this group was 42%. The leading surgical causes were: cardiopulmonary bypass, sepsis following abdominal surgery, abdominal aortic surgery, biliary surgery and acute pancreatitis.

Olsen *et al.*[5] reported 656 patients requiring abdominal aortic surgery, of whom 81 (12%) developed ARF. Of these, 32 were dialysed whilst 49 were not. The mortality was 58% irrespective of dialysis. Of 35 patients who developed ARF 0–14 days after cardiopulmonary bypass, the mortality was 74%. The mean creatinine was 362 mmol/l at time of diagnosis and all underwent haemofiltration. The only factor which affected mortality was the number of failed organs.[5]

Acute renal failure complicates acute pancreatitis in 6–10% of patients. The mortality is, however, over 80% when dialysis is required. Of 267 patients with acute pancreatitis reported by Tran *et al.*, 16% had acute renal failure as defined by oliguria and a creatinine of > 500 mmol/l. No patient requiring dialysis survived. Pre-existing renal disease and cardiovascular abnormality were found to be the main risk factors.[8]

In jaundiced patients with sepsis and liver dysfunction, as with patients with acute severe pancreatitis, the effects are predominantly intrinsically renal, resulting from the action of circulating vasoactive amines on the renal vasculature as well as the prerenal effect of hypovolaemia. In some instances a failing cardiac output adds to the injury. Increasing concentrations of bilirubin, *per se* have very little deleterious effect on renal function.

Diagnosis

Two main questions are posed. First, is the cause intrinsically renal or does renal failure result from pre- or postrenal factors, such as failing cardiac output, a diminished blood volume or urinary tract obstruction? Second, what is the precise cause of the intrinsic renal pathology. Is it acute tubular necrosis? Is there renal artery thombosis? Was there significant renal disease prior to surgery? Furthermore, is there a possibility of ureteric obstruction or damage.

The clinical history, symptoms and signs having been elicited, the fluid change is now carefully evaluated in the light of the biochemical findings.

The first question to be answered is: *is there fluid retention or fluid overload?* The second: *is there evidence of intrinsic renal dysfunction?*

THE DIURETIC TEST

In an adequately hydrated patient the response to 12.5 g of mannitol, infused in 300 ml of dextrose saline over 30 min, will generally clarify the clinical situation and give valuable therapeutic guidance. In acutely progressive intrinsic renal failure there is no appreciable response in the rate of urine flow. In hypovolaemia there is an oncotically driven response with a brisk increase in urine excretion over the ensuing 3 hours, thus indicating the patient's need for plasma, blood or crystalloid.

Frusemide, 10–20 mg given intravenously over 5 min with an infusion of 300 ml of saline, may achieve the same diuresis but is less useful diagnostically. Here diuresis results from a 'poisoning' of tubular sodium reabsorption and thus points less directly to therapeutic volume expansion. Nevertheless, a lack of response to frusemide certainly signals intrinsic renal failure and is thus a valuable diagnostic tool, particularly as the risk of circulatory overload is less than with mannitol.

Apart from the extrarenal possibilities, a severe urinary tract infection with pyelonephritis and systemic effects may cause creatinine elevation, but rarely by more than 100 mmol/l. Dehydration, particularly in the elderly, rarely results in serum creatinine levels greater than 500 mmol/l. In acute renal failure serum creatinine may rise over 150 mmol/l/ day.

Consideration of the rate of potassium rise is also important. A value of 6.5 mmol/l in a blood specimen drawn at 09.00 may indicate a rise to over 7 mmol/l by midnight with dire consequences. Extrarenal causes, unless concomitant with absorption of a collection of blood in the peritoneal cavity or the bowel, are unlikely to cause a continuous rise in the potassium level.

Having made a diagnosis of intrinsic renal damage, steps must be taken to establish its cause.

ULTRASOUND

Ultrasound has become the primary diagnostic procedure. This investigation non-invasively establishes the physical presence of both kidneys, their size and shape, and also the presence of any adjacent fluid collection or hydronephrosis. When combined with a Doppler facility, or even without one, the presence of pulsation in the renal arteries may be detected. Flow in the renal vein is detected with less certainty.

PERFUSION SCAN

A perfusion scan using radioactive ^{99m}technetium (^{99m}Tc) linked to DTPA (diethylpentaacetic acid) or DMSA (dimethylcaptosalycylic acid) may be of great value. It provides the definitive answer to the crucial question: are the kidneys perfused with blood, and if so, to what degree (i.e. perfusion index)? When ^{99m}Tc Mg$_3$ or ^{123}Iodine Hippuran are used, some functional values (such as GFR) can be established. Most helpful, too, is the establishment of a functional baseline which can be used when charting recovery after acute injury.

PERCUTANEOUS BIOPSY

A percutaneous biopsy of the kidney has a place in management only when recovery of a perfused kidney is significantly delayed. The presence of tubular regeneration (Fig. 8.1) gives hope for eventual recovery, whilst fibrosis and chronic degenerative changes will speed the decision to refer the patient for chronic renal replacement therapy or for transplantation. The investigation is not free from risk, and should always be done under ultrasound control.

PERCUTANEOUS ARTERIOGRAMS AND VENOGRAMS

Both percutaneous arteriograms or venograms are seldom indicated. The information which they provide is more safely obtained by the use of Doppler ultrasound.

Treatment

There are two main components of treatment. The first is the treatment of varying degrees of established acute tubular necrosis (ATN) causing acute renal failure, as defined by oliguria or anuria, together with a rapidly rising serum creatinine. The second component, which is far more rewarding therapeutically, is the prevention of renal damage by targeting the surgical situations in which it is most likely to occur and by taking the appropriate steps when possible.

Established acute tubular necrosis

Effective treatment is the successful exercise of a policy in damage limitation, especially for damage which has been or can be brought about by inappropriate medication and management. Treatment after diagnosis deals with the persisting causal factors which can increase or perpetuate the damage, combined with supportive measures which must be instituted whilst tubular healing, hopefully, takes place.

Two classically described phases of ATN are 'oliguric' and 'diuretic'. The latter represents the immediate recovery phase when increasingly large filtrates pass into tubules which are not yet able to reabsorb sodium and potassium and thus properly concentrate the urine. A third phase, described as the late recovery phase, is a reflection of the irretrievable damage which the kidneys have sustained. It may last for months before the full degree of recovery can be assessed.

Treatment of oliguric phase

ESTABLISH PROPER FLUID BALANCE

To do this effectively a careful study of the fluid chart after full clinical assessment is vital and frequently decisive. Major disparity betwen input and output becomes apparent. Commonly, fluid overload is present. Restriction of intake to 500 ml of normal saline every 24 hours is a useful rule of thumb.

If fever is present, an additional 200 ml for every 1°C rise above normothermia is a reasonable adjustment. If, less commonly, fluid depletion is found, replacement with normal saline is effective. Daily weighing of the patient is valuable in the monitoring of fluid balance. Loop diuretics, such as frusemide during this period may be harmful.

TREAT HYPERKALAEMIA

If the serum potassium is above 5.5 mmol/1, but below 6.5 mmol/1, calcium resonium 30 g in methylcellulose solution is given either as an enema to be retained for 9 hours or by mouth in a dose of 15 g tid. The side-effects of the former route are commonly constipation and, rarely, rectal ulceration. By mouth it is unpleasant to take and nausea may be a problem.

Reduction of the raised potassium level may take several hours. The medication may be continued for some days, providing the serum potassium remains stable and the electrocardiogram confirms the absence of the cardiac effects of hyperkalaemia.

In instances when a rapid decrease of serum potassium is necessary, e.g. to cover an operative procedure, a rapid but transient reduction may be achieved by infusion of 50 g of glucose covered by 10–15 units of soluble insulin. The potassium is driven intracellularly but this effect lasts for a few hours only. Persisting levels of potassium above 6.5 mmol/l are usually an indication for dialysis.

CONTROL INFECTION

Ongoing sepsis is a potent perpetuating factor preventing recovery from ATN. Its treatment is complicated by the need to select antibiotics, antifungal or antiviral agents which have the least nephrotoxicity. Particularly nephrotoxic agents include the aminoglycosides (e.g. gentamicin), non-steroidal anti-inflammatory agents, septrin, most sulphonamides, amphotericin, fluconazole, acyclovir and gancyclovir. Assiduous control of blood levels is mandatory when the clinical situation makes their use unavoidable.

PREVENT STRESS ULCERS

H_2-Antagonists such as ranitidine, 150 mg bd, should be prescribed routinely. They have been beneficial in the prevention of peptic ulceration, haematemesis and melaena.

TREAT ANAEMIA

Blood replacement for postsurgical anaemia poses not only the problem of fluid overload but also that of producing a very rapid hyperkalaemia due to the high potassium level of stored blood. A request for blood which has been banked for not longer than a few days helps the latter problem, whilst judicious gauging of fluid balance prevents the former.

NUTRITION

As a supplement, the use of a protein-free 49% glucose-containing oral fluid such as Hycal® to provide at least 2000 calories per day has been of proven benefit[9] in the maintenance of physiological stability during renal failure.

Dialysis

Dialysis can take the form of haemodialysis, ultrafiltration, continuous arteriovenous haemofiltration (CAVH), continuous venovenous haemofiltration (CVVH) and peritoneal dialysis – intermittent or continuous.

When renal function is absent, is at a very low level or the complications of its deficiency are apparent, extrarenal support is instituted. It consists of *haemodialysis* when the blood volume and composition are altered as a result of filtration through an artificial membrane, or *peritoneal dialysis* when a similar effect is achieved by using the peritoneum.

Haemodialysis is life saving when promptly instituted. If used inappropriately, or in excess, it may even be detrimental.[10] This is not only because hypotension may sometimes occur but also because the contact between the blood and some of the artificial membranes used may lead to complement and leucocyte activation and thus prolong oliguria.[11]

INDICATIONS

The absolute indications for haemodialysis are:

- a serum potassium greater than 6.5 mmol/l, particularly in the presence of ECG changes;
- the symptoms or signs of pulmonary oedema;
- anuria for longer than 36 hours when associated with a creatinine of > 500 mmol/l and acidosis;
- encephalopathy;
- uraemic pericarditis.

Relative indications include:

- unresponsive diastolic hypertension;
- blood urea > 30 mmol/l;
- the need for volume space for intravenous medication or blood replacement.

Commonly, haemodialysis treatment is intermittent with the patient being connected to the dialysis machine for 5–8 hours, three to five times a week depending on their needs. Fluid, electrolyte and molecular flux takes place as a result of concentration gradients between the plasma and the dialysate compartments, the two being separated by the interposed membrane. Modern dialysis machines allow monitored removal of both fluid and electrolytes by alterations of pump filtration pressure, thus ensuring *ultrafiltration* to be carried out simultaneously with dialysis. Expertise is required in running these machines. Furthermore, the rapid shifts of both fluid and electrolytes may cause hypotension, imposing a stress on myocardial function and cardiac output. Rapid fluid shifts may also directly lead to the so-called 'disequilibrium syndrome' and cerebral oedema.

Continuous arteriovenous haemofiltration

This form of haemofiltration (CAVH) has had a very significant impact on the speed and ease with which haemodialysis can be instituted. It is available in many intensive care units and has significantly decreased the number of patients referred to specialist renal units.[14]

The essence of the technique is the use of a continuous flow of blood through a membrane of smaller pore size than that used in standard haemodialysis. This permits large volumes of fluid to pass continuously through the membrane over a 24-hour period but necessitates precise calculation of volume replacement to keep the patient in proper fluid balance. These volumes may be of the order of 30–60 litres every 24 hours.

Arterial pressure alone sometimes drives the fluid through the membranes. Far more commonly, though, pumps are required. Continuous venovenous haemofiltration, using a percutaneously inserted double-lumen right atrial catheter, is being increasingly used as it avoids the need for arterial cannulation (Fig. 8.2).

All forms of haemodialysis require the use of pumps with heparin to a greater or lesser extent. Coagulation is therefore impaired. Immediate reversal by simultaneous protamine sulphate infusion is only partially effective. The use of prostacyclin, whilst effective, has the drawbacks of hypotension and the need for continuous infusion as well as expense. In surgical conditions, where bleeding may be a major problem, the anticoagulation effects imposed by all forms of haemodialysis must be appreciated both postoperatively and when planning any further surgical procedures.

Vascular access

A flow of 200–300 ml blood/min is necessary for efficient dialysis. Percutaneous insertion of a single- or double-lumen catheter into the right atrium using the Seldinger technique has replaced direct surgical cannulation of a suitable peripheral limb artery and vein. The internal jugular vein, preferably the right, is usually the best choice despite the awkward external 'lie' of the catheter. Subclavian vein cannulation provides better positioning but pneumothorax is a complication which may have serious results in a patient already in acute pulmonary overload. Percutaneous insertion of a catheter into the inferior vena cava via the femoral vein is reserved for emergency

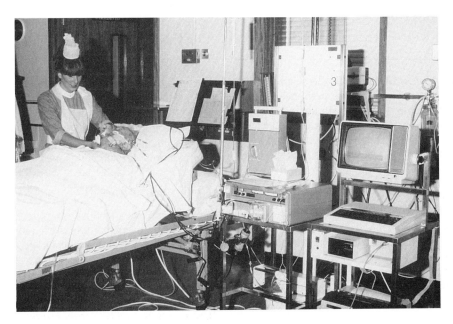

Fig 8.2 A patient is undergoing CVVH through a double lumen neck line inserted into the right atrium via the right internal jugular vein. Note the presence of a driving pump and also of the heparin infusion.

situations when the previously mentioned sites are not accessible due to lack of expertise or other factors.

Intermittent peritoneal dialysis

After percutaneous insertion of a radio-opaque Teflon® catheter into the peritoneal cavity, volumes of 2–3 litres of warm sterile dialysate fluid are introduced and removed in 30-min cycles, either mechanically or (labour intensively) by hand. The fluid used contains sodium 132 mmol/l, potassium 0 mmol/l, calcium 1.75 mmol/l, magnesium 0.75 mmol/l and lactate 35 mmol/l, as well as glucose, either as a 1.36% or a 3.86% solution, the latter being used when urgent removal of excess fluid is desirable. A well functioning catheter may allow many weeks of such dialysis. The disadvantages of this technique, compared with haemodialysis, is that in surgical practice the utilizable peritoneal surface may be considerably reduced. Furthermore, it may be breached in places, inflamed, or else be the seat of numerous adhesions thus rendering the technique impractical. In addition, the splinting effect of the peritoneal fluid on the diaphragm adds to any pulmonary embarrassment which may be present. Some albumin loss occurs also and both fluid and electrolyte control is slower and also less predictable than with haemodialysis. On the other hand, the fluid and electrolyte shifts are gentler and there is far less likelihood of hypotension with little haemodynamic stress on the circulation. Crucially, too, in the surgical context, the administration of heparin is not necessary.

INDICATIONS

Mild-to-moderate electrolyte imbalance is an indication in surgical patients in whom the peritoneal cavity is judged to be suitable. Patients with acute pancreatitis may constitute a favourable group in that the added possible benefit of removing ascitic fluid containing proteolytic enzymes is simultaneously achieved.

DIURETIC PHASE

Treatment is directed towards the replacement of fluid and electrolyte loss. Volumes which may exceed 10 litres/day are passed as the tubules gradually recover their reabsorbing capacity.

PREVENTION OF ACUTE RENAL FAILURE

1. Target the likely patient.
2. Target the likely procedure.
3. Institute prophylactic measures early.

Likely patient

It is obvious that elderly patients with compromised renal function are at risk during a surgical procedure which may impose any of the factors previously outlined. It is less obvious that a 60-year-old patient whose serum creatinine is 160 mmol/l has a renal function which is less than 50% of normal. If significant blood loss and hypotension are imposed during surgery, the possibility of renal damage is twice that of a similarly aged patient whose serum creatinine is 110 mmol/l. Thus a raised serum creatinine and the absence of proteinuria must be noted carefully and their importance in the preoperative assessment realized.

Likely procedures

Aortic aneurysm surgery

Compromise of the origin of the renal artery by aortic disease, together with aortic clamping and reduction or temporary arrest of renal inflow during the insertion of the graft, are the major pathophysical factors. In addition, release of vasoactive amines on removal of the aortic clamps, and the blood loss associated with the surgery for the condition, have resulted in the relative high incidence of renal failure following aortic surgery of between 10 and 33%.

In a recent report of 61 patients, in whom fluid loading and pulmonary wedge pressure monitoring was carried out, six (10%) had renal failure (variously defined) compared with 29 of 87 (33%) patients in whom special measures were not undertaken. Ligation of the left renal vein to enable aortic occlusion is not followed by an increased need for dialysis but it does result in creatinine levels higher than in a group in which this measure is not applied.[12]

Cardiopulmonary bypass

Patients aged over 70 with a pre-existing elevation of the serum creatinine are particularly at risk. In some reports renal failure necessitating dialysis was present in 20% of cases, the mortality in that subgroup being 50%[13]

Biliary procedures

When complicated by sepsis or preoperative jaundice the risk to patients is significant. In a large series of patients who had surgical procedures for obstructive jaundice, the overall mortality was 16%; 9% of the patients developed actue renal failure and of these, 76% died.[15] All patients requiring operation for obstructive jaundice should receive the prophylactic measures outlined below.[16]

All surgical procedures with massive blood loss

Anticipation of severe blood loss is a function of good communication between surgeon and anaesthetist and is a key feature in the prevention of renal failure.

All surgical procedures in which large masses of tissue are ischaemic for lengthy periods

Tissue ischaemia, either of organs or of tissues, is one of the basic factors producing renal failure. A special entity of muscle necrosis is the occurrence of rhabdomyoglobinuria.[17] The crush syndrome and pelvic procedures are usual antecedent causes.

Prophylaxis of acute tubular necrosis

The fluid maintenance of the 'at-risk' patient is hampered by the 8 hour 'nil by mouth' requirement imposed by an impending general anaesthetic, as well as by the difficulty in accurate monitoring of the circulatory volume.

An effective strategy for the 'at-risk' patient includes:

- Intravenous hydration and central venous pressure monitoring *prior* to going to theatre, the position of the line to be confirmed by X-ray, and the reading to be above 6 cm H_2O.
- If a urinary catheter is not in place, it should be inserted prior to surgery. The risk and consequence of a postoperative urinary tract infection are minimized by the use of a suitable antibiotic and are far less dangerous than renal failure.
- Mannitol 12.5 g given intravenously before the induction of general anaesthesia.
- Methyldopamine infusion at a dose of 2–5 µg/kg body wt/min instituted prior to anaesthesia and continued during surgery.
- Emptying of the urine bag and measuring urine output during the course of the operation. A flow of over 75 ml/h guarantees an acceptable cardiac output and an adequate circulatory volume.
- Central venous pressure maintained at 5–10 cm H_2O during positive pressure anaesthesia together

with a urine output of over 75 ml during the procedure. This may require the use of frusemide 20 mg given as an intravenous infusion over 5 min.

Although nephrotoxic antibiotics must be avoided, a *single dose* of 80 mg gentamicin with 500 mg metronidazole is an effective prophylactic measure.

The most effective way of preventing renal ischaemia is to reduce the core temperature of the kidney and thus its oxygen requirement. At normothermia, interruption of the arterial blood supply for 30–40 min results in an incidence of acute tubular necrosis of greater than 50%. A warm ischaemic interval of greater than 60 min in the human leads to inevitable acute renal failure. A minority of patients, depending on age and other factors, will recover with the support of maintenance dialysis.

When the kidney is cooled, the oxygen needs are greatly decreased. For example, at a core temperature of 20°C, only 10% of the normal oxygen requirement is necessary.[18] If after sustaining a 15-minute period of ischaemia the kidneys are cooled by intra-arterial infusion of an ice-cold crystalloid solution such as hyperosmolar citrate.[19,20] or the Wisconsin solution,[21] the recovery after a further 6 hours of cold ischaemia is likely to be nearly 100%. Furthermore, in over 50%, immediate life-supporting function can be expected.

Unfortunately, in most theatres, neither the technique nor the expertise necessary to institute such cooling is usually available at short notice. With due planning prior to surgery, however, relatively simple cooling techniques may be used which provide dramatic protection from acutely imposed ischaemic damage.[22] Thus, surface cooling of the human kidney to a core temperature of 20°C will allow recovery after a 4-hour interruption of arterial blood flow. If more technically exacting cooling via the renal artery, using 200 ml of ice-cold solution, can be instituted, then protection of function for 6 hours is possible with safety.[21]

PHARMACOLOGICAL PRESERVATIVES

For obvious reasons measures involving preservative solutions are more convenient. Apart from mannitol and diuretics, the most convenient pharmacological agent is methylprednisolone, An infusion of 1 g over 10 minutes prior to the imposition of the ischaemia should, on theroretical grounds,[23] provide protection for 90 minutes of warm ischaemia. Dopamine infusion at a rate of 2–5 µg/kg/min certainly increases renal blood flow and is likely to provide a safe 60 minutes of warm renal ischaemia.

TECHNIQUE OF KIDNEY COOLING

The two provisos which need to be observed are that (1) vascular isolation of the kidney by ligation of tributaries must first be performed so that the only inflow is through the renal artery or arteries and the venous outflow only through the renal vein or veins and (2) kidneys with more than one artery make the technique unduly complicated.

Intra-arterial perfusion

A 14-gauge intracath is bent to a right angle and introduced into the renal artery and the needle removed, leaving the cannula in place. Then 200 ml of ice-cold hyperosmolar citrate is infused from a height of 120 cm above the patient, a bull-dog clip having arrested arterial inflow from the aorta. The renal vein entrance into the inferior vena cava, having been similarly previously occluded, a small incision is made in the gonadal vein on the left side, or the renal vein itself on the right. The cold venous effluent is sucked out as it emerges. Clearing of the intrarenal blood thus takes place with the kidney assuming a pale colour. An ice-cold swab is then placed around the kidney and is left *in situ*. At the end of the procedure the small hole in the renal artery is sutured using 6/0 prolene, as is the incision in the right renal vein. The left gonadal vein is ligated.

Surface cooling

After complete isolation of the kidney has been achieved by dissection, the patient must be heparinized to prevent intrarenal clotting. Occlusion of the renal artery and the vein is then instituted. A large ice-cold saline-soaked swab is placed posterior to the dissected kidney surface and two sterile bags containing frozen saline are placed on the anterior and posterior surfaces of the kidney. This method is far less efficient than intra-arterial cooling. A cumbersome method, in which a cooling coil is placed around the dissected kidney, was described by Wickham but is rarely used.[24]

Autotransplantation

In some conditions, appropriate nephrectomy, extracorporeal cooling using hyperosmolar citrate or Wisconsin solution, and hypothermic storage in a plastic bag surrounded by sterile ice, can be undertaken. Autotransplantation into the right or left iliac fossae, or both, can then be carried out after the main surgical procedure has been completed. Protection of the kidney for 24 hours can be achieved with resulting good renal function after routine transplantation techniques.[20] Abdominal aneurysms involving the renal arteries[25] or more rarely dissection of the aorta in Marfan's syndrome[26] may be indications for these specialized procedures which are best carried out with the cooperation of a transplant team.

This chapter has reviewed some aspects of a very serious complication of general surgery, namely acute renal failure. The high mortality and morbidity often associated with it can be significantly reduced by three cardinal steps:

- early diagnosis of intrinsic renal failure by the use of the mannitol test;
- early institution of fluid restricton and dialysis;
- the identification of patients who are likely to be at high risk from acute renal failure and the careful planning and institution of available therapeutic measures to prevent it.

References

1. Wheeler DC, Feehally J, Walls J. High risk acute renal failure, *Quart J Med* 1986; **61**(234): 977–84.
2. Urschel JD, Antkowiak JG, Takita H. Acute renal failure following pulmonary surgery. *J Cardiovasc Surg* 1994; **35**(3): 215–8.
3. Svensson LG, Coselli JS, Safi HJ *et al.* Appraisal of adjuncts to prevent acute renal failure after surgery on the thoracic or thoracoabdominal aorta. *J Vasc Surg* 1989; **10**(3): 230–9.
4. Turney JH, Marshall DH, Brownjohn AM *et al*, The evolution of acute renal failure, 1956–1988. *Quart J Med* 1990; **74**(273): 83–104.
5. Olsen PS, Schroeder T, Perko M *et al.* Renal failure after operation for abdominal aortic aneurysm. *Ann Vas Surg* 1990; **4**(6): 580–3.
6. Slapak M, Dalton W, Lee HM, Hume DM. Variations of glomerular filtration rates after renal homotransplantation in the human being and the dog as measured by the blood clearance of $CO_{57}B_{12}$. *Surg Forum* 1965; **16**: 260.
7. Kolff WJ, De Kunstmatige Nier (The Artificial Kidney) MD thesis, University of Groningen, The Netherlands. 1946.
8. Tran DD, de Fitier CW, Van der Meuten J. Acute renal failure in patients with acute pancreatitis. *Naeph Dial Trans* 1993; **8**(4): 79–84.
9. Leurs PB, Mulder AW, Fiers HA. Chronic renal failure after cardiovasular surgery. *Eur Heart J* 1989; **10**(4): 38–42.
10. Conger JD. Does haemodialysis delay recovery from renal failure? *Semin Dial* 1990; **3**: 146–8.
11. Hakim RH, Wingard RL, Parker RA. Effects of the dialysis membrane in the treatment of patients with acute renal failure, *N Engl J Med* 1994; **331**: 1338–42.
12. Huber D, Harris J, Walker PJ *et al.* Does division of the left renal vein during aortic surgery

adversely affect renal function? *Ann Vasc Surg* 1991; **5**(1): 74–9.

13. Baudouin SVW, Wiggins J, Keogh BF *et al.* Continuous veno-venous haemofiltration following cardio-pulmonary bypass. Indications and outcome in 35 patients. *Intens Care Med* 1993; **19**(5): 290–3.

14. Mason JC, Cowell TK, Hilton PJ, Wing AJ. Continuous arteriovenous haemofiltration (CAVH) as complete replacement therapy in acute renal failure: management of fluid balance assisted by computer monitoring. In: Sieberth HG, Mann H (eds) *Continuous Arteriovenous Hemofiltration (CAVH).* International Conference on CAVH, Aachen 1984. Basel: Karger, 1984: 37–44.

15. Walt RB, Kahng KU. Renal failure complicating obstructive jaundice (see comments). *Am J Surg* 1990; **159**(4): 256–63.

16. Thompson JN, Edwards WH, Winearls CG *et al.* Renal impairment following biliary tract surgery. *Br J Surg* 1987 **74**(9): 843–7.

17, Palmer SH, Graham G. Tourniquet-induced rhabdomyolysis after total knee replacement, *Ann Roy Coll Surg* 1994; **76**: 416–17.

18. Harvey RB, Brothers AJ, Allen JG. Effect of temperature on function of isolated dog kidney. *Am J Physiol* 1959; **197**: 181–6.

19. Slapak M, Wilson A, Clyne C *et al* Hyperosmolar citrate vs Perfudex: a functional comparison in clinical organ transplantation. *Transp Proc* 1979; **11**: 478–81.

20. Marshall VC, Jablonski P, Howden BO *et al.* Hypothermic preservation of the rat kidney for transplantation using flushing solutions: effects of glucose (Abstract number 85). *Cryobiology* 1983; **20**: 720–1.

21. Wahlberg J, Love R, Landegaard L. 72 hour preservation of the canine pancreas. *Transplantation* 1987; **43**: 5.

22. Slapak M. New ideas and techniques for vital organ procurement and exchange. *Transp Proc* 1985; **17**(6): 88–91.

23. Chatterjee SN, Berne TV, Use of cellular membrane stablisers to prevent ischemic damage to the kidneys. *Surg Forum* 1975; **26**: 335–6.

24. Wickham J, Hanley HG, Joeke S. Regional renal hypothermia. *Br J Urol* 1967; **39**: 727–43,

25. Crawford ES, Coselli JS, Svensson LG *et al.* Diffuse aneurysmal disease (chronic aortic dissection Marfan and mega aorta syndromes) and multiple aneurysm. *Ann Surg* 1990; **211**: 521–37.

26. Thomson SD, Chmura A, Slapak M. Aortic dissection in Marfan Syndrome – the role of renal autotransplantation. *J Roy Soc Med* 1995; **88**: 532–3.

CHAPTER 9

Surgery and the patient with diabetes

M J SAMPSON, JS YUDKIN

Diabetes offers a serious bar to any kind of operation, and injuries involving open wounds, haemorrhage or damage to the blood vessels are exceedingly grave in subjects of this disease. A wound in the diabetic patient will probably not heal. . . . Gangrene readily follows an injury in diabetes and such patients show terrible proneness to the low form of erysipelas and cellulitis (Treves 1896).[1]

Introduction

Treves' description was written a quarter of a century before the discovery of insulin, when diabetic patients were chronically malnourished and suffered a commonly fatal disease. The morbidity and mortality associated with surgery in diabetic patients is now due mostly to the complications associated with diabetes, but the perioperative management of these patients still causes a great deal of uncertainty among medical and nursing staff.

This chapter focuses on why diabetic patients form such a large part of the surgeon's workload and why they have an increased perioperative morbidity; it also discusses practical and widely used methods for perioperative care.

Perioperative morbidity and mortality in patients with diabetes

There have been few adequate data on perioperative mortality in diabetic patients until recently – most previous studies have been retrospective and uncontrolled, and, of course, predate modern surgical techniques and diabetic care.

Brown and Rowen[2] prospectively studied 231 elderly patients undergoing non-cardiac surgery (predominantly vascular reconstruction). Diabetes was 2.5 times more frequent in patients suffering a perioperative cardiac event, and the majority of the patients who had such events were diabetic (10 of 19; 54%). This excess was partly explained by an excess of pre-existing coronary disease in the diabetic patients. In a similar though larger study, Velanovich[3] reported data from 514 patients undergoing elective non-cardiac surgery. Diabetes, even when well controlled with standard glucose and insulin regimen, was associated with a 4.5-fold increased risk of a cardiac event (19.2 vs 4.3% in non-diabetics; p < 0.0001), and this relationship was still apparent after age and other variables had been controlled for in multivariate analysis.

However, in these studies the diabetic and non-diabetic groups were not necessarily matched for pre-existing cardiac disease. Hjortrup *et al.*[4] did control for this when they studied 224 diabetic patients and 224 non-diabetic controls undergoing vascular reconstruction, elective abdominal surgery or surgery for femoral neck fractures. These groups were matched for previous cardiac failure, coronary disease and hypertension. This important study demonstrated that there was no difference in the morbidity between the two groups.

In summary, unselected diabetic patients have a 2.5- to 4.5-fold increased risk of suffering a perioperative cardiac event compared with non-diabetics. This risk is not related to glycaemic control at the time of the procedure but entirely to pre-existing vascular disease.

Perioperative sepsis and healing in the diabetic patient

Patients with diabetes are generally felt to be more at risk of sepsis than those without. However, other than a few uncommon infective processes, the clinical evidence for this in patients with reasonable glycaemic control is rather thin.

In the largest available studies, diabetes has *not* been independently linked to postoperative sepsis on multivariate analysis.[3, 4] Similarly, there is little evidence that diabetic patients in reasonable glycaemic control have an increased risk for failed healing. Eneroth and Persson[5] studied the risks associated with poor wound healing in 177 elderly patients undergoing lower limb amputations for vascular disease. Diabetes and preoperative blood glucose had no influence on healing rates.

In summary, there is little evidence that randomly selected diabetic patients, treated with modern standard regimen pre- and postoperatively, have an increased rate of sepsis or poor wound healing.

Surgically relevant complications of diabetes

AUTONOMIC NEUROPATHY

Autonomic dysfunction in diabetic patients is very common when formal autonomic function tests are carried out,[6] but the severe clinical syndrome is fortunately rare. In its most extreme form patients can have disabling postural hypotension, intermittent nocturnal diarrhoea, gastroparesis and urinary retention.[7] There are two reasons why it is important to detect autonomic neuropathy in diabetic patients. First, it is associated with an increased mortality from coexisting coronary artery disease and nephropathy[8] and second, it may be associated with an increased frequency of cardiorespiratory arrests and death, particularly perioperatively.[9–11] These deaths do not appear to be due to occult coronary artery disease, which is often absent at autopsy.[12] There is little direct evidence that these episodes are due to disordered respiratory reflexes or autonomic control of breathing,[13] and a more physiologically likely mechanism is cardiac QT interval prolongation leading to ventricular arrythmias.[14] Attention to perioperative cardiac monitoring and electrolyte balance is necessary, but it is impossible to predict which patients are likely to suffer cardio-respiratory arrests, although those with the most severe autonomic disease are at greatest risk.

DIABETIC NEPHROPATHY

The majority of diabetic patients over the age of 45 with significant renal impairment have both coronary artery[15] and hypertensive heart disease.[12] These abnormalities may not be clinically apparent, and the risk of fluid overload or perioperative hypotension is greatest in these patients. In addition, diabetic patients with nephropathy have a high prevalence of low renin hypoaldosteronism which makes hyperkalaemia a particular risk in these patients.

PERIPHERAL VASCULAR DISEASE

Peripheral vascular disease develops in the diabetic patient at an earlier age and diabetic patients tend to have more triple vessel disease below the knee, increasing the indications for distal or pedal grafting in diabetic populations.[16] Patients with end-stage renal disease have a very high rate of peripheral vascular insufficiency and a high amputation rate.[17] The factors leading to premature peripheral vascular

Table 9.1 Risk factors for coronary and peripheral arterial disease in diabetes

Hypertension
   Common in NIDDM patients
   Common in all diabetics with nephropathy
Central obesity
   Common in NIDDM patients
Dyslipidaemia
   Low HDL and high triglycerides common in obese
     NIDDM
   High triglycerides common when diabetic control is
     poor
   More atherogenic LDL particles
High plasma fibrinogen levels
Microalbuminuria/diabetic renal disease
Enhanced platelet aggregation and adhesiveness
Endothelial damage
   Due to hyperglycaemia?
Hyperinsulinaemia?
Smoking

NIDDM: non-insulin dependent diabetes mellitus; HDL: high density lipoproteins; LDL: low density lipoproteins.

Table 9.2 Preoperative assessment of the diabetic patient

IDDM or NIDDM ?
   IDDM patients have an absolute requirement for
     insulin and are at risk of ketoacidosis.
   NIDDM patients are insulin resistant, may need large
     doses of insulin but rarely develop ketoacidosis.
Autonomic neuropathy present if:
   Postural drop in systolic blood pressure of > 30 mmHg
     after 2 minutes standing
   Classical symptoms of gustatory sweating, nocturnal
     diarrhoea, impotence
   Peripheral neuropathy must be present.
   Bladder paresis rare
Nephropathy present if:
   Albustix® positive proteinuria is present
   Urinary protein excretion more than 500 mg/day
   Serum creatinine may be elevated.
Coronary artery disease
   ECG on all patients regardless of history
Assess blood pressure and cardiac status
Assess peripheral vascular disease and peripheral
neuropathy
   Foot pulses and tendon reflexes
Assess glycaemic control preoperatively
   Outpatient HbA1
   Glucose profile on ward
Assess hypoglycaemia
   How frequent and at what time?
   Hypoglycaemic awareness still present?

IDDM: insulin-dependent diabetes mellitus; NIDDM: non-insulin dependent diabetes mellitus.

disease are broadly the same as those leading to the excess of coronary disease in diabetic patients. Some of these factors are summarized in Table 9.1.

Preoperative assessment of the diabetic patient

The preoperative assessment of the diabetic patient should be geared towards detecting those with an increased risk of perioperative morbidity (Table 9.2). Ideally, diabetic patients should be admitted 48 hours preoperatively for assessment, but this is not always practicable nowadays. The use of preadmission outpatient assessment by junior staff would be useful for dealing with diabetic patients undergoing elective surgery.

History and examination should detect clinically apparent vascular disease and autonomic dysfunction. Some diabetic patients lose awareness of hypoglycaemia after many years of diabetes, and this must therefore be specifically asked for.

All diabetic patients should have a 12-lead ECG – if there are any abnormalities, thallium myocardial scintigraphy is a quick and accurate predictor of those at highest risk of perioperative myocardial infarction.[2] Potassium abnormalities and renal func-

tion should be clearly documented preoperatively. Blood glucose profiles (preprandial and 1–2 hours postprandial) can be taken on the ward, and can be left to the patients to do themselves if they are experienced.

Endocrine response to surgery

The hormonal and metabolic responses to surgical trauma are well described. These responses are greater in patients suffering the greatest surgical trauma, and begin as surgery commences. Plasma adrenocorticotropic hormone (ACTH) and cortisol levels rise immediately, as do catecholamine levels. There is also a glucagon and growth hormone response to trauma, and these 'stress responses' to injury lead to a state of insulin resistance. Moderate surgical trauma leads to a 35–50% reduction in insulin-mediated glucose disposal.[18] The clinical implications of this are that glycaemic control is likely to deteriorate and that there will be increasing requirements for insulin or hypoglycaemic drugs.

Insulin is a major anabolic hormone, and resistance to its action, together with the increase in catabolic stress hormones, promotes the development of protein breakdown, lipolysis and ketone body formation, increased levels of plasma free fatty acids and hyperglycaemia.

Principles of diabetes treatment during surgery

It is essential that there are clear, concise guidelines for the management of diabetic surgical patients. These guidelines should be drawn up in consultation with a diabetologist who has an interest in this area, and should be distributed to all surgical wards and junior staff, particularly the house surgeons, who are usually delegated the task of dealing with diabetes perioperatively. Senior or middle-grade staff from the diabetic department should be available for advice where appropriate. In general, these guidelines must take into account the pressures in any busy surgical ward, and should be:

1. As simple as possible – the more complex a regimen is, the more likely it is to go wrong. The simpler a regimen, the more confident junior medical and nursing staff will feel with diabetes management.
2. As practical as possible – applicable to all patients, with a minimum number of interventions needed.

Aims of diabetes treatment perioperatively

MAINTAINING BLOOD GLUCOSE BETWEEN 6 AND 10 MMOL/L

As there is no convincing evidence that perfect glycaemic control perioperatively reduces morbidity or mortality, it is sensible simply to aim for acceptable glycaemic control. The upper limit of 10 mmol/l is arbitrary, but concentrations above this will lead to heavy glycosuria, osmotic diuresis and volume depletion. In addition, blood glucose concentrations below 10 mmol/l in insulin-dependent patients are likely to

reflect a state where lipolysis is not excessive and ketone body formation is minimal.

AVOIDANCE OF HYPOGLYCAEMIA

Hypoglycaemia is unlikely to occur if blood glucose concentrations are above 6 mmol/l. Hypoglycameia can easily be missed under general anaesthesia.

APPROPRIATE TRANSFER TO USUAL REGIMEN POSTOPERATIVELY

Failure to transfer patients to their normal regimen postoperatively at the appropriate time, or in the appropriate way, is a common cause for delayed discharge.

Regimen for insulin-treated patients

A proportion of these patients will be older non-insulin dependent patients who now require insulin treatment, but *all* insulin-treated patients should be managed similarly. They should all be treated as if they have an obligatory requirement for insulin, and should receive both glucose and insulin infusions perioperatively.

Many regimen in the past have suggested changing insulin treatment before surgery, by reducing the amounts of long-acting insulin for several days before the operation. In our experience this is more trouble than it is worth, and increases the risk of cancelled or delayed surgery. It is sensible to reduce by one-third the amount of evening or night-time long-acting insulin taken the night before surgery if the glucose concentration is normally less than 8 mmol/l pre-breakfast. Otherwise, it should be left alone. Subcutaneous insulin regimen with sliding scales are problematic and should not be used. There are two classes of insulin/glucose regimen, one where glucose insulin and potassium are infused separately (dual infusion) and one where glucose, potassium and insulin are infused through the same line.[19]

DUAL INFUSION

This method is effective, practical and widely used. A typical regimen is shown in Table 9.3. Many patients on this regimen reach a 'steady state', where the insulin infusion rate does not need to be changed, and monitoring can be less intense. Nursing staff

Table 9.3 Dual infusion regimen

Start 10% glucose infusion with 20 mmol KCL (1 litre over 16 hours) at 07.30 if on morning list.
Continue infusion at this rate.
Start human soluble insulin (i.e. Actrapid®/Velosulin®/Humulin S®) infusion at 2 units/h through same line (50 units in 50 ml saline at 2 ml/h via syringe pump).
Monitor test strip glucose hourly and serum potassium 12-hourly.
If glucose concentration is above 10 mmol/l then increase infusion rate by 1 unit/h (each hour) until glucose is below 10 mmol/l. Call doctor if above this level on two occasions, and immediately if glucose above 15 mmol/l.
If glucose is approaching or below 6 mmol/l, decrease insulin infusion by 1 unit/h (each hour) and repeat this decrement until above 6 mmol/l
Call doctor if glucose below 4 mmol/l.

are usually quite happy to supervise these regimen under direction, as the only input needed is to change the insulin infusion rate, measure the glucose concentration and inform the doctor when necessary. There are some complicated algorithms for insulin infusion rates with this system,[20] but these are usually of academic use only.

A theoretical problem with these regimen is that hypoglycaemia can occur if the glucose infusion 'tissues' or is disconnected. This is unlikely to occur if the insulin infusion is 'piggy backed' on to the glucose infusion.

Table 9.4 GIK regimen

Add 15 units of human soluble insulin (i.e. Actrapid®/Velosulin®/Humulin S®) to 500 ml 10% glucose with 10 mmol/l of KCl and infuse over 5 hours.
Start this infusion at 07.30 if on morning list and monitor test strip glucose concentration hourly.
If glucose concentration above 10 mmol/l increase insulin to 20 units/500 ml and repeat this increment until less than 10 mmol/l. *Change the bag with each insulin change.* Call doctor if above this level on two occasions, and immediately if glucose above 15 mmol/l.
If glucose below 6 mmol/l, decrease insulin content to 10 units/500 ml and repeat this decrement if necessary.
Change the bag
Call doctor if glucose below 4 mmol/l.
Monitor serum potassium concentration 12-hourly.

GLUCOSE–INSULIN–POTASSIUM (GIK) METHOD)

This is the other commonly used method and is generally safe and effective.[19] A typical regimen is shown in Table 9.4. The advantage of this method is that glucose is always infused with insulin, so the risks of hypoglycaemia are less, and monitoring of infusion rates can be less intensive. The disadvantage of this method is that it can be quite labour intensive, with frequent changing of bags and infusion lines. Elementary errors are not uncommon – such as giving increasingly large amounts of insulin into progressively smaller volumes of glucose, rather than changing bags. Finally, it can also involve infusing large volumes of fluid over 24 hours (2.5 l or more) rather than the usual 1.5 l in a dual infusion system. This may be important in older patients or those with cardiac disease.

Regimen for non-insulin dependent patients

The first decision to make with non-insulin dependent diabetes mellitus (NIDDM) patients is whether they can be managed conservatively or whether they need one of the regimen already described. Generally, NIDDM patients undergoing minor surgery, or surgery where the patient is likely to be eating fairly soon after the operation, do not need insulin. Patients with NIDDM undergoing more extensive or traumatic surgery are best managed with one of the above regimen. A reasonable approach is outlined in Table 9.5.

Table 9.5 Management of NIDDM patients

Change long-acting agents (chlorpropamide, glibenclamide) to short-acting agents *before* admission.
Omit long-acting agent on the night before operation if this has not been done.
If conservative management has been planned, monitor glucose test strips 2-hourly. Be flexible: start glucose–insulin infusion if in any doubt.
If glucose concentration more than 17 mmol/l preoperatively, always start glucose–insulin infusion.

Troubleshooting

DISCONTINUING THE INSULIN INFUSION

It is tempting to turn off the insulin infusion if the patient's glucose test measurements are declining rapidly or below 5 mmol/l, but this can be dangerous, as complete insulin deficiency is almost immediate and renders the patient prone to ketosis. As a general rule, glucose should always be given with insulin and vice versa. Transiently increasing the glucose infusion rate and restarting the insulin at the lowest infusion rate is the appropriate response to this situation. There is a mistaken belief among some medical staff that many anaesthetists discontinue insulin infusions as soon as the patient is in theatre, which would of course render patients prone to ketosis.

POSTOPERATIVE HYPOTENSION

Diabetic patients have a 2.5- to 4.5-fold risk of a coronary event perioperatively. Hypotension in this period should lead to a prompt 12-lead ECG and chest radiograph before colloid or saline replacement is undertaken.

POSTOPERATIVE CONFUSIONAL STATES IN DIABETIC PATIENTS

Apart from the usual causes of postoperative confusion, diabetic patients are more prone to hypoglycaemia, and to metabolic acidosis with hyperglycaemia, both of which would can cause confusion. In addition, postoperative diabetic patients often receive large amounts of glucose which can cause hyponatraemia.

CONVERSION TO A SUBCUTANEOUS REGIMEN

Many insulin-dependent diabetes mellitus (IDDM) patients can be converted directly to their normal insulin regimen as soon as they are eating, but the glucose and insulin infusion should be continued until they can eat adequately. Sick, febrile or complicated IDDM patients are sometimes more easily managed with a multiple-dose subcutaneous insulin regimen until they improve. The same applies to NIDDM patients. Patients should be converted back to their normal regimen before the day of discharge, and clear follow-up arrangements should be made with the diabetic team. The first insulin subcutaneous insulin injection should be given 15 minutes before the intravenous insulin is stopped to maintain plasma insulin levels.

UNDETECTED KETOACIDOSIS

It is surprising how quickly IDDM patients can develop ketoacidosis after surgical stress – sometimes within hours. The diagnosis can be made by the presence of heavy ketonuria, hyperglycaemia (which is not always severe), and a reduced arterial pH (less than 7.34) or reduced arterial bicarbonate (less than 20 mmol/l). These patients should be managed in collaboration with the medical team and diabetes specialists.

NIL BY MOUTH

Diabetic control during prolonged periods of nil by mouth can be managed by the various regimen described above. However, these regimen do not supply salt or adequate nutrition. Saline (or colloid) and parenteral nutrition may need to be considered after 24–48 hours.

CARDIAC SURGERY

Diabetic patients undergoing cardiac surgery become extremely insulin resistant because of the degree of surgical trauma, inotropic drugs, cardioplegia and glucose infusions that many of these patients experience. Insulin requirements may increase ten-fold perioperatively[21,22] and adequate glucose control is essential. Poor glycaemic control increases plasma levels of free fatty acids which may promote arrhythmias.[23] These patients must be managed be a dual infusion system.

Conclusions

High quality perioperative diabetes care depends on assessing the patient fully before surgery to detect those at risk, in collaboration with diabetes specialists if necessary, and on developing clear management protocols for diabetic patients. Maintaining acceptable glycaemic control is all that is necessary and should be achievable in all patients. The gloom and anxiety associated with surgical diabetes care should be a thing of the past.[1]

References

1. Treves F. *System of Surgery*. London, 1896: 268.
2. Brown KA, Rowen M. Extent of jeopardized viable myocardium determined by myocardial perfusion imaging best predicts perioperative cardiac events in patients undergoing noncardiac surgery. *J Am Coll Cardiol* 1993; **21**: 325–30.
3. Velanovich V. The effects of age, gender, race and concomitant disease on postoperative complications. *J Roy Coll Surg* 1993; **38**: 225–30.
4. Hjortrup A. Influence of diabetes mellitus on operative risk. *Br J Surg* 1985; **72**: 783–5.
5. Eneroth M, Persson BM. Risk factors for failed healing in amputation for vascular disease. A prospective, consecutive study of 177 cases. *Acta Orthop Scand* 1993; **64**: 369–72.
6. Ewing DJ, Martyn CN, Young RJ, Clarke BF. The value of cardiovascular autonomic function tests: 10 years experience in diabetes. *Diab Care* 1985; **8**: 491–8.
7. Ewing DJ, Campbell D, Clarke BF. The natural history of diabetic autonomic neuropathy. *Quart J Med* 1980; **49**: 95–100.
8. Sampson MJ, Wilson S, Karragiannis P *et al*. Progression of diabetic autonomic neuropathy over a decade in insulin dependent diabetics. *Quart J Med* 1990; **278**: 635–46.
9. Page MM, Watkins PJ. Cardiorespiratory arrest and diabetic autonomic neuropathy. *Lancet* 1978; **i**: 14–16.
10. Srinivasan G, Sanders G. Cardiorespiratory arrest in diabetes. *Lancet* 1978; **1**: 505.
11. Garcia-Bunuel L. Cardiorespiratory arrest in diabetic autonomic neuropathy. *Lancet* 1978; **1**: 504–5.
12. Sampson MJ, Chambers JB, Sprigings DC, Drury PL. Interventricular septal hypertrophy in diabetic patients with microalbuminuria or early proteinuria. *Diab Med* 1990; **7**: 126–31.
13. Catterall JRI, Calverly PM, Ewing DJ *et al*. Breathing, sleep and diabetic autonomic neuropathy. *Diabetes* 1984; **33**: 1025–7.
14. Chambers JB, Sampson MJ, Sprigings DC, Jackson G. QT interval prolongation in on the electrocardiogram in diabetic autonomic neuropathy. *Diab Med* 1990; **7**: 105–11.
15. Manske CL, Thomas W, Wang Y, Wilson RF. Screening diabetic transplant candidates for coronary artery disease: identification of a low risk subgroup. *Kidney Int* 1993; **44**: 617–621.
16. Schneider JR, Walsh DB, McDaniel *et al*. Pedal bypass versus tibial bypass with autogenous vein: a comparison of outcome and hemodynamic results. *J Vasc Surg* 1993; **17**(6): 1029–39.
17. Peters C, Sutherland DER, Simmons RL *et al*. Patients and graft survival in amputated versus non-amputated diabetic primary renal allograft recipients. *Transplantation* 1981; **32**: 498–503.
18. Nordenstrom J, Sonnenfeld T, Arner P. Characterisation of insulin resistance after surgery. *Surgery* 1989; **105**(1): 28–35.
19. Husband DJ, Thai AC, Alberti KGMM. Management of diabetes during surgery with glucose–insulin–potassium infusion. *Diab Med* 1985; **3**: 69–74.
20. Meyers EF, Albert D, Gordon M. Perioperative control of blood glucose in diabetic patients: a two step protocol. *Diab Care* 1986; **9**: 40–5.
21. Elliot MJ, Gill G, Home PD *et al*. A comparison of two regimens for the management of diabetes during open heart surgery. *Anesthesiology* 1994; **60** 364–8.
22. Thomas DJ, Hinds CJ, Rees GM. The management of insulin dependent diabetes during cardiopulmonary bypass and general surgery. *Anaesthesia* 1983; **38**: 1047–52.
23. Kurlen VA, Oliver MF. A metabolic cause for arrhythmias during acute myocardial hypoxia. *Lancet* 1970; **1**: 813–15.

CHAPTER 10

Resuscitation of the critically ill (including trauma)

TOM DIAMOND, BRIAN J ROWLANDS

Introduction

There are many causes of collapse or coma which result in a patient being brought to an emergency department in a critically ill state. The spectrum ranges from medical conditions, such as hypoglycaemia, through to surgical problems such as hypovolaemia due to gastrointestinal bleeding and trauma resulting in direct central nervous system (CNS) damage or indirect CNS depression via haemorrhage and hypovolaemic shock. In each situation, the receiving doctor is faced with the same problem – a critically ill patient who requires immediate assessment and resuscitation. Despite the diversity of possible aetiologies, it is important that time is not wasted in attempting to determine the exact aetiology but that a rapid sequence of steps for assessment and resuscitation is followed in every case so that life-threatening situations can be detected and rectified.

There have been various sequences devised, usually based on an ABC mnemonic, but the system most widely adopted in recent years is that of the Advanced Trauma Life Support (ATLS) course of the American College of Surgeons.[1] This aims to establish assessment and management priorities and divides these into four main phases: primary survey; resuscitation phase; secondary survey; definitive care phase. In practical terms, many aspects of the primary survey and the initial resuscitation phase occur simultaneously and it is useful to consider them together in terms of assessment (primary survey) and management (resuscitation) components. The components will be discussed separately and the various practical skills necessary in each described.

Primary survey plus initial resuscitation

The standard sequence of the primary survey involves:

Airway (plus cervical spine [C-spine] control)
Breathing
Circulation
Disability – a rapid neurological status assessment
Exposure – the patient should be completely undressed and examined.

Airway (plus C-spine control)

In all trauma victims it is essential to avoid an iatrogenic injury to the cervical spine during manoeuvres to secure an airway. This must, therefore, be kept in mind from the very beginning of the primary survey sequence and it must be assumed that a cervical spine fracture is present in any patient with multiple trauma, particularly with a blunt injury above the clavicles. The neck should not be hyperextended or hyperflexed. The head and neck should be immobilized using an appropriately sized hard collar or sand bags and adhesive tapes. This immobilization should be maintained until it is felt appropriate to discontinue it, based on clinical judgement, later C-spine X-rays (to include the C7–T1 interspace) and neurosurgical or orthopaedic consultation, if appropriate.

AIRWAY ASSESSMENT

The patency of the airway may be assessed by talking to the patient (confusion or agitation may indicate hypoxia), listening (stridor or gurgling may indicate a compromised airway), feeling, for warm air flow against the hand and whether the trachea is the midline and looking to see whether chest movements are adequate.

BASIC AIRWAY MANAGEMENT

In a patient with an altered level of consciousness the tongue falls backwards and obstructs the hypopharynx. Several manoeuvres are available to obtain an airway and maintain it, thereby providing initial basic life support.

Chin lift

The fingers of one hand are placed under the mandible while the thumb of the same hand depresses the lower lip and incisors to open the mouth. The mandible is then gently lifted upwards to bring the chin anteriorily. During this chin lift manoeuvre the neck should not be hyperextended.

Jaw thrust

This is performed by grasping the angles of the mandible, one hand on each side, and displacing the mandible forwards. When this is used with a face mask to deliver oxygen, the mask can be held with the thumbs and forefingers and a good seal can be obtained.

Suction

Having obtained the airway and opened the mouth (e.g. with the chin lift), a rigid sucker (and finger, if necessary) should be used to clear blood, secretions, vomitus and foreign bodies.

Oropharyngeal airway

If the gag reflex is diminished, the patient will tolerate an oropharyngeal (Guedel) airway. This may be inserted by putting it into the oral cavity upside-down initially, so that the concavity is directed cephalically. As it is further inserted it is rotated through 180° so that the concavity faces caudally and it slips over the tongue into the hypopharynx.

Nasopharyngeal airway

If a Guedel airway is not tolerated and obstruction to breathing is still present, a nasopharyngeal airway may be inserted, following lubrication, into the nostril that appears unobstructed.

Once an airway has been obtained and secured, oxygen should be given, via a face mask with a reservoir device, delivered at 10–15 l/min to provide 85% inspired oxygen.

ADVANCED AIRWAY MANAGEMENT

Endotracheal intubation

If none of the basic airway manoeuvres is successful in obtaining and securing an airway, endotracheal intubation should be performed, if possible. An endotracheal tube may be inserted via the oral or nasal routes. Oral endotracheal intubation requires extension of the neck and should not be attempted if cervical spine instability is suspected and has not been excluded. If there is an immediate need for an airway in this situation a nasoendotracheal intubation should be attempted. In other circumstances, oral tracheal intubation should be used as it is the easier technique to perform.

Orotracheal intubation is performed in the standard way using a laryngoscope in the left hand. During insertion, an assistant should manually immobilize the head and neck.

Nasotracheal intubation is more difficult and is used in patients in whom a cervical spine injury exists or cannot be ruled out. It involves inserting a lubricated tube, via the nose, and advancing it while listening for airflow emanating from the end of the tube. When airflow is maximal, suggesting that the tip of the tube is at the opening of the trachea, the tube is advanced quickly, during inhalation. Gentle pressure on the thyroid cartilage may help passage of the tube into the trachea.

SURGICAL AIRWAY MANAGEMENT

A surgical airway is indicated when oedema of the glottis, fracture of the larynx or severe oropharyngeal injury or haemorrhage prevents placement of an endotracheal tube.

Needle cricothyroidotomy and jet insufflation

A needle cricothyroidotomy using a large calibre (12- or 14-gauge) needle inserted through the cricothyroid membrane may be used to obtain an immediate airway in the emergency situation. This can then be connected to a standard wall oxygen supply at 15 litres/min with a Y-connector or side hole cut in the tubing. Intermittent ventilation can be achieved by placing the thumb over the open end of the Y-connector or side hole (1 second on and 4 seconds off). This technique can only be used to ventilate for

approximately 30 minutes as carbon dioxide accumulates due to inadequate exhalation.

Surgical cricothyroidotomy

This may be performed by making an incision over the cricothyroid membrane which penetrates the skin and the membrane (Fig. 10.1). An artery clip is then insinuated and opened to dilate the opening. A small (5–7 mm) endotracheal or tracheostomy tube can then be inserted. Alternatively, a Seldinger-type Minitrach® is available, which involves insertion of a Seldinger wire into the trachea, via a needle cricothyroidotomy and subsequently dilating a tract around this to allow insertion of a small (5–7 mm) tube. The principle is similar to the Seldinger technique for insertion of a central venous line. This technique, however, takes slightly more time than the incision and artery clip technique. The latter is, therefore, probably the best to use in an extreme emergency. When using the above techniques the cervical collar may be loosened but head and neck immobilization should be maintained by an assistant. After the airway has been obtained the cervical collar may be reapplied.

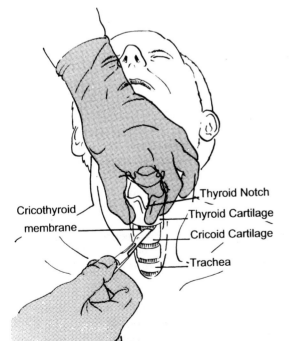

Fig. 10.1 Anatomical landmarks for surgical cricothyroidotomy.

Cricothyroid membrane

Thyroid Notch
Thyroid Cartilage
Cricoid Cartilage
Trachea

Breathing

BREATHING AND VENTILATION ASSESSMENT

Breathing and lung ventilation may be assessed by the following methods. *Observing*, for cyanosis and distension of the neck veins. If the neck veins are distended, the possibility of a tension pneumothorax, cardiac tamponade, myocardial contusion or pulmonary embolus should be considered. In addition, observing for movement of the chest wall – paradoxical movement of a segment of the chest wall may be present with a flail segment, where three or more consecutive ribs are each fractured in two or more places. *Feeling*, for the position of the trachea – deviation to one side may be caused by a tension pneumothorax on the opposite side. *Counting*, the respiratory rate – this should normally be 12–20/min. *Auscultating*, for air entry or lack of it. If there is decreased or absent air entry on one side, percussion will help further elucidate whether or not there is a pneumothorax on that side. It is important to remember that a severe asthmatic may have lack of air entry on each side due to extreme airway narrowing.

BREATHING AND VENTILATION MANAGEMENT

The primary aim of breathing and ventilation is to achieve maximum cellular oxygenation and prevent hypercarbia, cerebral vasodilatation and a consequent increase in intracranial pressure. This is especially important in trauma patients if they have sustained a head injury.

Oxygenation and ventilation

In a patient who is hypoxic and/or apnoeic oxygenation and ventilation must be performed for at least 3 minutes before intubation is attempted. Adequate oxygenation cannot be provided in such a patient with nasal cannulae or a simple oxygen face mask. It is essential to use a tight fitting, oxygen reservoir face mask connected to an oxygen flow of 10–15 litres/min. This can deliver an inspired oxygen concentration of 85%. Ventilation may be achieved using a mouth to face mask or, preferably, a bag valve face mask, connected to an oxygen flow of 10–15 litres/min. The aim of oxygenation and ventilation is to keep the blood gas oxygen tension above 10 kPa (80 mmHg) and the carbon dioxide tension below 5.5 kPa (40 mmHg). It is essential, therefore, that in an apnoeic/hypoxic patient oxygenation and ventilation are commenced immediately and continued until adequate tissue oxygenation, with disappearance of cyanosis, has been achieved. Intubation can then be attempted but prolonged attempts at intubation should be avoided. A useful rule is that the doctor attempting intubation should take a deep breath and when he or she finds it necessary to breath again the attempted intubation should be stopped and the patient oxygenated and ventilated. When intubation is achieved, oxygenation and ventilation should continue using a similar bag technique or a mechanical positive-pressure ventilator. When this situation has been achieved, the arterial oxygen tension (paO_2) should be measured by taking blood into a heparized syringe from the radial or femoral artery. If facilities allow, tissue oxygen saturation may be monitored continuously using a pulse oximeter, thus giving an estimation of tissue perfusion and oxygenation.

In virtually all collapsed or traumatized patients oxygen should be delivered to achieve an inspired concentration of 85%. One exception is in a patient with chronic obstructive airways disease (COAD) in whom the actual drive to respiration is hypoxia rather than hypercarbia and administration of excess oxygen may remove their respiratory drive.

Circulation

Assessment and management of the circulation is the third priority in resuscitation, after airway plus C-spine control and breathing plus ventilation.[2]

CIRCULATION ASSESSMENT

Assessment of the circulatory system principally involves the recognition and diagnosis of shock, which is defined as an abnormality of the circulatory system which results in inadequate organ perfusion. The early signs include anxiety, tachycardia (100–120 beats/min), tachypnoea (20–30 breaths/min) and skin pallor or mottling, with a prolonged capillary refill time (more than 2 seconds). A drop in systolic blood pressure, which is often considered to be one of three key features of shock, does not usually occur until later in the pathophysiological sequence. For example, in haemorrhagic shock, a drop in systolic blood pressure does not occur until an adult has lost approximately 1.5–2 litres of blood (30–40% of the circulating blood volume). At this stage in the development of shock the patient is generally ashen in colour because of markedly reduced tissue perfusion in the extremities and the level of consciousness is decreased because of inadequate cerebral perfusion.

CIRCULATION MANAGEMENT

Immediate control of obvious profuse haemorrhage should be achieved by direct pressure, with limb elevation where appropriate. Securing pressure dressings *in situ* by bandaging frees an assistant to help with other initial management steps. The most important step in circulation management is then to obtain access to the venous system to allow rapid infusion of fluids. Flow rate through a tube is proportional to the fourth power of the radius and inversely proportional to the length (Poiseuille's law). Thus, in a hypovolaemic or severely traumatized patient, short, wide-bore cannulae (14-gauge or larger) should be used. Two cannulae should be inserted. The sites used depend on those available and the experience and skill of the doctor involved in circulation management. Initially, attempts should be made to insert a wide-bore cannula in each antecubital fossa. If this is not possible, usually due to collapse of the veins, a venous cutdown is a safe and quick procedure to use to achieve venous access.

Technique for venous cutdown

The best vein to use is the long saphenous vein where it originates, just anterior to the medial mallelolus. Blunt dissection (e.g. with an artery clip) is used to expose the long saphenous vein. The vein is tied distally with a suture (e.g. 2/0 Vicryl®) and controlled proximally with a loose suture. A transverse incision is made in the anterior third of the circumference of the vein and a wide-bore cannula is inserted. If there is difficulty in inserting the cannula, this may be facilitated by using an injection needle, with the bevel bent backwards, to act as a hook which can elevate the upper edge of the venotomy. Following insertion of the cannula, it is secured using the proximal suture. The basilic vein at the elbow may also be used by making a 2 cm incision anterior to the medial epicondyle and employing the above technique.

Intraosseous infusion

This simple technique may be used in children. A specifically designed intraosseous cannula is inserted through the centre of the bone into the marrow. The site used is two finger breadths distal to the tibial tuberosity on the anteromedial surface of the tibia.

Central venous cannulation

Central venous cannulation is associated with well-recognized complications, particularly when performed by inexperienced staff in an emergency situation. Complications include pneumothorax, which may prove fatal in an already compromised, severely traumatized patient. It should, therefore, not be used by inexperienced staff in the initial phase of resuscitation. However, when very experienced staff are available in the early phase of resuscitation or in the later phase when central vein cannulation to allow central venous pressure monitoring is indicated, it is an extremely useful technique. In a severely shocked patient the route can be used to obtain wide-bore access (e.g. 8F cannula used for later insertion of a Swan–Ganz catheter). This will allow rapid transfusion of fluids or blood.

Subclavian vein cannulation (Fig. 10.2)

1. The patient is tilted head down by approximately 20°. This helps fill the vein and reduces the risk of air embolus. A sand bag is placed between the shoulders so that they lie more posteriorly – this should not be performed if there is a possibility of a spinal fracture.
2. The skin is cleansed with antiseptic solution. The right subclavian vein is usually the chosen site. Remember that if there is chest trauma or a pneumothorax on one side, central vein cannulation should be performed on that side as use of the other side introduces the chance of producing another pneumothorax.
3. A small stab incision is made on the skin 2 cm inferior to the midpoint of the clavicle. A needle is introduced into this with the right hand and advanced towards the tip of the index finger which is placed in the suprasternal notch. The needle may strike the inferior surface of the clavicle – if this occurs it should be eased under the clavicle and advanced, with a negative pressure in the syringe chamber, until it enters the subclavian vein and a flashback is obtained. If the patient is conscious, local anaesthetic should be inserted before these steps.
4. The syringe is then removed and a Seldinger wire is inserted, via the needle. The needle is removed and a dilator is passed over the wire. This is removed and the cannula is inserted. The guidewire is then removed. Blood is aspirated from the cannula to check that it is in a vein and an intravenous infusion set is attached.
5. The central line is secured in position using silk sutures and a Steridrape® dressing.
6. Radiological confirmation of correct siting is then obtained.

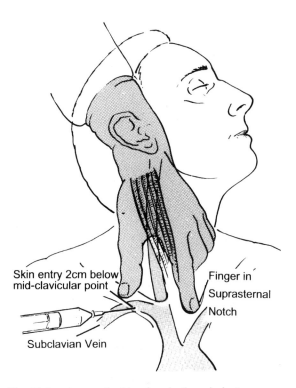

Fig. 10.2. Anatomical landmarks for subclavian venous cannulation.

Internal jugular vein cannulation

Internal jugular vein cannulation (Fig. 10.3) may be performed as above except that in step 3 the anatomical landmarks are as follows: a stab incision is made in the centre of the triangle formed by the two heads of the sternomastoid muscle and the clavicle. A needle is introduced, with the bevel upwards, and advanced caudally, parallel to the saggital plane, at a 30° posterior angle with the frontal plane. A negative pressure is applied in the syringe chamber and the needle is advanced until it enters the internal jugular vein and a flashback is obtained.

Resuscitation fluid–crystalloid, colloid or blood?

The success of the initial resuscitation in the acutely hypovolaemic or traumatized patient depends more on the speed of achievement of good venous access and adequacy of repletion rather than upon the type of fluids which are used. Remember that anaemia is tolerated better than hypovolaemia! There is much debate as to which is the best solute for initial resuscitation – colloid or crystalloid? In the majority of clinical studies the type of fluid administered did not influence the outcome. There are, however, two facts which are not disputed. First, approximately 50–70% less colloid than crystalloid is required to achieve a given endpoint in terms of intravascular volume expansion. Second, unlike crystalloids, colloids are associated with allergic reactions, although these are rare. One other important factor is that crystalloid solutions are significantly less expensive than colloids. In practice, combined therapy using both crystalloids and colloids is often used and the policy will differ from one institution to another. The ATLS course of the American College of Surgeons recommends the use of isotonic electrolyte solutions for initial resuscitation (e.g. Ringer's lactate).

It is important to remember that the above guidelines refer only to the initial resuscitation fluids and it is extremely important to assess the response to initial fluid administration and, if indicated, then give the most effective replacement fluid – blood. If a patient responds rapidly to initial fluid administration, with normalization of their pulse and blood pressure, and remains stable, it is likely that they have lost less than 20% of their circulating blood volume. In such patients, no further fluid bolus or immediate blood transfusion is indicated and the fluid infusion can be slowed. However, if the response is only transient or there is minimal or no response to initial fluid administration, administration of blood is indicated. Early administration of blood is also indicated in patients where injuries are such that excessive blood loss is most likely (e.g. severe trauma due to a road accident or bomb blast). When giving blood, fully cross-matched blood is preferable. However, in most blood banks, this may take up to an hour to obtain and in patients with life-threatening hypovolaemic shock situations type-specific blood should be used. This is compatible for ABO and Rhesus blood types. If type-specific blood is unavailable, type O, Rhesus negative packed cells may be used for patients with exsanguinating haemorrhage.[3]

Blood warmers, blood filters and pressure bags

Iatrogenic hypothermia is a significant risk during resuscitation of a severely hypovolaemic or traumatized patient. This may exacerbate coagulopathy and must be avoided. A blood warmer should always be used. Crystalloid solutions should always be warmed to 39°C before rapid infusion. The use of a blood filter is also indicated, when whole blood is being given, to remove clots and debris. The use of pressure bags is indicated to allow transfusions of fluids or blood at fast flow rates.

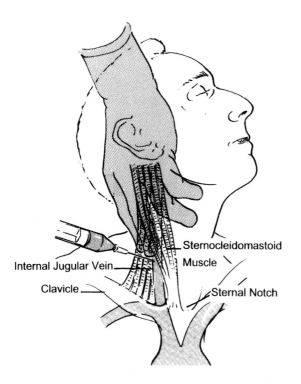

Internal Jugular Vein

Clavicle

Sternocleidomastoid Muscle

Sternal Notch

Fig. 10.3. Anatomical landmarks for internal jugular venous cannulation.

Disability

This fourth part of the ABCDE system is used during the initial examination to allow a brief and rapid neurological assessment. The mnemonic used in the ATLS course is AVPU:

A – **A**lert
V – responds to **V**erbal stimuli
P – responds to **P**ainful stimuli
U – **U**nresponsive

In addition, the pupillary size, equality and response should be assessed. Unilateral or bilateral dilatation and unresponsiveness of the pupils may indicate a localized cerebral lesion or generalized cerebral oedema with increased intracranial pressure. Alternatively, bilateral small pupils denote opiate toxicity.

Exposure

This part of the mnemonic is to emphasize that in a severely traumatized or acutely ill patient a complete examination of the body is essential. This necessitates removal of all clothing, taking care to protect the cervical spine.

Monitoring

During the initial assessment and resuscitation phases it is important that ongoing monitoring of the vital signs and simple clinical and physical measurements is performed in order to assess response to treatment or detect any significant deterioration which may suggest a sudden event such as a pneumothorax or progression of a particular problem which may have been overlooked or missed initially.[4]

PULSE, BLOOD PRESSURE AND PULSE PRESSURE

A fast pulse (tachycardia) is one of the earliest signs of a circulatory shock. Thus, in an injured patient who is cool, tachycardia should be taken to indicate shock until proven otherwise. The normal heart rate varies with age, being greater than 160/min in an infant, approximately 140 in a pre-school child, 120 from school age to puberty and less than 100 in an adult. An elderly patient may not be able to develop a tachycardia because of attenuated cardiac response

to catecholamine release or because of medications such as β-blockers (e.g. propranolol).

In contrast to the pulse, change in the blood pressure is not a good early indicator of shock as compensatory mechanisms usually result in maintenance of the systolic blood pressure until the patient has lost 30% or more of the circulating blood volume. The *pulse pressure* (systolic pressure minus the diastolic pressure) is a more accurate measurement – a narrowed pulse pressure suggests significant blood loss and involvement of compensatory mechanisms. The narrowing, or decrease, of the pulse pressure is due initially to a rise in the diastolic pressure secondary to vasoconstriction. Later, after loss of 30% of the circulating blood volume, the pulse pressure decreases further due to a fall in the systolic blood pressure.

Monitoring of the pulse and blood pressure, however, provide a useful and simple way to monitor the patient for deterioration or response to therapy – restoration of the blood pressure and reduction of tachycardia, with maintenance of these, indicate that initial control of bleeding and resuscitation have been adequate.

RESPIRATORY RATE

The normal range for this is 12–20 breaths/min. Like the pulse, it rises early with blood loss or hypoxia and is a very useful indicator of the patient's clinical state.

CAPILLARY REFILL TIME

This is the time taken for blood to return to a compressed nailbed on release of the pressure. The normal is 2 seconds but this increases early in shock, in association with cutaneous vasoconstriction, usually following approximately 15% loss of blood volume.

URINARY OUTPUT

Measurement of urinary output is a very good indirect method of assessing haemodynamic status as it is related to renal perfusion. Urine output should be measured on an hourly basis in all severely traumatized or critically ill patients. In trauma patients, a urinary catheter should be inserted at an early stage in the assessment and resuscitation (after the primary survey). A contraindication to insertion of a catheter is the presence of blood at the external urethral meatus. This may indicate a urethral injury which may be exacerbated by urinary catheterization. In such patients, catheterization should not be attempted until a urethrogram has been performed. The normal output in the adult is 1 ml/min or 60 ml/h. The minimal obligatory output is 30 ml/h – in a child it is 1 ml/kg/h.

CENTRAL VENOUS PRESSURE

This is measured, in centimetres of water, via a central venous catheter. The manometer is placed on a stand so that the zero mark is level with the patient's right atrium. Alternatively it may be measured and recorded continuously using a pressure transducer. The normal central venous pressure (CVP) is approximately 3–5 cm above the angle of Louis (sternal notch) with the patient at 45° to the horizontal. The CVP will be low if the patient is hypovolaemic and will rise to normal with satisfactory correction of the intravascular volume deficit. This provides a satisfactory way of monitoring fluid replacement. The CVP will rise above normal with over-transfusion. The CVP will also rise above normal if there is dysfunction of the right side of the heart and in such cases it cannot be used as an indicator of filling of the systemic circulation. It may also be raised for mechanical reasons such as a tension pneumothorax or cardiac tamponade.

ARTERIAL BLOOD GASES

Measurement of the arterial blood gases gives an assessment of the adequacy of oxygenation and ventilation. During resuscitation a blood gas tension above 10 kPa (80 mmHg) and carbon dioxide tension below 5.5 kPa (40 mmHg) should be achieved. Arterial blood is sampled, using a heparinized syringe, from the radial or femoral artery.

BLOOD SUGAR

In all patients with an altered level of consciousness, obviously not due to trauma, blood sugar estimation should be performed using a reagent strip, to avoid missing hypoglycaemia. This should be followed by a laboratory estimation.

Secondary survey

The aim of the secondary survey, which follows the primary survey and resuscitation phases, is to discover a cause for the patient's collapse and, in a trauma case, to document the exact extent of injuries. In addition, an important aim of this phase is to detect occult injury which may not have been obvious on initial assessment during the primary survey. This phase should, therefore, involve a full head to toe examination. During this examination it is important to keep an open mind to all diagnostic possibilities.[5] During this phase in a trauma patient, a cervical collar should be kept on.

HEAD

The secondary survey commences with examination of the head. The eyes should be re-examined to check for pupillary size and reaction and conjunctival haemorrhage or evidence of penetrating injury (including visualization of the fundus). Each external auditory meatus should be checked for bleeding. Intraoral examination should be performed to check for laceration of the tongue, dislocation of the teeth or other injuries. The bony structures of the face should be palpated to detect maxillofacial injuries and if there is any bruising or other suspicion of this, X-rays should be arranged. Patients with facial fractures may have associated fractures of the cribriform plate. In these patients, nasogastric intubation should not be performed (the oral route should be used, if necessary) as the tube may pass into the cranial cavity!

NECK AND CERVICAL SPINE

Examination of the neck involves visual inspection and palpation. Inspection may reveal haematomas or lacerations and palpation may reveal subcutaneous crepitus if there is a laryngeal or tracheal injury. All patients with blunt trauma, particularly above the clavicles, should be presumed to have a cervical spine fracture and the neck should be protected by a collar or sand bags and tape, until this is ruled out.

CHEST

Visual examination of the chest (anterior and posterior) should be performed initially to detect any large wounds (e.g. sucking wound) or flail segment. Complete examination of the entire thoracic cage involves palpation of individual ribs, the clavicles and the sternum. Pressure on the sternum or pressure from each side (springing the chest) will produce pain if fractures are present. Auscultation and percussion should then be performed. These may reveal signs of a pneumothorax (decreased breath sounds, hyperresonance) or cardiac tamponade (distant heart sounds). Following clinical examination, a chest X-ray should be performed.

ABDOMEN

An abdominal injury is potentially very dangerous and it is extremely important that it should not be missed. At this stage of assessment, determination that an abdominal injury is present is the most important factor rather than determination of the specific type of injury – this can be undertaken later by radiological investigation or at laparotomy. The suspicion of an intra-abdominal injury may be so high (e.g. gross, tense distension in the presence of bruising over the splenic area) that a diagnosis of intra-abdominal injury is obvious. In less obvious cases, particularly in blunt abdominal trauma, peritoneal lavage is indicated. In cases of penetrating abdominal injury the general rule used by most emergency departments in the UK is that all patients with gunshot or stab wounds to the abdomen, anterior to the mid-axillary line should undergoe exploratory laparotomy.

RECTUM

Digital rectal examination forms an integral part of the secondary survey. The presence of blood in the bowel lumen should be sought and anal sphincter tone should be assessed. The prostate should be examined – a high riding prostate will indicate the presence of a rupture of the membranous urethra.

LIMBS/EXTREMITIES

All limbs should be visually examined and palpated (with rotational or three-point pressure) to check for tenderness, crepitation or abnormal movement. Posterior pressure on each anterior superior iliac spine may detect a pelvic fracture. All peripheral pulses and neurological function should be assessed.

X-RAYS IN THE SECONDARY SURVEY

X-rays are indicated according to the clinical findings and the sites of injury detected in the secondary survey. However, the three most important X-rays – which should be performed in all cases of severe trauma – are the cervical spine (to exclude a fracture), the chest (to exclude potentially life-threatening injury such as pneumothorax or mediastinal injury) and the pelvis (a pelvic fracture is a serious injury from which a patient can bleed catastrophically – it also indicates a very significant degree of trauma to the body).

Conclusion

The above outline provides the basic elements of assessment and resuscitation of a critically ill or severely traumatized patient. It is important for each individual involved in resuscitation to have a background theoretical knowledge as documented above but it is equally important that each individual, particularly a trainee, has the necessary confidence and clarity of thought to convert theoretical knowledge efficiently into action. Obviously, experience such as that obtained in a busy accident and emergency department is the best way to improve skills and enhance confidence, but it is important that each individual, even an experienced person, has their own mental sequence of steps and events to be followed. Mental energy, therefore, instead of concentrating on basic sequences, can be used to best effect and provide the best chance of making correct decisions and prevent the individual from making hasty or preconceived conclusions – something which is very easy to do under pressure in a tense situation. This ultimately provides the best chance of improving patient survival.

In addition to the very strict sequences of the primary and secondary surveys, the clinician must also be aware of other factors which may adversely affect a patient's prognosis. For example, a patient must not be allowed to become cold and must not be left unobserved, particularly when initial stability has been achieved and a false sense of security has been reached. This is particularly important during investigations in poorly equipped places such as an X-ray or CT scanner room. It is also important to keep clear, precise records of the resuscitation sequence, particularly details of drugs and fluids administered.

References

1. *Advanced Trauma Life Support Course Manual.* Chicago: American College of Surgeons, 1993.
2. Evans TR. *ABC of Resuscitation.* London: British Medical Association, 1990.
3. Donaldson MDJ, Seaman MJ, Park GR. Massive blood transfusion. *Br J Anaesthes* 1992; **69**: 621–30.
4. Messinger G, Segal E, Perel A. Monitoring of hypovolaemia. *Curr Opin Anaesthesiol* 1993; **6**: 393–9.
5. Rowlands BJ. Management of major trauma. In: Russell RCG (ed.) *Recent Advances in Surgery.* London: Churchill Livingstone, 1988: 1–17.

PART III

Perioperative principles

CHAPTER 11

Preoperative assessment for abdominal surgery

ALLEN EDWARDS, HOWARD YOUNG

Introduction

Prior to surgery all patients require assessment by both surgeon and anaesthetist. The aim of this assessment is to establish the diagnosis, identify any special risk factors which might affect the outcome of surgery or anaesthesia, as well as provide the patient with a detailed explanation of their diagnosis, treatment options, likely outcome and possible complications to enable the patient to give fully informed consent to treatment.

The investigation, treatment and management of specific surgical diseases will be covered elsewhere in this book. This chapter will be confined to the general principles of preoperative assessment which are applicable to all patients undergoing abdominal operations.

There is a high incidence of medical conditions in patients requiring surgery and they should actively be sought in the preoperative phase. Clinical evaluation remains the single most important aspect of preoperative assessment with the history alone able to identify 56% of patients with significant problems. Examination will identify a further 17% of problems and laboratory investigations will yield only a further 1%.[1] Questionnaires for patients to complete prior to examination may help in the assessment process, and are mainly used to select patients suitable for day-case surgery.[2] Joint assessment clinics run by anaesthetists and surgeons can identify problems likely to delay surgery at an earlier stage and enable appropriate referrals and investigations to be performed as an outpatient.

History

CARDIOVASCULAR SYSTEM

Ischaemic heart disease is common and symptoms of exertional chest pain may give a clue to undiagnosed angina. Myocardial infarction within 6 months of surgery is one of the chief predictors of postoperative cardiac morbidity and mortality and operation should be delayed where possible. The risk of perioperative myocardial infarction is around 27% within 3 months of infarction, 11% between 3 and

6 months and 6% after 6 months.[3] The incidence of myocardial infarction in the general surgical population is only 0.2%. Symptoms and signs of uncompensated heart failure are particularly worrying and patients should be specifically questioned about ankle swelling, orthopnoea and paroxysmal nocturnal dyspnoea to assess the degree of cardiac failure. Nocturnal cough may be the only symptom of early cardiac failure. There is a 20% cardiac mortality in patients with untreated heart failure which falls to 5% if appropriate preoperative measures are instituted.

A history of previous deep vein thrombosis (DVT) and pulmonary embolus (PE) will indicate patients at risk of thromboembolism in the peri- and postoperative phase allowing appropriate antithrombotic measures to be taken.

RESPIRATORY SYSTEM

Dyspnoea may be a symptom of both heart and lung disease. Exertional dyspnoea should be graded by asking about common activities such as climbing stairs or running for a bus. The presence of dyspnoea at rest indicates more advanced cardiorespiratory disease. Productive cough or haemoptysis might suggest underlying chest infection, malignancy or left heart failure. An occupational history might uncover individuals liable to coal worker's and slate worker's pneumoconiosis and asbestosis, while farmers are prone to many forms of allergic lung disease. Wheeze and persistent non-productive cough may indicate asthma.

Smokers are at increased risk of chest infection as well as being prone to atherosclerosis. Smoking increases mucus production by the airways as well as decreasing mucociliary transport. Ideally, smokers should abstain for 4 weeks prior to elective surgery.

URAEMIA

Renal disease carries a high risk of postoperative complication. Symptoms of uraemia include lethargy, headache, fits, oedema of hands, face and ankles.

ENDOCRINE

Diabetes is common in the overweight and symptoms of polyuria and polydipsia should be sought. Recovery from anaesthesia is delayed in those with hypothyroidism and enquiries about appetite, weight and temperature preference may indicate thyroid dis-

ease. The possibility of unrecognized pregnancy should be considered in all young women and elective surgery deferred if possible.

PREVIOUS SURGERY

Previous operations may have important implications if further surgery is required. Nephrectomy in a patient who has undergone previous contralateral nephrectomy would have obvious disastrous consequences. Abdominal surgery may lead to intra-abdominal adhesions which might lengthen and complicate later procedures. Adhesions may make laparoscopic surgery impossible. Some individuals are particularly prone to postoperative nausea and vomiting which patients often rate worse than postoperative pain. The anaesthetist should be made aware of this problem since he or she may need to modify their technique or consider the use of a prophylactic anti-emetic such as ondansetron. A history of excessive bleeding at dental extractions or previous surgery may alert the clinician to an unrecognized bleeding tendency.

Altough pseudocholinesterase deficiency and malignant hyperpyrexia are rare, adverse events during previous anaesthetics and problems in family members should be recorded. Surgery should be delayed whenever any doubt exists and appropriate investigations initiated.

DRUG HISTORY

Many drugs can interfere with anaesthetic agents and a detailed drug history is essential. Drugs of particular concern are steroids, insulin, antihypertensives, calcium antagonists, antipsychotics, tranquillizers, monoamine oxidase inhibitors, anticoagulants and the oral contraceptive.

Excess alcohol intake poses special problems. Liver enzymes may be induced which might mean that larger doses of anaesthetic agents will be required as well as an increased requirement for postoperative analgesia. In advanced alcoholic liver disease the opposite may occur and all drugs must be titrated carefully. Postoperative confusion may be due to acute alcohol withdrawal. This is particularly common in the elderly who may deny excess alcohol intake. Drug abuse is becoming more common and may again interfere with anaesthetic agents. Intravenous drug users have a particularly high risk lifestyle. They will be at risk of hepatitis B, C and D as well as HIV infection. This poses a risk to the operating staff and others who come into contact with their body fluids and appropriate precautions will be required.

INTUBATION

Of particular interest to the anaesthetist are loose teeth and dental work which should be noted along with the state of the mouth. Patients with rheumatoid arthritis pose special problems as they may be unable to open their mouths wide enough to admit an airway even when anaesthetized. Additionally, they may have unstable cervical spines which may lead to a myelopathy during forcible neck extension. An awake fibre optic intubation may be required.

The anaesthetist will also pay attention to the state of superficial veins and peripheral arteries during the preoperative consultation as this may aid in planning vascular access.

Examination

Physical examination often generates valuable information about the patient's general condition including their nutritional state. All patients should be weighed before operation to assess nutritional status and allow calculation of drug doses where required. Anaemia, cyanosis, obesity, jaundice and other signs of chronic liver disease are obvious and will dictate further investigations. Signs of renal failure include a sallow appearance with oedema of hands, face and ankles.

Between 5 and 7% of all postoperative complications are due to respiratory disease. This complication rate is doubled in patients undergoing abdominal procedures, trebled in smokers and quadrupled in the presence of chronic obstructive airways disease. Twenty-five percent of postoperative deaths are due to pulmonary problems and pulmonary complications are implicated in a further 25% of deaths. Clinical examination of the respiratory system may give a good idea of respiratory reserve and function. A simple clinical assessment consists of observing a patient climb a flight of stairs. Patients who can achieve this without stopping and without becoming excessively short of breath are likely to withstand surgery. Another bedside test is the Sabrasez breath-holding test. Healthy individuals should be able to hold their breath for 25 seconds or longer. If this is reduced to less than 15 seconds it implies diminished cardiorespiratory reserve.

Unfortunately heart disease may not always be symptomatic, even when severe. Murmurs may be functional and of no significance; however, their presence should be taken seriously. A diastolic murmur invariably indicates significant heart disease. Systolic murmurs may be functional but in general terms if the murmur extends up to the second heart sound it is likely to represent organic disease. A thrill always indicates significant disease. Aortic stenosis is always worrying and should be further investigated. Patients with aortic stenosis are at risk of sudden death and are unable to cope with the widespread peripheral vasodilation which may occur in spinal anaesthesia. Although mitral stenosis is less hazardous, patients are prone to fluid overload and are best managed by keeping them slightly underhydrated. They are also at risk of atrial fibrillation and may require anticoagulation. In general, patients with incompetent valves are at less risk than those with stenotic lesions. It should always be remembered that patients with valvular heart disease or prosthetic valves are prone to endocarditis and appropriate antibiotic prophylaxis should be used, especially during dirty abdominal procedures.

Hypertension can be asymptomatic and blood pressure must always be checked prior to surgery. A diastolic pressure greater than 110 mmHg carries a high risk of postoperative cardiovascular events.[4] The first reading may be spuriously high through anxiety and should be repeated. Where possible hypertension should be treated prior to operation and surgery delayed if possible. Congestive heart failure carries an increased risk of postoperative complications. Signs of heart failure include a raised jugular venous pressure, gallop rhythm, basal crepitations and ankle swelling.

Investigations

All patients should undergo urinalysis; it is cheap and simple and proprietary dipsticks can provide a wealth of information about the presence of blood, protein, ketones and bile in the urine. It is unlikely that urinalysis will be normal in the presence of significant renal disease.

Routine haematological screening of all surgical patients is unjustified on account of the low yield of abnormal results and the cost of unnecessary tests. All diagnostic tests carry a risk of false positive results which might subject patients to unnecessary and potentially harmful further investigation. Blery investigated 3866 consecutive general surgical patients who all underwent a battery of blood investigations.[5] Prior to the study an agreed protocol for investigations was agreed on the basis of clinical history and signs. In the patients who would not have warranted laboratory investigation there were clinically significant abnormalities in only 0.4% of cases. There were no deaths or adverse clinical events in this group and it is unlikely that the results would have altered the clinical management. Even in the elderly, routine testing will only alter clinical management in a small proportion of patients.[6] Laboratory testing is therefore only indicated for confirming and quantifying clinically suspected disease. It may be used for screening only where there is clear evidence of clinical benefit. Protocols for ordering preoperative investigations can successfully be used to selectively order tests with obvious resource implications and do not appear to put patients at risk or miss important diagnoses. There have been numerous attempts to educate house staff about the appropriateness of blood tests but these programmes appear to have had little effect on request patterns. Each unit should draw up specific protocols, agreed between surgeon and anaesthetist, on who should be tested and what investigations to perform. A further source of overinvestigation is the unnecessary duplication of tests. Laboratory tests ordered in the outpatient department as part of the diagnostic workup may be valid for up to 4 months.[7]

HAEMATOLOGICAL SCREENING

The full blood count is a simple way of detecting anaemia and abnormalities of platelet count. Anaemia places patients at increased risk from general anaesthesia.[8] The accepted level of haemoglobin for anaesthesia is 10 g/dl although there is little scientific evidence to support this figure. Indeed patients with chronic renal failure are often accepted for surgery at much lower levels. Knowledge of the preoperative haemoglobin does, however, provide a baseline on which blood loss can be estimated and transfusion requirements determined. In patients undergoing ambulatory surgery, where blood loss is minimal and where there are no concomitant diseases, the full blood count can be safely omitted.

Patients of Afro-Caribbean descent are at risk of sickle cell disease which makes anaesthesia hazardous through the risk of a sickle cell crisis occurring during hypoxia, hypotension or hypovolaemia. Although the full blown homozygous form of the disease is uncommon in the UK it is sensible to test all Afro-Caribbean patients as the incidence of the trait is high. In those with the homozygous form, arterial PaO_2 should be kept as high as possible. In those with the trait the risks are less, although hypoxia and hypotension should still be avoided. Tourniquets should be avoided wherever possible.

Routine coagulation screening is of little benefit in those without a history of bleeding as there is a high incidence of false positive results.[9] Abnormal results occur in only 7% of patients with a history of bleeding and are very uncommon in patients with no history of bleeding problems.[10] Excessive bleeding at previous operations or during dental extractions provides a clue. All patients on anticoagulants and with evidence of liver disease, particularly if jaundiced, should undergo coagulation screening.

BIOCHEMICAL SCREENING

Abnormalities of electrolytes, particularly potassium, can adversely affect anaesthesia and lead to fatal arrhythmias. Hyperkalaemia can lead to arrhythmias and arrest especially if suxamethonium is used. As with haematological screening, routine biochemical screening is unjustified. The yield of abnormal results is low, at around 1% and these abnormalities are rarely unexpected or alter clinical management. Even in the over-sixties the yield of abnormalities is only 5%.[11] Diabetes is common but can be detected by urinalysis. Renal disease serious enough to produce electrolyte disturbance is unlikely to be clinically unapparent and there will be evidence of disease on urinalysis. The same applies to significant liver disease. One of the principle indications for electrolyte estimations appears to be those taking digoxin, diuretics, steroids or other drugs likely to cause electrolyte disturbance.

ELECTROCARDIOGRAPHY (ECG)

Severe heart disease may be asymptomatic and further investigation of cardiovascular status is important. The resting ECG is simple and particularly in the elderly there is a high yield of abnormalities; however, whether these abnormalities are clinically significant is unclear. Gold has suggested that only 2% of patients with abnormal ECGs will have serious postoperative cardiac problems.[12] Indeed, the ECG may well be normal even in the presence of severe coronary atherosclerosis.

One of the major determinants of outcome following surgery is a myocardial infarction in the 6 months prior to surgery. The main purpose of the ECG is therefore to detect evidence of previous myocardial infarction which may have been silent. Although it gives no indication of when infarction occurred it may identify patients who warrant further investigation. The chief indication for preoperative ECG is patients with symptomatic cardiovascular disease including hypertension, symptomatic respiratory disease and patients over 60 years of age.

Table 11.1   Guidelines for preoperative chest radiography

1.	Chronic cardiorespiratory disease where a chest X-ray has not been performed within previous 12 months
2.	Acute cardiorespiratory symptoms or signs
3.	Possible primary or secondary malignancy
4.	Immigrants from countries where tuberculosis is endemic if a chest X-ray has not been performed within previous 12 months

Arrhythmias carry a high risk of postoperative cardiovascular events and their preoperative detection and correction is important. Major abnormalities are non-sinus rhythm, premature ventricular ectopics and heart block. Unfortunately, transient arrhythmias may be missed on a standard 12-lead ECG but the use of 24-hour Holter tape monitoring may improve the detection of preoperative arrhythmias. Unfortunately Holter monitoring is expensive and impractical for routine use. Arrhythmias detected by Holter monitoring are associated with postoperative congestive heart failure but not with an increased incidence of ischaemic events or arrhythmias.[13]

CHEST RADIOGRAPHY

The preoperative chest X-ray has been the subject of numerous audits and the Royal College of Radiologists has issued guidelines on the indications for preoperative chest radiography. It is no longer acceptable to write 'preop. check' on a request form and in our own hospital these forms are rapidly returned to the ward with a copy of the departmental guidelines (Table 11.1).

The preoperative chest X-ray establishes the extent of cardiorespiratory symptoms and measures heart size. The chest X-ray provides valuable information on the presence of metastases in patients with suspected or proven malignant disease. In one study it was estimated that 27% of chest X-rays are unreported by a radiologist prior to operation, while a more recent study suggested that many of these X-rays were not even looked at by the requesting doctors or anaesthetists.[14,15] Reducing preoperative chest radiography does not lead to an increase in postoperative problems.[16]

Assessment of risk

Cardiorespiratory complications are common following surgery and are increased in those with pre-existing cardiorespiratory disease. Although surgery may be unavoidable in patients with cardiorespiratory dis-

ease, its recognition may allow institution of appropriate treatments or dictate postoperative therapies such as mechanical ventilation.

CARDIOVASCULAR

The preoperative ECG can be unreliable and may be normal even in the presence of severe coronary atherosclerosis. Chest wall mapping using electrodes at sites other than the classic 12-lead has proved of little use in clinical practice.

Dynamic tests of cardiac function provide useful additional information on underlying cardiac disease and can be used to select patients who may require further invasive investigations. A high proportion of patients with normal resting ECGs show abnormalities on exercise and a significant proportion who will do so without experiencing chest pain. In patients undergoing peripheral vascular reconstruction the degree of ST-segment depression and heart rate can be used to assess the cardiac complication rate. In patients with > 1 mm ST depression and who failed to achieve a heart rate > 85% of predicted there was a 33% cardiac complication rate.[17] In patients with claudication or severe respiratory disease exercise may not be possible. In these instances dipyridamole-thallium scanning (DTS) is useful. Thallium detects areas of myocardial underperfusion or redistribution blood flow. The test is performed initially at rest and then following injection of the vasodilator dipyridamole. Areas of underperfusion that appear on stress represent areas liable to ischaemia. Around 50% of patients who show an abnormality with DTS will have a perioperative myocardial infarct.[18] One drawback is that patients with long-standing hypertension often have abnormal scans but little risk of postoperative infarction.

Coronary angiography is the gold standard for diagnosing surgically correctable coronary artery lesions and may be combined with angioplasty of significant lesions. However, the technique is hazardous and should only be considered in those with

Table 11.2 Goldman cardiac risk index

Risk factor	Score
Third heart sound, raised JVP	11
Myocardial infarct < 6 months old	10
More than five ventricular ectopics per minute	7
Non-sinus rhythm	7
Over 70 years old	5
Emergency	4
Intraperitoneal, thoracic or aortic surgery	3
Aortic stenosis	3
Poor general condition	3
PaO_2 < 60 mmHg, $PaCO_2$ >50 mmHg	
K+ <3.0 mmol/l, HCO_3 <20 mmol/l	
BUN >50 mg/100 ml, creatinine > 300 mg/ 100 ml	
elevated transaminases	
signs of chronic liver disease	
patient bedridden from non-cardiac causes	

JVP: Jugular blood pressure. BUN: Blood, urea, nitrogen.

symptoms which are severe enough to warrant coronary artery bypass.

Left ventricular function is a useful predictor of cardiac status. Most studies of left ventricular ejection fraction (LVEF) have been performed in patients undergoing aortic aneurysm repair or peripheral vascular reconstruction. In one British study of radionuclide ventriculography, patients undergoing aortic surgery were divided into two groups with ejection fractions greater than or less than 30%. In patients with low ejection fractions there was a 75% cardiac death rate as opposed to 2.7% in those with LVEFs above 30%.[19] In patients with peripheral vascular disease the risk of perioperative myocardial infarction is high when the LVEF is < 40%. Patients with LVEFs between 40 and 50% may

benefit from further investigation including angiography.[20] It is now possible to measure LVEF non-invasively using echocardiography, and in many centres LVEF is measured routinely prior to aortic surgery.

GOLDMAN CARDIAC RISK INDEX

Goldman retrospectively studied 1001 patients undergoing non-cardiac surgery and devised a risk index based on the history, physical examination, resting ECG and the type of surgical procedure (Table 11.2).[21] Goldman identified nine factors that gave a good indication of the risk of postoperative cardiac events. He gave weightings to these factors and when weightings are added together they yield a risk score; the higher the score, the higher the risk of postoperative cardiac problems (Table 11.3). The index does not apply to all patients, and patients undergoing abdominal aortic aneurysm repair or peripheral vascular surgery have more cardiac events than the risk index predicts. There have been a number of modifications to the system in recent years but the main determinants of outcome remain the same among all the systems, namely preoperative myocardial infarction, congestive cardiac failure and preoperative arrhythmias.

Respiratory

Not all patients require detailed investigation of the respiratory system. In general, patients under 40 years with no obvious respiratory symptoms or signs do not require detailed preoperative pulmonary function testing. The principle risk factors for postoperative lung problems are chronic lung disease, smoking and the type of surgery planned.

Table 11.3 Goldman cardiac risk index (when weightings are added together the score predicts the risk of complications or death)

Points	Class	Risk of complications %		
		Minor	Life-threatening	Cardiac death
0–5	I	1	0.7	0.2
6–12	II	7	5	2
13–25	III	14	11	2
> 25	IV	78	22	56

Table 11.4 The American Society of Anesthesiologists (ASA) physical status score

ASA I	Normal healthy patient
ASA II	Patient with mild systemic disease: mild organic heart disease, mild hypertension, diabetes, anaemia, old age, obesity, mild chronic obstruction airways disease
ASA III	Severe systemic disease that limits activity but is not incapacitating: angina, old myocardial infarction, severe diabetes, heart failure
ASA IV	Severe, incapacitating systemic disease which is a constant threat to life: severe heart failure, unstable angina, myocarditis; advanced renal, liver, respiratory and endocrine failure
ASA V	Moribund patient unlikely to survive more than 24 hours even with surgery. Little or no anaesthesia is required.

Emergency operations carry greater risk and are denoted by the letter E.

Patients with a persistent cough or spinal and chest wall deformities as well as the obese and elderly may also deserve more involved testing. Upper abdominal surgery leads to a 40–50% reduction in forced vital capacity (FVC) which may last up to 72 hours and is associated with a higher risk of postoperative lung complications than lower abdominal surgery. The principal determinant of this decrease in lung mechanics is site of the incision. This may explain why patients undergoing laparoscopic cholecystectomy fare better than those undergoing open surgery although the intraperitonal dissection is just as extensive. In surgical patients with chronic lung disease there is a 60% risk of postoperative lung problems. The importance of identifying these patients is that with appropriate preoperative physiotherapy, antibiotics and broncho-

Table 11.5 Mortality rates for individual ASA grade

ASA	Mortality (%)	Increased mortality (over ASA I)
I	0.08	–
II	0.27	3.4
III	1.8	22.5
IV	7.8	97.5
V	9.4	117.5

dilators this can be reduced to 20%.[22] Unfortunately, there is no one test that accurately predicts the likelihood of chest problems and a battery of tests is required.

ARTERIAL BLOOD GASES

Arterial blood gases (ABGs) vary with age. As one becomes older the lungs stiffen and the PaO_2 declines. It is therefore difficult to define an absolute figure at which problems may occur. Average PaO_2 can be estimated from the following formula.

$$PaO_2 \text{ (mmHg)} = 100 - 0.54 \times \text{age}$$

Because of the variability in ABGs between individuals, ABGs on air should be determined preoperatively wherever possible to give a baseline for postoperative management. A low PaO_2 denotes poor ventilation/perfusion match and a high $PaCO_2$ represents poor alveolar ventilation. PaO_2 < 60 mmHg and a $PaCO_2$ > 50 mmHg places the patient at increased risk of pulmonary problems.

SPIROMETRY

Spirometry can be performed at the bedside or in the clinic before and after inhaling a bronchodilator to determine the degree of airways disease, its pattern and reversibility. No single test appears to accurately predict the risk of surgery and most studies have used a variety of tests to predict outcome. In patients undergoing abdominal operations if FEV_1/FVC is less than 65% and FVC less than 70% of predicted value there is nearly a 100% risk of postoperative pulmonary complications.[23] Other indicators of a poor outcome are a maximal ventilation volume (MVV) of < 50 l/min. (FEV_1: forced expiratory volume in first second).

Risk stratification

PHYSICAL STATUS SCORE

The American Society of Anesthesiologists' (ASA) physical status score is a simple system of classifying patients according to their general health and provides an indication of risk and outcome (Table 11.4). As a bedside system it has gained wide acceptance, although anaesthetists may differ on the classification of individual patients. Its main drawback is that it fails to take account of asymptomatic severe coronary artery disease. It has, however, been adopted by the National Confidential Enquiry into Perioperative Deaths (NCEPOD) as part of the audit reporting mechanism regarding patients who have undergone surgery and subsequently died in the postoperative period. Although the ASA score was not originally designed as a prognostic index its simplicity has led to its rapid adoption by the medical community and there does appear to be a correlation between ASA grade and outcome (Table 11.5).

APACHE SCORE

The APACHE (Acute Physiology and Chronic Health Evaluation) is a more detailed assessment of physical status which takes account of chronic health problems. It is an objective score based on 34 physiological variables and provides an objective and reproducible measure of a patient's physical status. It is complicated and requires the measurement of a large number of parameters and has therefore found little use in routine preoperative assessment, although it does have obvious applications as an audit tool. In one study of patients undergoing major upper abdominal surgery an APACHE II score > 8 was associated with a 46% incidence of postoperative complications and death in 13% of patients.[24]

Informed consent

All patients should be provided with enough information about their condition, proposed treatment and alternatives, a realistic assessment of their prognosis and the likely complications of treatment to enable them to make an educated decision regarding treatment. A major complaint of patients who perceive that they have been badly managed is that they were not given enough information about their condition and were not fully informed regarding their progress. The decision on what to tell patients and how much is a difficult one and there is a worry that too frank a discussion of complications may unduly worry patients and raise anxiety levels. A recent study compared anxiety levels in patients given a standard cursory explanation by house staff and a more detailed multi-page document and 'American-style' explanation of their treatment. Patients given the more detailed explanation had less anxiety.[25] Patients entered into clinical research protocols (which must *always* have full approval of the local Ethics Committee) must be given more detailed information and never 'coerced' into participating.

Preoperative preparation

FLUID RESTRICITION

Traditional preparation for theatre dictated that all patients should receive nothing by mouth after midnight on the day before surgery and that for emergency cases there should be a 6-hour fast wherever possible. This view is being challenged and particularly in children it is acceptable to allow clear fluids for up to 2 hours before surgery. In adults the midnight rule could safely be replaced with a regimen allowing fluids up to 4 hours before surgery.[26]

SHAVING

Shaving hair from the site of incision often makes placement of incisions easier and avoids the problem of hairs becoming tangled up in the wound during closure and acting as a nidus for infection. Patients shaved on the ward often arrive in theatre with multiple cuts and scratches. The danger is that these superficial wounds will become colonized with hospital pathogens and there is some evidence to suggest that shaving may increase wound infection. Shaving in the anaesthetic room and prior to entry into theatre with safety razors or electric shavers does not appear to increase infection risk.[27]

ANTISEPTIC WASHES

Antiseptic washes confer no advantage over a simple shower to achieve social cleanliness. There is a theoretical danger that killing off normal skin commensals will allow colonization with hospital pathogens. Any obvious wounds should be swabbed to allow choice of antibiotics. There is no benefit in the routine swabbing of nose, perineum or other sites unless there is specific evidence of infection. (e.g. fear of MRSA – methicillin-resistant staphylococci – which carries high risk, including mortality and necessitates closure of wards and theatres).

BOWEL PREPARATION

Patients undergoing large bowel resection should have bowel preparation wherever possible. Patients with obstruction or impending obstruction are obvious exceptions. Patients are usually admitted a few days prior to surgery and started on a low residue diet and then given a purgative to clear the bowel. Herculean washout has fallen into disrepute due to the dangers of circulatory collapse in frail elderly patients. Oral antibiotics have been popular in the US but have found little place in British practice. (See also Chapter 5.) More recently bowel preparation has become very much simpler with the introduction of preparations such as Picolax® and Kleanprep.® Patients can now be admitted the day before surgery and bowel preparation started on the evening prior to operation. There is some evidence, however, that bowel preparation is unnecessary. Often with poorly prepared bowel the presence of semi-liquid faeces washing around the abdomen is more unacceptable that that of solid pieces of faeces which can be easily controlled and removed from the operative field.[28]

DVT PROPHYLAXIS

All patients undergoing all but the most minor forms of surgery should have some form of DVT prophylaxis. At its simplest this will consist of making sure the patient is as medically fit as possible and is not dehydrated. All patients should have anti-embolic elasticated stockings and, when in theatre, calves should be raised on a heel bar and pneumatic stockings fitted. The role of pharmacological prophylaxis is more complicated. However, all patients who fall into a high risk group should receive pharmacological prophylaxis in the form of mini-heparin. High risk groups include those with a history of previous DVT and PE, patients undergoing pelvic surgery or surgery for malignancy and anyone who shows signs of general debilitation.

Conclusion

A good history and physical examination together with appropriate investigations provide the basis for minimizing postoperative complications. The use of risk assessment may be important as well as providing an audit tool. Wasteful use of resources, coupled with unnecessary investigations, must be avoided and the introduction of preoperative assessment clinics can minimize the inpatient stay. This is beneficial to the psychological wellbeing of the patient as well as enabling appropriate planning for the patient's surgery. The introduction of patient hotels may require a radical reconsideration of patient assessment and preparation for surgery.

References

1. Sandler G. Costs of unnecessary tests. *Br Med J* 1979; **2**: 21–4.
2. McKee RF, Scott ME. The value of routine preoperative investigations. *Ann Roy Coll Surg Engl* 1987; **69**: 160–2.
3. Steen PA, Tinker JN, Tarhan S. Myocardial reinfarction following anaesthesia and surgery. *JAMA* 1978; **239**: 2566–70.
4. Goldman L, Caldera DC. Risks of general anaesthesia and elective operations in hypertensive patients. *Anesthesiology* 1979; **50**: 285–92.
5. Blery C, Charpak Y, Szatan M *et al.* Evaluation of a protocol for selective ordering of preoperative tests. *Lancet* 1986; **1**: 139–41.
6. Domoto K, Ben R, Wei JY *et al.* Yield of routine annual laboratory screening in the institutionalised elderly. *Am J Public Health* 1985; **75**: 243–5.
7. McPherson DS, Snow R, Lofgren RP. Preoperative screening: value of previous tests. *Ann Intern Med* 1990; **113**: 969–73.
8. Lunn JN, Elwood PC. Anaemia and surgery. *Br Med J* 1970; **3**: 71–3.
9. Burk CD, Miller L, Handler SC, Cohen AR. Preoperative history and coagulation screening in children undergoing tonsillectomy. *Pediatrics* 1992; **89**: 691–5.
10. Rohrer MJ, Michelotti MC, Nahrwold DL. A prospective evaluation of the efficacy of preoperative coagulation testing. *Ann Surg* 1988; **208**: 554–7.
11. Campbell IT, Gosling P. Preoperative biochemical screening. *Br Med J* 1988; **297**: 803–4.
12. Gold BS, Young ML, Kinman JL *et al.* The utility of preoperative electrocardiograms in the ambulatory surgical patient. *Arch Intern Med* 1992; **152**: 301–5.
13. Mangano DT, Browner WS, Hollenberger M *et al.* Association of perioperative myocardial ischaemia with cardiac morbidity and mortality in men undergoing non-cardiac surgery. *N Engl J Med* 1990; **323**: 1781–8.
14. National study by the Royal College of Radiologists. Preoperative chest radiology. *Lancet* 1979; **2**: 83–6.
15. Walker D, Williams P, Tawn J. Audit of requests for preoperative chest radiography. *Br Med J* 1994; **309**: 772–3.
16. Roberts CJ, Fowkes FGR, Ennis WP, Mitchell M. Possible impact of audit on chest X-ray requests from surgical wards. *Lancet* 1983; **2**: 446–8.
17. McPhail N, Calvin JE, Shariatmadar A *et al.* The use of preoperative exercise testing to predict cardiac complications after peripheral arterial reconstruction. *J Vasc Surg* 1988; **7**: 60–8.
18. Brewster DC, Okada RD, Strauss HW *et al.* Selection of patients for preoperative coronary angiography: use of dipyridamole-stress-thallium myocardial imaging. *J Vasc Surg 1985;* **2**: 504–10.
19. Moseley JG, Clarke JMF, Ell PJ, Marston A. Assessment of myocardial function before aortic

surgery using radionuclide angiocardiography. *Br J Surg* 1985; **72**: 886–7.

20. Jain KM, Patil KD, Docten NS, Peck SL. Preoperative cardiac screening before peripheral vascular operations. *Am Surg* 1985; **51** 77–81.

21. Goldman L, Caldera DL, Nussbaum SR *et al.* Multifactorial index of cardiac risk in non-cardiac surgical procedures. *N Engl J Med* 1977; **297**: 845–50.

22. Stein M, Cassara EL. Preoperative pulmonary evaluation and therapy for surgery patients. *JAMA* 1970; **211**: 787–90.

23. Latimer RC, Dickman M, Day WC *et al.* Ventilatory patterns and pulmonary complications after upper abdominal surgery determined by preoperative and postoperative computerised spirometry and blood gas analysis. *Am J Surg* 1971; **122**: 622–32.

24. Gagner M. Value of preoperative physiologic assessment in outcome of patients undergoing major surgical procedures. *Surg Clin N Am* 1991; **71**: 1141–50.

25. Kerrigan DD, Theuasagayam RS, Woods TO *et al.* Who's afraid of informed consent? *Br Med J* 1993; **306**: 298–300.

26. Editorial. How long should patients fast before surgery? Time for new guidelines. *Br J Anaesth* 1993; **70**: 1–3.

27. Court-Brown CM. Preoperative skin depilation and its effect on postoperative wound infection. *J Roy Coll Surg Edin* 1981; **261**: 238–41.

28. Irving AD, Scrimgeour D. Mechanical bowel preparation for colonic resection and anastomosis. *Br J Surg* 1987; **74**: 580–1.

CHAPTER 12

Local and regional anaesthesia in general surgery

LESLEY BROMLEY, MAIR DAVIES

Introduction

Local anaesthetics were first used when Koller applied cocaine to the conjunctiva in 1884.[1] Advances in techniques including local infiltration, nerve block, epidural and spinal anaesthesia led to, increased use of these methods during the first part of this century. Following World War II popularity of these fell due to improvements in general anaesthetic techniques. The notorious Wolley and Roe cases in the 1950s, where two patients became paraplegic on the same day following spinal anaesthesia, dramatically reduced the use of intrathecal spinal blocks for 20 years.

In modern practice, there has been a renewed interest in the use of local anaesthetic techniques by anaesthetists and surgeons. Local anaesthetics may provide the sole anaesthetic in a variety of procedures or may be employed in combination with general anaesthesia. The combination of general and local anaesthesia has the advantage of providing both intraoperative and postoperative analgesia. If the block is given before surgery commences, there is evidence that the need for postoperative analgesia is reduced.[2]

Pharmacology of local anaesthetics

MODE OF ACTION

Local anaesthetic drugs reversibly block the transmission of peripheral and neuraxis nerve impulses by blocking membrane depolarization. This is achieved by blocking the sodium channels thus preventing the influx of sodium into the nerve tissue following nerve stimulation and hence the action potential associated with nerve conduction is not sustained.[3,4]

Local anaesthetics in solution are weak bases. The nerve is penetrated by a local anaesthetic in its non-ionized form and subsequently ionizes within the acid inner environment. This ionized form enters the sodium channel thereby blocking it.[5] The degree of dissociation is related to the pH of the environment and the dissociation constant or pKa of the local anaesthetic. The pKa is derived from the Henderson–Hasselbalch equation:

$$pKa - pH = [BH^+]/[B]$$

where B = base.

In a relatively acid medium, for example in the presence of infection or haematoma, more of the local anaesthetic agent will be in the ionized form. As a result, the proportion of the local anaesthetic available in the non-ionized form to cross the nerve membrane will be reduced. This explains the commonly observed clinical finding that local anaesthetics are less effective in the presence of infection. Conversely, carbonated solutions of local anaesthetics have been used to speed the onset and improve the quality of the block, although the clinical efficacy of this technique is debatable.[6]

In myelinated nerves sodium channels are located at the nodes of Ranvier and two to three nodes must be blocked to prevent conduction. In larger nerves the nodes of Ranvier are further apart and as a consequence smaller nerves are more easily blocked than larger ones. It is important to recognize that the anaesthetic effect occurs when the local concentration of the drug is high. The concentration required to block a nerve is proportional to the diameter of the fibres and also to their degree of myelination. The sequence of the block is, therefore, first autonomic, then sensory and finally motor. The drug bupivacaine is used extensively in extradural anaesthesia and analgesia because at concentrations of 0.25% or less, good quality analgesia may be obtained with minimal motor block.[7]

STRUCTURE ACTIVITY RELATIONSHIP

Local anaesthetic structure consists of an aromatic (lipophilic) group and also a tertiary amine (hydrophilic) group. These are connected by an intermediate link. This link may be an ester or an amide and this difference forms the basis of the classification of local anaesthetics.[8] Esters are less chemically stable and cannot be heat sterilized. They are more likely to produce allergic reactions and are also metabolized more rapidly than the amide group.

Ester local anaesthetics	Amide local anaesthetics
Cocaine	Lignocaine
Benzocaine	Prilocaine
Procaine	Bupivacaine
	Ropivacaine

The potency of a drug is related to the lipid solubility of the non-ionized form since this determines the substance's ability to penetrate lipid cell membranes. Its duration of action,[9] however, depends on affinity of the molecule to bind to protein and is increased by reducing the rate of removal of local anaesthetic from the site of action. Reducing blood flow to the area of injection reduces the removal rate and the effect may be produced by the addition of vasoconstrictors such as adrenaline or felypressin.[10] Only cocaine and ropivacaine demonstrate intrinsic vasoconstrictive activity. On the contrary, most of the other agents cause vasodilatation.

Other factors may affect drug potency, onset, duration of action and toxicity.[11] The larger the dose the more rapid the onset and also the duration of action. The dose may be altered by changing either the concentration or volume. Changing volume is usually more effective in producing adequate anaesthesia. The site of the block will also influence onset time. This is almost immediate following infiltration anaesthesia and it progressively lengthens following spinal, peripheral nerve, epidural and brachial plexus block. This reflects the barriers around the nerve trunks at various sites. The dose of drug required also increases in the same manner.

ADDITION OF VASOCONSTRICTOR

Adrenaline has been used in combination with local anaesthetics since the beginning of the century.[12] Its action causes vasoconstriction and thereby both increases the duration action and also decreases toxicity of the drug and is thought to improve the efficacy of the block. The usual strength is 1:200 000, i.e. 5 µg/ml and the maximum recommended dose is 500 µg. Other recommendations state that a maximum of 10 ml of 1:100 000 adrenaline may be injected with safety in any 10-minute period if no hypoxia or hypercarbia is present, with a limit of 30 ml/h.[13] Absolute contraindications to its use include injection around end arteries (digits and penis) and also in total intravenous regional anaesthesia. Care must be taken if the patient is undergoing general anaesthesia using halothane, since the myocardium may be sensitized and the risk of arrhythmia is thereby increased. It should be avoided in patients on tricyclic antidepressants and also in those suffering from ischaemic heart disease and thyrotoxicosis.

METABOLISM AND ELIMINATION

The metabolic fate of local anaesthetics depends on their structure. Amides are extensively metabolized in the liver. Lignocaine has a liver clearance of 80%.[14] Prilocaine is the most rapidly metabolized of the amides and one of its metabolites, o-toluidine, is responsible for the methaemoglobinaemia and cyanosis which can occur approximately 6 hours after large doses of prilocaine. This usually resolves spontaneously.[15] Bupivacaine has a relatively low liver clearance and is only slowly metabolized.

The ester local anaesthetics are metabolized by plasma cholinesterase and also by esterases in tissues. The exception to this is cocaine which is relatively resistant to plasma cholinesterase and is largely metabolized in the liver.

Table 12.1 Maximum volume of lignocaine for patients of different weight

Drug	45 kg (45 × = 135 mg)	70 kg (70 × 3 = 210 mg)	85 kg (85 × 3 = 255 mg)
Lignocaine 0.5% (5 mg/ml)	27 ml	42 ml	51 ml
Lignocaine 1% (10 mg/ml)	13.5 ml	21 ml	25.5 ml
Lignocaine 2% (20 mg/ml)	6.75 ml	10.5 ml	12.75 ml

Remember 1% means 1 g in 100 ml

Individual drugs

LIGNOCAINE

Lignocaine was first produced in the 1940s by Lundqvist of Sweden. It has been used safely for many years and is considered to be the gold standard for local anaesthetic agents. It is very versatile and comes in a range of concentrations and may be used for topical, infiltrative, nerve and central neuronal blockade. As an amide it is stable during autoclaving and can be heat sterilized.

Lignocaine is presented in a 0.5%, 1% and 2% solution for use in local infiltration and nerve blocks. It is also available with adrenaline (1:200 000) as a vasoconstrictor. A 5% lignocaine preparation is also occasionally used for intrathecal anaesthesia. It has a rapid onset of action, within 3–5 minutes but its action is not instantaneous and patients will be appreciative if this is remembered! Its duration of action is also short, in the region of 1 or 2 hours with adrenaline. Onset and duration will vary depending on the site of use and the size of nerves that are to be blocked.

The maximum recommended dose of lignocaine for infiltration is 3 mg/kg alone and 7 mg/kg with adrenaline.

PRILOCAINE

Prilocaine is also one of the amide group of local anaesthetics. It has a lower toxicity than lignocaine, possibly due to its rapid redistribution. It is available as 0.5–2% concentration and because of its therapeutic ratio is the drug of choice for regional intravenous anaesthesia. It has a rapid onset of action, about 5 minutes, and its duration is of the order of 2 hours. It is metabolized in the liver, lungs and kidneys. At high doses, however, there is a risk of methaemoglobinaemia which can be treated with methylene blue. Its onset of action is rapid and its duration is 1–2 hours. The maximum recommended dose is 5 mg/kg without adrenaline and 8 mg/kg with adrenaline.

BUPIVACAINE

Bupivacaine has been in clinical use since 1963. It is four times as potent as lignocaine and when used in extradural block produces good sensory block with a minimum of motor block. Its onset of action is relatively slow, from 15 to 30 minutes depending on the site, but its duration is longer, in the order of 5 hours. However, in some patients it may be up to 16 hours and for this reason it has been used for intermittent 'top up' techniques for extradural pain relief in obstetrics and postoperative analgesia.[16] The addition of adrenaline does not increase the duration of action of

Table 12.2 Maximum volume of prilocaine for patients of different weights

	45 kg	70 kg	85 kg
Prilocaine 0.5% (5 mg/ml)	45 ml	70 ml	85 ml
Prilocaine 1% (10 mg/ml)	22.5 ml	35 ml	42.5 ml
Prilocaine 2%	11.25 ml	17.5 ml	21.25 ml

Table 12.3 Maximum volume of bupivacaine for patients of different weights

	45 kg	70 kg	85 kg
Bupivacaine 0.25% (2.5 mg/ml)	36 ml	56 ml	68 ml
Bupivacaine 0.5% (5 mg/ml)	18 ml	28 ml	34 ml

bupivacaine significantly although it may shorten the time of onset. Historically, bupivacaine was used in total intravenous regional anaesthesia because it provided several hours of postoperative analgesia. This use has been discontinued as a number of fatalities were reported with the technique.[17] Bupivacaine binds avidly with sodium channels producing a long duration of action. It will also bind to sodium channels in other excitable tissue as well as nerves and as a result it has a marked cardiac toxicity. Where bupivacaine inadvertently entered the circulation during regional intravenous anaesthesia, such cardiac toxicity, particularly intractable ventricular fibrillation and death resulted.[18] Bupivacaine is presented as a racemic mixture and the D-isomer is associated with this cardiac toxicity. The L-isomer will be available shortly.[19] The maximum recommended dose of bupivacaine is 2 mg/kg plain, and 5 mg/kg with adrenaline, although the addition of adrenaline does not confer any advantage.

ROPIVACAINE

Ropivacaine has only recently been available and is still undergoing clinical evaluation. It has a similar profile to bupivacaine but it is a vasoconstrictor in its own right. It has a slightly shorter duration of action, but having a more rapid clearance, repeated doses can be used safely.[20] It has been used in concentrations of 0.5 and 1% for epidural blockade. It has a similar margin of safety for seizures but its cardiotoxic potential is less than that of bupivacaine.[21]

Toxicity of local anaesthetics

Toxicity from local anaesthetic drugs is rare. It can result from intravenous injection or absolute overdosage of the drug resulting from significant vascular absorption. Either can cause systemic toxic reactions which, unless dealt with promptly, may be fatal. The risk of toxicity can be minimized by careful calculation of the correct dose for the weight of the patient and, when placing needles for injection of local anaesthetics, aspiration before injection to guard against intravenous injection. The risk of intravenous injection is minimized by continuous moving of the needles during injection and aspiration is particularly important prior to injection of large volumes.

When using local anaesthetic drugs to provide anaesthesia for surgery, risks of toxicity can be minimized if a full history, including any allergies or reactions to local anaesthetics, is established. Patients must be starved before having an operation under local anaesthesia in the same manner as for general anaesthesia, as the toxic effects may result in loss of consciousness with a consequent risk of aspiration of gastric contents into the lungs. Intravenous access with a cannula should be established before commencing any local anaesthetic technique, to allow for the treatment of toxicity should it occur.

Avoiding overdosage is more controversial since, although maximum permissible doses based on weight are quoted for a variety of agents, numerous other factors affect toxic vascular concentrations. These include age, site of injection and physical status. Absorption is rapid and peak blood concentrations may enter the toxic range following injections to vascular sites such as the intercostal space.

MECHANISM OF TOXICITY

Local anaesthetics, by blocking sodium channels, can stabilize the membranes of all excitable tissues. At high systemic concentrations they will suppress activity in the central nervous system and myocardium.[22] The brain is more susceptible than the heart to local anaesthetic effects. This is demonstrated by the fact that the dose and blood concentration of local anaesthetic required to cause toxic effects in brain tissue is lower than that required in myocardial tissue. It must be noted, however, that the treatment of myocardial toxicity is more difficult.

Initial symptoms include circumoral tingling, lightheadedness and dizziness followed frequently by visual and auditory disturbance, muscle twitching and tremors. Significant overdose will lead to convulsions, respiratory depression and respiratory arrest.[23] The potential toxicity of individual local anaesthetics may be influenced by the rate of injection and also whether either hypercapnia or acidosis is present.

The myocardial membrane stabilization produces a negative inotropic effect. This myocardial depression is dose dependent, and cardiovascular collapse may occur. Resuscitation has been shown to be more difficult under conditions of metabolic acidosis and hypoxia.

TREATMENT OF LOCAL ANAESTHETIC TOXICITY

The immediate management consists of basic life support with control of the airway, and ventilation if respiration has ceased. This may mean manual ventilation and/or intubation and giving oxygen whilst checking that the circulation is maintained. Control of convulsions can be achieved with intravenous diazepam or thiopentone. In the event of cardiovascu-

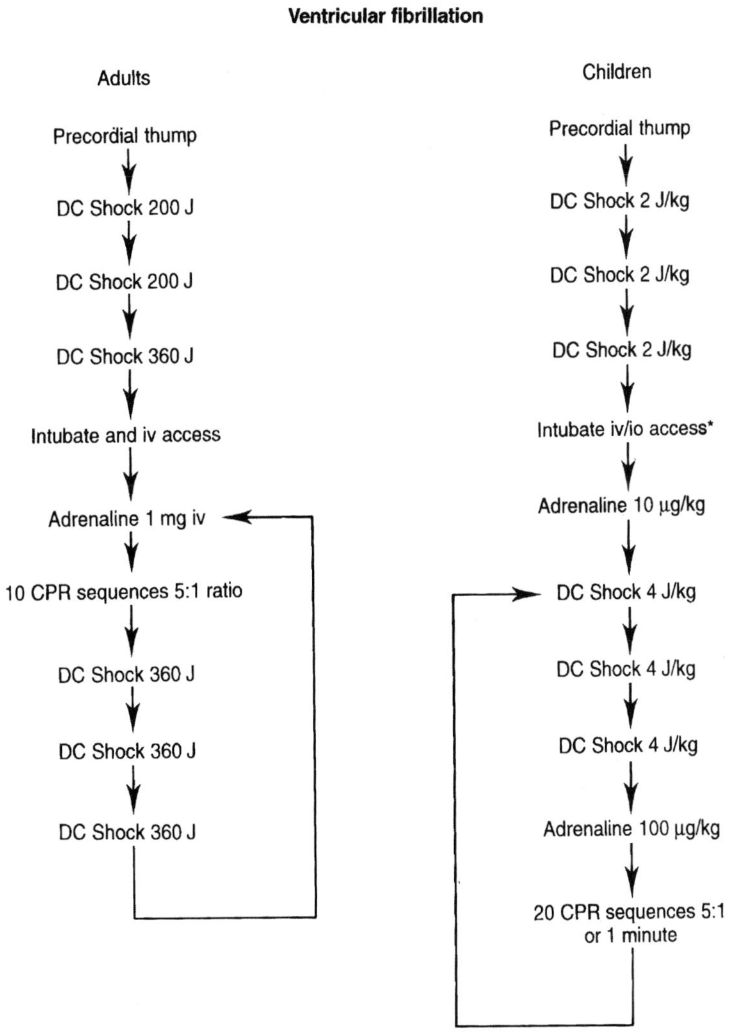

Ventricular fibrillation

Adults	Children
Precordial thump	Precordial thump
↓	↓
DC Shock 200 J	DC Shock 2 J/kg
↓	↓
DC Shock 200 J	DC Shock 2 J/kg
↓	↓
DC Shock 360 J	DC Shock 2 J/kg
↓	↓
Intubate and iv access	Intubate iv/io access*
↓	↓
Adrenaline 1 mg iv	Adrenaline 10 µg/kg
↓	↓
10 CPR sequences 5:1 ratio	DC Shock 4 J/kg
↓	↓
DC Shock 360 J	DC Shock 4 J/kg
↓	↓
DC Shock 360 J	DC Shock 4 J/kg
↓	↓
DC Shock 360 J	Adrenaline 100 µg/kg
	↓
	20 CPR sequences 5:1 or 1 minute

Fig. 12.1 Management of ventricular fibrillation in adults and children (*io: intra-osseus access).

lar collapse the arrhythmia is frequently ventricular fibrillation although asystole or complete atrioventricular dissociation may also be seen. Management of the arrhythmia (Fig. 12.1) following the resuscitation guidelines of the European Resuscitation Council should be undertaken.

The role of local anaesthesia

Local anaesthesia, infiltration and nerve blocks, and intravenous regional anaesthesia may be used as the sole anaesthetic technique for a number of procedures. In major surgery these techniques may be combined with light general anaesthesia in order to provide analgesia during the surgical procedure and also postoperatively.

The preoperative management of patients undergoing local techniques is the same as for those undergoing general anaesthesia. Patients must be assessed and prepared adequately with a full history and examination. It is necessary for the patient to lie still for the period of the surgery and any medical condition which makes this difficult should be treated before surgery. Consent must be gained for regional techniques, and an inability of the patient to understand the procedure, or any other difficulty in communication with the patient may make local techniques very difficult for both surgeon and patient. Intravenous access in a site not involved in the technique, using a good sized cannula, should be established before commencing the local anaesthesia. Local anaesthetic techniques should be carried out in a place where suction, oxygen and full resuscitation equipment are available. These techniques should *not* be regarded as necessarily a safe alternative to general anaesthesia.

ADVANTAGES OF LOCAL ANAESTHETIC TECHNIQUES

If local anaesthesia is used as the sole anaesthetic technique, the complications associated with general anaesthesia can be avoided. These may be significant in patients who are predicted to have a difficult airway or pose potential difficulties with intubation. For patients with severe respiratory disease avoiding general anaesthesia may have great advantages ranging from avoiding instrumentation of the airways in severe asthma to preventing loss of respiratory control in carbon dioxide retaining chronic obstructive pulmonary disease. Certainly the combination of avoiding atelectasis whilst providing good postoperative pain control would be advantageous to the respiratory cripple.[24] The place of local anaesthetic techniques is established in patients with ischaemic heart disease. The advantage lies in the avoidance of the negative inotropic effects of general anaesthetic drugs, together with the complication of pressor response to airway/laryngeal manipulation.

Local anaesthetic techniques are particularly applicable to day surgery.[25] In the case of local anaesthetic alone, the patient avoids a general anaesthetic and therefore has no residual effects and the case can be scheduled later in the day as no recovery time is required. In day surgery the use of local anaesthetics in combination with general anaesthesia provides good analgesia for the journey home.

Topical local anaesthetics can be used for painful diagnostic and therapeutic procedures. Nerve endings in the mucosa and conjunctiva can be easily and quickly anaesthetized by comparison with the skin. Eutectic mixture of local anaesthetic (Emla® cream) is a 50:50 mixture of lignocaine 25 mg/ml and prilocaine 25 mg/ml and has been used to provide topical skin anaesthesia before venepuncture in children.[26] This cream is applied under an occlusive dressing for 1 hour before the procedure. Emla cream has also been used for topical anaesthesia for dermatological procedures and plastic surgery.[27] It causes some blanching of the skin,[28] but this is rapidly reversed after the cream is removed, whereas the anaesthesia lasts for some time.

DISADVANTAGES OF LOCAL ANAESTHESIA

These techniques are not 100% reliable. Patients must be told that they may not work but the failure rate decreases with the familiarity and experience of the person performing the block. These techniques also take longer to perform. They require forward planning and good organization in order to maintain the smooth running of operating lists. If multiple blocks are required these may be very uncomfortable for the patient since they would require multiple needle stabs and the volumes and doses used may be close to the maximum recommended dose.

The role of epidural and spinal local anaesthetics

Local anaesthetic solutions can be placed in the epidural space, or into the cerebrospinal fluid (CSF) to produce neural blockade.

SPINAL OR INTRATHECAL ANAESTHESIA

The intrathecal or spinal local anaesthetic technique is used to provide anaesthesia for operation on the lower half of the body. It is a 'single shot' technique, where a fine needle 22-gauge or smaller is introduced into the CSF in the lumbar region and a small volume of local anaesthetic injected. The needle is then removed, and the patient rapidly becomes anaesthetized over the lower half of the body.[29] The shape of the vertebral column, with its lumbar lordosis, limits the upward spread of the local anaesthetic. In addition, the use of hyperbaric local anaesthetic solutions made up with dextrose to give it a higher specific gravity than CSF, limits the upward spread of the block.[30] Bupivacaine is commonly used and has a duration of over 2 hours.

Spinal anaesthesia is a suitable technique for operations on the lower limb, the lower abdominal wall and the pelvis. The innervation of the peritoneum is very variable and the ability to perform complex intra-abdominal surgery under spinal anaesthesia may be limited by inability to perform safely a block sufficiently high to anaesthetize the whole of the peritoneum.

As the dura is to be punctured it is important to establish the clotting status of the patient as bleeding into the intrathecal or epidural space can result in neurological damage.[31]

Advantages of spinal anaesthesia

Spinal anaesthesia is a useful technique commonly employed in orthopaedic surgery, urology and gynaecology. It has the advantage that it can give a very dense block, both sensory and motor, with a high success rate. It avoids all the complications of general anaesthesia and in patients with severe respiratory disease it has the advantage of avoiding the potential respiratory complications of a general anaesthetic.

In experienced hands this technique is simple and quick to perform with a high degree of reliability. It requires relatively simple equipment and it also provides postoperative pain relief. There is some evidence that the use of a spinal rather than a general anaesthetic may have a pre-emptive effect and may reduce the demand for postoperative analgesia.[32]

Disadvantages of spinal anaesthesia

The technique commonly used of a single shot injection of local anaesthetic requires experience to achieve a sufficient level of block. Piercing the dura carries a number of risks, including spinal headache,[33] infection and bleeding into the CSF.

The block produced by spinal anaesthetic captures sensory, motor and sympathetic fibres.[34] The loss of tone in the sympathetic nervous system results in peripheral vasodilation which has both advantages and disadvantages. Pooling of blood in the periphery will decrease the venous return and hence the cardiac output with a resultant fall in blood pressure. In cardiac patients the combination of low blood pressure and reflex tachycardia increases the work of the left ventricle which may already be critically ischaemic. Maintenance of adequate coronary perfusion pressure is crucial in patients whose coronary circulation is compromised.[35] A sudden fall in blood pressure or heart rate which may accompany central neural blockade may worsen pre-existing ischaemia. These effects can be minimized by preloading the patient with fluid before performing the spinal block.[36] There has been much discussion about the best fluid for preloading before spinal and epidural block; 1 litre of Hartmann's solution is generally used. Preloading patients who are in incipient heart failure is obviously unwise.

Spinal blocks have been used for producing moderate hypotension by this mechanism. The level of the block is directly related to the degree of hypotension as the sympathetic outflow ends at L2. Blocks which do not reach higher than L2 are unlikely to affect the blood pressure.[37]

Contraindications

Absolute contraindications to the spinal blockade are hypovolaemia, severe ischaemic heart disease including recent myocardial infarction and patients with uncontrolled heart failure. It is an absolute contraindication to use these techniques in patients with fixed cardiac outputs, i.e. in aortic or mitral stenosis or hypotrophic obstructive cardiomyopathy. In less severe ischaemic heart disease there may be some advantage to the drop in blood pressure as myocardial oxygen demand will fall because of a decrease in systemic vascular resistance and reduction in heart rate. This effect may outweigh the fall in pressure and therefore improve myocardial oxygenation.[38] However, the precise effects of the changes in blood pressure on the diseased myocardium are difficult to predict and other anaesthetic techniques may well be preferable.

Pre-existing abnormalities of the central nervous system also preclude patients from spinal anaesthesia. Mechanical problems such as abnormalities of the vertebral column may make spinal block difficult or impossible. Patients who cannot lie flat, for whatever reason, may be unsuitable for a spinal anaesthetic.

EPIDURAL LOCAL ANAESTHETICS

Local anaesthetics placed in the epidural space act on the spinal nerves as they pass through the space, producing a block which is segmental around the level at which the epidural is performed. This technique can also be performed as a 'single shot' technique but it is possible to place a catheter in the space and give continuous or intermittent boluses of local anaesthetic through it, thus allowing the block to be maintained for long periods. This technique has been used for the provision of analgesia and anaesthesia in obstetrics for more than 10 years. Epidural anaesthesia has been used as the sole anaesthetic in lower abdominal surgery, orthopaedics, and less frequently, for upper abdominal surgery. The technique involves passing a Touhy needle (a specially designed, usually 18-gauge, hollow needle with a blunt tip) through the ligamentum flavum into the epidural space. The epidural space is identified by loss of resistance either to air or saline. A catheter can then be passed through the needle and left in the space. The space can be identified at any level; cervical epidurals are used for monitoring the spinal cord during spinal surgery and thoracic epidurals are now used extensively in the management of postoperative pain following thoracotomy. Low thoracic and lumbar epidurals can be used for intraoperative anaesthesia or combined with a light general anaesthetic and postoperatively for analgesia. The caudal route can be used to enter the epidural space and 'single shot' and catheter techniques are used extensively in urology, both adult and paediatric.

Advantages of epidural local anaesthetics

The use of the epidural space to provide anaesthesia and analgesia for general surgery has grown over the past decade. Epidural anaesthesia offers the advantage of flexibility, as the dose of local anaesthetic can be varied in order to alter the intensity of the block. A full, dense, motor and sensory block can be produced which provides sufficient anaesthesia for surgery on the lower limb and lower abdomen, and may be titrated to reach sufficient height to block the peritoneum. An increasing number of caesarean sections are conducted under this type of anaesthesia as it has, in addition to other advantages, the ability to allow the mother to see the baby as soon as it is born. The use of epidural anaesthesia has the same advantages as spinal anaesthesia in terms of avoiding general anaesthesia, especially in the case of severe respiratory disease. The additional advantage is that the block can be 'topped up' via the catheter, thus extending the period over which the anaesthesia can be maintained and the operations which can be performed.

The epidural catheter can be left in place for a number of days postoperatively and can be used to provide postoperative pain relief.[39] Local anaesthetic solutions alone have been used for postoperative pain relief but their repeated use can be limited by tachyphylaxis. This can be overcome by using low doses of local anaesthetic in combination with opiates, given by continuous infusion.[40]

There is evidence from the use of epidurals in vascular surgery that establishing the block before surgery (so called 'pre-emptive analgesia') can be beneficial. Patients who had epidural blockade with a dense sensory block established for 24 hours before amputation of the lower limb had a dramatically reduced incidence of subsequent phantom limb pain.[41] This study was one of the first pieces of evidence for the clinical relevance of the phenomenon of pre-emptive analgesia.

Disadvantages of epidural anaesthesia and analgesia

Performing an epidural block requires a level of expertise and is complex and more lengthy than a spinal block. The onset of the block may be 20–30 minutes after the injection. It therefore requires more staff time and organization to use this technique and maintain the smooth running of lists. There is a failure rate with epidurals even in the best hands.

Dural puncture may complicate attempts to per-form an epidural; this may result in a postdural puncture headache which may persist and distress the patient for some days. It can be treated with an epidural blood patch but this carries its own risks and morbidity.[42]

Postoperative analgesia via an epidural can only be used in circumstances where suitable nursing expertise exists to manage it. Preferably, an acute pain team should be active in the surgical wards and suitable protocols for management by nurses and junior medical staff should be available.[43]

The cardiovascular effects described for spinal anaesthesia can also occur with lumbar epidural anaesthesia. The use of preloading can minimize this effect, but hypotension and tachycardia can result with concomitant deleterious effect on the cardiovascular system. By contrast, epidurals at the thoracic level can block the cardiac sympathetics and block the tachycardia, thus reducing myocardial work.[44]

Contraindications

Patients with abnormal clotting profiles should not have an epidural performed. The risk of puncturing an epidural vein and producing an epidural haematoma is unjustifiable. Epidural haematomas require urgent neurosurgical decompression, otherwise permanent paralysis can result. In patients who are receiving subcuticular heparin as prophylaxis against deep vein thrombosis, if an epidural is to be performed, the first dose of heparin should be withheld until the catheter has been placed. Lumbar epidural may be technically difficult in patients with congenital abnormalities of the vertebrae. Caudal epidural blocks are much easier in children than adults because the sacrococcygeal membrane becomes calcified with age.

Effects of using epidural analgesia on surgical outcome

STRESS RESPONSE TO SURGERY

It has been suggested that there is a causal relationship between the stress response to surgery and postoperative morbidity, although there is little direct evidence to support this. General anaesthesia allows the stress response to occur and, indeed, may exacerbate it.[45] Epidural local anaesthesia has been shown to ablate the stress response to surgery completely when performed below the umbilicus[46] but is only partly effective in surgery above the umbilicus. It has been suggested that the inability to completely block the innervation of the upper peritoneum, and thus noxious stimuli reaching the spinal cord, accounts for the partial effectiveness of this technique in upper abdominal surgery.[47] Epidural analgesia continued into the postoperative period continues to modify the stress response. This effect is not seen with patient-controlled analgesia using intravenous opiates despite adequate dosage.

CARDIOVASCULAR SYSTEM

The unpredictable effects of lumbar epidural anaesthesia on the cardiovascular system have already been discussed. There is some evidence, however, that an epidural in the thoracic region can be beneficial to the cardiovascular system. This is particularly true in the postoperative period, when pain and anxiety can activate sympathetic responses and thus increase myocardial oxygen demand. Thoracic epidurals have been shown to increase the myocardial blood flow to ischaemic areas.[48] Myocardial ischaemia occurring in the postoperative period is more frequent, more severe and more prolonged than either preoperative or intraoperative ischaemia.[49] Large randomized controlled trials on the use of postoperative epidurals and their effect on cardiac morbidity are in progress and this technique will undoubtedly become increasingly widespread in the future.

COAGULATION

Major surgery is associated with a hypercoagulable state which persists into the postoperative period and is associated with thromboembolic events. General anaesthesia with parenteral opiates has little effect *per se.*[50] Epidural anaesthesia and analgesia appears to reduce significantly the incidence of thromboses of vascular grafts and of deep vein thrombosis and pulmonary embolism in patients undergoing hip replacement.[51] Lumbar epidural anaesthesia followed by 24 hours of analgesia with bupivacaine has been shown to produce a 2.5- to 5-fold reduction in the incidence of deep vein thrombosis and a 3-fold reduction in pulmonary embolism.[52] As thromboembolic phenomena almost certainly start intraoperatively it is probably the combination of epidural anaesthesia and analgesia that confers protection. This is underlined by the fact that the use of spinal anaesthesia has also been shown to reduce the incidence of postoperative deep vein thrombosis.

RESPIRATORY SYSTEM

General anaesthesia may exacerbate surgery-induced pulmonary dysfunction.[54] By contrast, epidural anaes-

thesia has a minimal effect on pulmonary function.[55] The effects of general anaesthesia, however, are short lived and probably do not contribute significantly to postoperative morbidity. It is probably due to the superior pain relief produced by postoperative epidural analgesia that a reduced incidence of postoperative pneumonia, respiratory failure and radiological markers of pulmonary morbidity results.[56,57]

GASTROINTESTINAL SYSTEM

Postoperative ileus is a major cause of surgical morbidity. The pathophysiology of ileus is ill defined, but surgical stress, pain and sympathetic stimulation are all contributors. High epidural block not involving the sacral routes can block sympathetic innervation whilst sparing parasympathetic innervation. In theory this should reduce the incidence of postoperative ileus. Postoperative analgesia with local anaesthetics given via a thoracic epidural has to be continued until bowel function returns for benefit to be obtained.[58]

IMMUNE SYSTEM

Epidural anaesthesia, by suppressing the stress response to surgery also reduces the immunosuppressive effects of surgery.[59] Clinical studies have suggested that the combination of epidural anaesthesia and postoperative analgesia is associated with a lower incidence of postoperative wound sepsis as well as postoperative chest infections.[60] There have been no clinical studies evaluating the effectiveness of epidural anaesthesia and analgesia in oncological surgery to date.

CONCLUSIONS

Epidural and spinal anaesthesia and analgesia provide an alternative to general anaesthesia for a number of surgical procedures. They both require anaesthetic expertise but they have advantages in the postoperative period and contribute to the reduction of postoperative morbidity.

References

1. Koller C. *Klin Mbl Augen* 1884; **22**: 60.
2. Tverskoy MM, Cozacov C, Ayache M *et al.* Postoperative pain after inguinal herniorrhaphy with different types of anaesthesia. *Anesthes Analges* 1990; **70**: 29–35.
3. Cahalan MD, Almers W. Interactions between quarternary lidocaine, the sodium channel gates and tetradotoxin. *Biophys J* 1979; **27**: 57–74.

4. Ritchie JM. Mechanism of action of local anaesthetic agents and biotoxins. *Br J Anaesthes* 1975; **47** 191–8.

5. Covino BG. Pharmacology of local anaesthetic agents. *Br J Anaesthes* 1986; **58**: 701–16.

6. Catchlove RFH. The influence of CO_2 and pH on local anaesthetic agents. *J Pharmacol Exp Ther* 1972; **181**: 298–309.

7. Franz DN, Perry RS. Mechanisms of differential block among single myelinated and nonmyelinated axons by procaine. *J Physiol* 1974; **236**: 193–201.

8. Ritchie JM, Ritchie B, Greengard P. The active structure of local anaesthetics. *J Pharmacol Exp Ther* 1965; **150**: 160–4.

9. Swerdlow M, Jones R. The duration of action of bupivacaine, prilocaine, and lignocaine. *Br J Anaesthes* 1970; **42**: 335–9.

10. Braid DP, Scott DB. The effect of adrenaline on the systemic adsorption of local anaesthetic drugs. *Acta Anaesthes Scand* 1966; Suppl 23 334–46.

11. Covino BD. Pharmacokinetics of local anaesthetic drugs. In: Prys-Roberts C, Hugg CC (eds) *Pharmacokinetics of Anaesthesia*. Oxford: Blackwell, 1984: 270–92.

12. Braun H. *Arch Klin Chir* 1902; **69**: 541.

13. Cotton BR, Henderson HP, Achola KJ, Smith G. Changes in plasma catecholamine concentrations following infiltration with large volumes of local anaesthetic solution containing adrenaline. *Br J Anaesthes* 1986; **58**: 593–7.

14. Boynes RN. A review of the metabolism of amide local anaesthetic agents. *Br J Anaesthes* 1975; **47**: 225–30.

15. Scott DB, Jebson PJR, Braid DP *et al.* Factors affecting plasma levels of lignocaine and prilocaine. *Br J Anaesthes* 1972; **44**: 1040–9.

16. Moore DC, Bridenbaugh LD, Bridenbaugh PO, Tucker GT. Bupivicaine hydrocholide: laboratory and clinical studies. *Anaesthesiology* 1970; **32**: 78–83.

17. Heath M. Deaths after intravenous regional anaesthesia. *Br Med J* 1982; **285**: 913.

18. Reiz S, Nath S. Cardiotoxicity of local anaesthetic agents. *Br J Anaesthes* 1986; **58**: 736–46.

19. Toxicological and local anaesthetic effects of optically active isomers of two local anaesthetic compounds. *Acta Pharmacol Toxicol* 1972; **31**: 273–86.

20. Akerman B, Hellberg I-B, Trossvik C. Primary evaluation of the local anaesthetic properties of the amino amide agent ropivacaine. *Acta Anaesthes Scand* 1988; **32**: 571–8.

21. Reiz S, Haggmark S, Johansson G, Naith S. Cardiotoxicity of ropivicaine, a new amide local anaesthetic. *Acta Anaesthes Scand* 1989; **33**: 93–8.

22. Reynolds F. Adverse effects of local anaesthetics. *Br J Anaesthes* 1987; **59**: 78–95.

23. Scott DB. Toxic effects of local anaesthetic agents on the central nervous system. *Br J Anaesthes* 1986; **58**: 732–5.

24. Wildsmith JAW, Armitage EN. *Principles and Practice of Regional Anaesthesia*. Edinburgh: Churchill Livingstone, 1987.

25. Dawson B, Reed WA. Anaesthesia for adult surgery outpatients. Anaesthesia for day case surgery; a symposium in four parts. *J Can Anesthes Soc* 1980; **27**: 409.

26. Hallen B, Carlsson P, Uppfeldt A. Clinical study of lignocaine:prilocaine cream to relieve the pain of venepuncture. *Br J Anaesthes* 1985; **57**: 326–8.

27. Hjort N, Harring M, Hahn A. Epilation of upper lip hirsutism with a eutectic mixture of lignocaine and prilocaine used as a topical anaesthetic. *J Am Acad Dermatol* 1991; **25**: 809–11.

28. Pepall LM, Cosgrove MP, Cunliffe WJ. Ablation of whiteheads by cautery under topical anaesthesia. *Br J Dermatol* 1991; **125**: 256–9.

29. Barker AE. A report on experience with spinal anaesthesia in 100 cases. *Br Med J* 1908; **7**: 453–5.

30. Wildsmith JAW, McClure JH, Brown DT, Scott BD. Effects of posture on the spread of isobaric and hyperbaric amethocaine. *Br J Anaesthes* 1981; **53**: 273–8.

31. Kane RE. Neurologic defects following epidural or spinal anesthesia. *Anesthes Analges* 1981; **60**: 150–61.

32. Shir Y, Raja SN, Frank SM. The effect of epidural versus general anaesthesia on postoperative pain and analgesic requirements in patients undergoing radical prostatectomy. *Anesthesiology* 1994; **80**: 49–56.

33. Flaaten H, Rodt SA, Vamnes J *et al.* Postdural puncture headache. A comparison between 26- and 29-gauge needles in young patients. *Anaesthesia* 1989; **44**: 147–9.

34. Galindo A, Hernandez J, Benavides O *et al.* Quality of spinal extradural analgesia: the influence of spinal nerve root diameter. *Br J Anaesthes* 1975; **47**: 41.

35. Reiz S, Blfora E, Sorenson MB *et al. Reg Anaesthes* 1982; **7**: 8–18.

36. Baron J-F, Coriat P, Mundler O *et al.* Left ventricular global and regional function during lumbar epidural anaesthesia in patients with angina pectoris. The influence of fluid loading. *Anesthesiology* 1987; **66**: 621.

37. Sjorgren S, Wright B. Circulatory changes during continuous epidural blockade. *Acta Anaesthes Scand* 1972; **16**: 5.

36. Reiz S, Nath S, Rais O. The effects of thoracic block and prenatolol on coronary vascular resistance and myocardial metabolism in patients with coronary artery disease. *Acta Anaesthes Scand* 1980; **24**: 11.

39. Schug SA, Fry RA. Continuous regional analgesia in comparison with intravenous opioids administration for routine postoperative pain control. *Anaesthesia* 1994; **49**: 528–32.

40. Paech MJ, Westmore MD. Postoperative epidural fentanyl infusion – is the addition of 0.1% bupivicaine of benefit? *Anaesthes Intens Care* 1994; **22**: 9–14.

41. Bach S, Noreng MF, Tjellden NU. Phantom limb in amputees during the first 12 months following limb

amputation, after preoperative lumbar epidural blockade. *Pain* 1988; **33**: 287–301.

42. Di Giovanni AJ, Dunbar BS. Epidural injection of autologous blood for postlumbar puncture headache. *Anesthes Analges* 1970; **49**: 268–71.

43. Schug SA, Torrie JJ. Safety assessment of postoperative management by an acute pain service. *Pain* 1993; **55**: 387–91.

44. Reiz S, Haggmark S, Rydvall A, Ostman M. Betablockers and thoracic epidural analgesia. Cardioprotective and synergistic effects. *Acta Anaesthes Scand* 1980; **76**: 54.

45. Weissman C, Hollinger I. Modifying systemic responses with anaesthetic techniques. *Anesthes Clin N Am* 1988; **6**: 221–35.

46. Kehlet H. The stress response to surgery: release mechanisms and the modifying effect of pain relief. *Acta Chir Scand* 1988; **550** (Suppl): 22–8.

47. Naito Y, Tamai S, Shingu K *et al*. Responses of plasma adrenocorticotropic hormone, cortisol, and cytokines during and after upper abdominal surgery. *Anesthesiology* 1992; **77**: 426–31.

48. Blomberg S, Emanuelson H, Kvist H *et al*. Effects of thoracic epidural anaesthesia on coronary arteries and arterioles in patients with coronary artery disease. *Anesthesiology* 1990; **73**: 840–7.

49. Mangano DT, Browner WS, Hollenberg M *et al*. Association of perioperative myocardial ischaemia with cardiac morbidity and mortality in men undergoing noncardiac surgery. *N Engl J Med* 1990; **323**: 1781–8.

50. Christopherson R, Beattie C, Frank SM *et al*. Perioperative morbidity in patients randomised to epidural or general anesthesia for lower extremity vascular surgery. *Anesthesiology* 1993; **79**: 422–34.

51. Sharrock N, Rainawat C, Urquhart B, Peterson M. Factors influencing deep vein thrombosis following total hip arthroplasty under epidural anaesthesia. *Anesthes Analges* 1993; **76**: 756–71.

52. Modig J, Maripuu E, Sahlstedt B. Thromboembolism following total hip replacement; a prospective investigation of 94 patients with emphasis on the efficacy of lumbar epidural anaesthesia in prophylaxis *Reg Anesthes* 1986; **11**: 72–9.

53. Sorenson R, Pace N. Anaesthetic techniques during surgical repair of femoral neck fractures. *Anaesthesiology* 1992; **77**: 1095–104.

54. Pansard J-L, Mankikian B, Bertrand M *et al*. Effects of thoracic extradural block on diaphragmatic electrical activity and contractility after upper abdominal surgery. *Anesthesiology* 1993; **78**: 63–71.

55. Hendolin H, Lahtinen J, Lansimies E *et al*. The effect of thoracic epidural analgesia on respiratory function after cholecystectomy. *Acta Anaesthes Scand* 1987; **31**: 645–51.

56. Yeager MP, Glass DD, Neff RK, Brinck-Johnson T. Epidural anaesthesia and analgesia in high risk surgical patients. *Anesthesiology* 1987; **66**: 729–36.

57. Hasenbos M, Van Egmond J, Gielen M, Crul J. Post-operative versus intramuscular nicomorphine after thoracotomy. Part III the effects of per- and post operative analgesia on morbidity. *Acta Anaesthes Scand* 1987; **31**: 608–15.

58. Scheinen B, Asantila R, Orko R. The effects of bupivacaine and morphine on pain and bowel function after colonic surgery. *Acta Anaesthes Scand* 1987; **31**: 161–4.

59. Tonnesen E, Wahlgreen C. Influence of extradural and general anaesthesia on natural killer cell activity and lymphocyte subpopulations in patients undergoing hysterectomy. *Br J Anaesthes* 1988; **60**: 500–7.

60. Hjorstso NC, Neumann P, Frosig F. A controlled study on the effect of epidural analgesia with local anaesthetic and morphine on morbidity after abdominal surgery. *Acta Anaesthes Scand* 1985; **29**: 705–16.

CHAPTER 13

Surgical access to the abdomen

V JAFFE, I TAYLOR

Introduction

The surgical incision and resultant wound represent a major part of the morbidity of abdominal surgery. Surgeons have long recognized that they must, therefore, balance their need for access to perform safe and effective procedures against the trauma to the abdominal wall and other viscera that they incur in so doing. Before the advent of minimally invasive techniques, optimal access could only be achieved at the expense of large, high morbidity incisions. Endoscopic and laparoscopic technology has, however, revolutionized these concepts facilitating 'patient friendly' access to even the most remote of abdominal organs. What is not yet fully evaluated is to what extent safe and effective surgery can be prosecuted when such access is obtained in this way.

It can be fully appreciated that, when considering the need for surgery to a particular intra-abdominal organ, balanced appraisal is made of the various modalities available – open, laparoscopic and endoscopic. Whether an open or laparoscopic technique is employed, it will be obvious that careful planning of placement of the incision or laparoscopic ports will be paramount in ensuring optimal access with minimum morbidity. This chapter will discuss the general principles on which such decisions are made for both open and laparoscopic surgery before considering the various incisions and approaches that are in popular usage.

General principles

OPEN SURGERY

Length of incision

Although, as discussed above, the surgeon should try to minimize the surgical trauma to the abdominal wall, it is his or her prime responsibility to perform safe and effective surgery. To do so at an open operation requires adequate exposure. It should be a salutary lesson to the surgical trainee that their senior, when called in to help out at a difficult laparotomy, will almost always enlarge the original incision. It is also perhaps appropriate to restate two old surgical adages 'Little surgeons make little incisions' and 'Big mistakes are made through small holes'.

The eventual size of the opening in the abdominal wall is directly related to the length of the incision and this is important to bear in mind if lateral retraction will be needed in vertical incisions (or craniocaudal retraction in transverse incisions). The quality of retraction will be an important factor in determining the extent of exposure for a given length of incision. With the help of the anaesthetist effecting complete muscle relaxation and using specialized ring retractors (Codman®, Omnitrac®, Buckvolt®) it is possible to successively retract a wound in different directions enabling fairly extensive surgery to be performed through relatively short but well-placed incisions.

Orientation

The target organ and the shape of the patient's abdomen should help determine in which direction to orientate the incision. In general a vertical incision is more suitable for the long thin abdomen and a transverse incision for the broader shorter one. Midline vertical incisions are quick to make, easy and safe to close, and permit exploration of all four quadrants by cranial or caudal extension. This makes them particularly suitable for emergency or exploratory procedures. Paramedian vertical incisions, although rarely used nowadays, were very popular in the era of 'closure in layers', but they still have a place when access to laterally placed organs is required.

Transverse incisions are usually more time-consuming, involving muscle cutting which results in increased blood loss. They tend to give relatively poor access to the upper and lower reaches of the abdomen and pelvis, but can be suitable for laterally placed organs such as the kidneys, ureters or adrenals. In neonates and infants the subdiaphragmatic and pelvic recesses are comparatively shallow and in these patients a transverse incision will permit adequate access to the upper and lower abdominal viscera.

Patient factors

It has been well established that the upper abdominal wall is an important ventilatory muscle and that upper midline incisions cause significant falls in vital capacity. Furthermore, midline incisions are said to be more painful because they cross several dermatomes. For these reasons some surgeons prefer to use transverse incisions in patients who may be at risk of postoperative respiratory embarrassment. However, with the advent of local and regional anaesthetic regimen, as well as with more effective analgesic techniques, the current view is that these factors are less important than is the need for optimal access.

In the abdomen that has had previous surgery it may be safer to make at least part of the incision in 'virginal' abdominal wall so as to reduce the risk of damage to underlying adherent structures. Care must be taken to avoid 'tramline' or 'acute angle' incisions (Fig. 13.1) which could lead to the devascularization of tissue. It is also beneficial to the patient if incisions are kept as remote as possible from established or proposed stoma sites.

Finally, most patients are concerned about the eventual appearance of their abdominal scar, irrespective of their shape or medical condition. Consideration should be given, wherever possible, to siting incisions in natural skin creases or along Langer's lines. Good cosmesis helps patient morale.

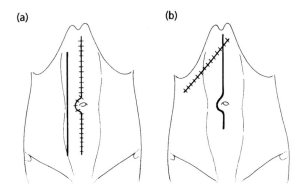

Fig. 13.1　(a) Tramline incision. (b) Acute angle incision.

LAPAROSCOPIC SURGERY

It is beyond the scope of this chapter to analyse the role of laparoscopic techniques in abdominal surgery. However, it is perhaps relevant, when discussing access, to emphasize that minimally invasive surgery minimizes the trauma of access not only by avoiding the need for a significant wound but also by permitting the execution of the procedure in an isolated physiological environment. Only when one observes the rapid recovery from successful major laparoscopic surgery does one appreciate the extent to which trauma to the abdominal wall, in addition to the handling and retraction of abdominal viscera, contributes to postoperative surgical morbidity.

Laparoscopic equipment

The rapid advance in technology – particularly in camera chips, high resolution monitors, automatic powerful light sources and telescope optics – has enabled the surgeon to view with remarkable clarity remote areas of the closed abdomen.

Pneumoperitoneum

The normal peritoneal cavity is a potential space only and a pneumoperitoneum is essential to provide a working cavity for the laparoscope and its associated instruments. Successful laparoscopy can, therefore, only be performed if the peritoneal cavity can be safely and effectively insufflated. If the cavity has been obliterated as a result of previous severe peritonitis or multiple surgical procedures or if there is a large hiatus or external hernia, then a safe and workable pneumoperitoneum may be impossible to establish. General anaesthesia with muscle relaxation will facilitate a steady and reliable pneumoperitoneum. Larger insufflation volumes produce a larger cavity and thereby reduce the potential danger of trocar, or other, damage to the underlying viscera. However, this must be balanced against the potential cardiovascular sequelae (reduced venous return and splanchnic blood flow) of a persistent high pressure pneumoperitoneum.

Trocars/ports

These permit the repeated passage of telescope and working instruments through the abdominal wall. Progressively more complex procedures can be performed within the peritoneal cavity as a result of refinement of these working instruments, which obviously must traverse the narrow ports. It is an axiom of laparoscopic surgery that all ports, except the first, and all instruments, should be placed under direct laparoscopic vision.

Retraction

In laparoscopic surgery instrumentation is small and there are no operator's or assistant's hands to impede the view. As a consequence, the exposure required around the target organ is reduced and the need for retraction is likewise lessened. Simple tilting of the patient may provide excellent unimpeded access to the pelvis and other areas. Laparoscopic forceps, Babcock's probe and fan retractors all provide an excellent method of retracting mobile viscera to ensure optimal access.

Suitability or contraindications

It is now technically possible to perform a wide range of intra-abdominal procedures entirely laparoscopically or laparoscopically assisted. However, the most suitable procedures are those where the actual surgical procedure is relatively small by comparison with the large incision and mobilization required to gain open exposure. Remote and confined areas, such as the pelvis or the subphrenic space are particularly suitable in this respect.

In the opinion of some experts there are no absolute contraindications to laparoscopic abdominal surgery. However, there are several relative contraindications of which the wise operator should be aware. Patients with considerable intraperitoneal adhesions or large hernias (particularly hiatus hernias) make the generation of a safe and workable pneumoperitoneum very difficult and sometimes dangerous. Pregnancy, coagulopathies and morbid obesity (particularly in the male) are, likewise, all relative contraindications.

Surgical incisions in the anterior abdominal wall

GENERAL TECHNIQUE

Shaving

Although the old 'nipples to knees' shave is no longer fashionable, adequate shaving of the incision area is important. There is some doubt as to whether wound infection rates are reduced by shaving but a hairless wound is certainly much easier to manage after surgery.

Shaving should be carefully performed, preferably on the day of surgery, with an electric shaver, and the patient should shower or wash thereafter to remove loose hairs. If there is substantial delay between shaving and surgery, bacterial colonization of the minute abrasions may occur, and this may lead to an increased risk of wound infection.

Skin preparation

Many skin antiseptic preparations are available and selection is often based on personal preference. Microbiologists recommend that the preparations, particularly alcohol-based ones, are allowed to dry in order to effect maximum antisepsis. Towels or drapes are then placed so as to isolate the planned wound – provision should be made for possible incision extension. Adhesive skin drapes may further help to isolate the wound from skin contaminants and are specially indicated if prosthetic materials are used.

Alcohol-based solutions must be used with great care when diathermy is used. Severe flash burns have been caused by ignition of such solutions by sparks.

The incision

Surgical dissection is greatly facilitated by ensuring that the tissues are under sufficient tension. The operator's non-dominant finger or thumb and the swab-covered hand of an assistant can be used to stretch the skin and subcutaneous tissue and this will allow a clean and accurate incision. Whenever possible, the incision should be perpendicular to the skin surface and pass through the subcutaneous fat with a single cut. The scalpel blade remains the most popular cutting instrument. Blood loss can be reduced, however, by utilizing a diathermy spatula on 'cutting', 'high coagulation' or 'blend' modes. Bleeding vessels are picked up with fine haemostats and coagulated or ligated.

Once the linea alba, rectus or oblique muscle sheath is reduced the fat is cleared for a few millimetres on either side. This will help with identification of the correct layers on closure. This clearance of fat should not be too excessive, as there is some evidence that this may lead to significant devascularization of the sheath.

SPECIAL INCISIONS

Midline

Suitability

The midline incision will give access to most intra-abdominal areas. In the emergency situation it has taken over from the right paramedian as the 'incision of indecision'. It combines ease and speed of access with flexibility and security of closure. In the upper abdomen it gives reasonable access to the viscera in the supracolic compartment. When combined with bilateral oblique incisions ('Mercedes Benz') it gives excellent access to the liver, stomach and pancreas (see below). In the lower abdomen access can be gained to the infracolic compartment and to the pelvis. For all the above reasons the midline incision has become the most popular in open abdominal surgery.

Technique

In order to ensure correct midline siting of the skin and sheath incisions it is important to delineate the xiphisternum, umbilicus and pubic symphysis as midline landmarks. The skin is then incised with the umbilicus skirted. If there is a stoma *in situ* or planned, then the incision should be taken to the contralateral side. The incision is then continued through the subcutaneous fat until the linea alba is reached. This can be accurately identified by its decussating fibres. If there is difficulty in defining the linea, the first cut in the sheath should be close to the umbilicus which is always, itself, in the midline. A few millimetres of fat should be cleared from the sheath to ensure accurate identification of the layer on closure. The linea alba is placed under tension by elevating and separating the skin and subcutaneous tissues with the swab-covered hands of the operator and assistant. This not only facilitates division of the linea, but will reduce the potential danger of damage to underlying intraperitoneal viscera. In the upper two-thirds of the abdomen there may be a separate posterior sheath which will need division. The bulging extraperitoneal fat is swept clear. It often contains some troublesome vessels which are best coagulated before division. The peritoneum is then exposed, picked up between two fine haemostats, 'tented', and then incised. The smallest incision is followed by an inrush of air and allows the intra-abdominal contents to fall away. The incision in the peritoneum is completed using scissors – using the inside blade and fingers as elevators to further protect the underlying viscera.

Extension

When the midline incision is extended inferiorly to the pubic symphysis, care must be taken not to injure the bladder when dividing the lowermost peritoneum. Preoperative placement of a catheter is the best preventative measure, but if this has not been done then careful division under direct vision is mandatory.

Superior extension may involve the xiphisternum and this often results in a painful wound. Although many older manuals recommended skirting the cartilage it is probably less traumatic to divide it with heavy scissors. The resulting wound is said to be much more secure and less painful.

Paramedian

Suitability

The role of the rectus muscle in buttressing the closure of this type of incision was said to be a great advantage in the era of 'closure in layers'. With the advent of mass closure with high tensile monofilament sutures this is no longer a significant factor. On the contrary, the paramedian incision has the definite potential to denervate or devascularize the medial segment of the rectus muscle. In general the 'paramedian' is laborious, difficult to extend superiorly (limited by the costal margin) and does not give good access to contralateral structures. As a result of these disadvantages the paramedian incision, much used and beloved by many surgeons, has become unfashionable. It is still used, occasionally, for planned surgery to laterally placed structures – particularly the lateral paramedian variant.

Technique

The skin, subcutaneous fat and anterior sheath are all incised in a line two to three finger breadths from the midline (Fig. 13.2). (In the 'lateral' variant the incision is made one finger's breadth medial to the linea semilunaris.) The medial cut edge of the sheath is then elevated along its length with haemostats and the tendinous intersections released. This is best accomplished using a sharp scalpel blade and diathermy forceps to coagulate the vessels which cross at these points. The rectus muscle is then displaced laterally. In the lower abdomen care is taken to avoid avulsing or dividing the inferior epigastric vessels as they course lateromedially behind the muscle belly. An alternative quicker, but bloodier, method is to split the muscle in the line of the incision. The posterior sheath and peritoneum is then elevated and divided between haemostats and the peritoneal cavity is

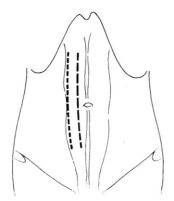

Fig. 13.2 A-A: Paramedian incision; B-B: lateral para-median incision.

entered through an incision in line with the original skin incision. In the upper abdomen the falciform ligament will be encountered at this point on the right side and it is safest to formally ligate and divide this structure to avoid later troublesome haemorrhage.

Transverse/oblique incisions

These incisions have limited flexibility and extensibility in the event of unexpected or remote pathology and are, therefore, usually reserved for elective operations where the precise location and procedure has been fully defined preoperatively. The incisions tend to lie in the natural skin creases or Langer's lines and achieve a much more acceptable cosmetic result.

Transverse

Suitability

Unilateral transverse incisions are appropriate for laterally placed viscera, e.g. right colon. They can be used for extraperitoneal approaches to the posterior abdominal wall, e.g. ureters, iliac vessels or sympathetic chain. Bilateral transverse incisions give excellent exposure for aortic surgery, and tend to be less painful postoperatively than long midline incisions. A very short right upper transverse incision has been used for gall bladder surgery – the minicholecystectomy. The incision is centred directly over the gall bladder and is no longer than 5–6 cm. No attempt is made to introduce the hand through the wound and good retraction and instrumentation is therefore vital to its success. The morbidity (e.g. pain and gastrointestinal upset) is minimized by the 'minimally invasive' technique and patients leave hospital and return to normal activity very rapidly.

Technique

The anterior sheath or external oblique is divided in

the line of the incision. The rectus muscle is best divided using a diathermy spatula with an assistant picking up the traversing vessels as they are encountered. More laterally the underlying internal oblique and transversus muscle may be split or cut. At this stage it is possible either to enter the peritoneal cavity or to develop the extraperitoneal plane laterally by mobilizing the peritoneum off the adherent transversus fascia.

Kocher's

This is classically described as an incision two finger breadths below and parallel to the costal margin. Its medial end is the midline and it extends laterally to the tip of the 9th costal cartilage (Fig. 13.3).

Suitability

On the right side this incision gives good access to the liver and biliary tract and on the left to the normal sized spleen. Its advantages include a sound and cosmetic result but is rather laborious to make and is very inflexible.

Technique

This is essentially a transverse muscle cutting incision, as described above, but carried out obliquely. Laterally the oblique muscles are carefully divided or split in order to try to identify and preserve the 9th, and occasionally the 8th, intercostal nerve branch.

Rooftop (Mercedes Benz)

This is a slightly more complex incision comprising two (left and right) less acutely angled Kocher incisions (see Fig. 13.4). It is particularly suitable for patients with a wide costal margin and for major liver, biliary or pancreatic surgery. The Mercedes Benz variant consists of bilateral low Kocher's incisions

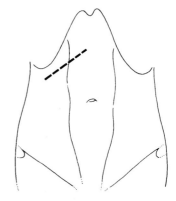

Fig. 13.3 Kocher's incision.

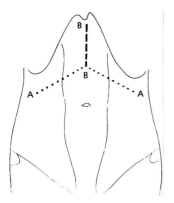

Fig. 13.4 A. . .A: Rooftop incision; B. . . .B: Mercedes Benz extension.

with an upper midline limb up to and through the xiphisternum (Fig. 13.4). This gives excellent access to all the upper abdominal viscera and, in particular, to all the diaphragmatic hiatuses. These incisions do involve considerable surgical trauma to the abdominal wall and an understandably poor cosmetic result. When making the incision it is useful to place strong sutures on the inferior margins of the midline incision which can then be used to retract the 'flaps' upwards and outwards, and also to aid correct apposition or wound closure.

Gridiron (McBurney)

Definition

Originally described by McBurney as 'an inch or so medial to the anterior superior iliac spine (ASIS) at right angles to a line drawn from the umbilicus to the ASIS' (Fig. 13.5).

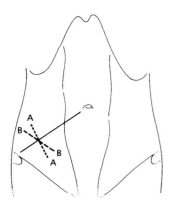

Fig. 13.5 A— —A: McBurney's incision; B— B: skin crease incision.

Suitability

This incision is principally used for appendicectomy. It is popular because the appendix can almost always be delivered even with quite small incisions and because it can easily be enlarged medially or laterally should difficulty or unexpected pathology be encountered. Many modifications exist and nowadays the incision is usually made along the lines of Langer – the 'skin crease' incision. It is centred on the point two-thirds along a line from the umbilicus to the ASIS (Fig. 13.5). The Lanz incision is also made in the skin crease, but is lower and is said to produce an improved cosmetic result. The muscle-splitting incision in either iliac fossa can be used to gain access to the peritoneal cavity for small procedures such as inserting a dialysis catheter or raising a loop stoma. It can be performed under local anaesthetic.

Technique

The exact position and length of incision will be determined by several factors including the site of maximal tenderness, the presence of a palpable mass and the size and obesity of the patient. The incision should be lateral to the rectus muscle (which can usually be palpated) and should lie in a skin crease. The skin, subcutaneous tissues and the external oblique are incised in the same line, and the internal oblique and transversus abdominis are split in the line of their fibres. This splitting is more easily accomplished by first making a small 'nick', as medially as possible, in the thin fascial covering of the internal oblique. Medially, the muscle bellies are at their thinnest and permit the insertion of the tips of straight Mayo scissors which can be gently opened until a glimpse of the white, glistening peritoneum is seen. Full splitting can then be achieved with the use of retractors or fingers. It is helpful to obtain good haemostasis prior to opening the peritoneum. Fine haemostats are used to 'tent' the peritoneum, which is then palpated between finger and thumb to ensure that underlying structures are distracted. The peritoneum is then incised between the haemostats in the line of the incision. It is helpful to place two further marker haemostats on the medial and lateral corners of the peritoneum to aid identification on closure, but these may need to be removed if the main procedure proves difficult.

Pfannenstiel

Definition

A transverse suprapubic incision parallel with the suprapubic skin crease and just below the 'hair line' (Fig. 13.6).

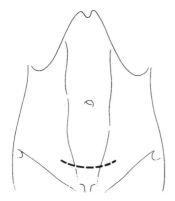

Fig. 13.6 Pfannenstiel incision.

Suitability

It provides excellent access to the pelvis – particularly the broader female pelvis. It is therefore the 'workhorse' incision of gynaecological surgery, but it also gives good access, extraperitoneally, to the bladder and prostate for urological surgery and to the groin hernial orifices for bilateral hernia repair. It gives excellent cosmetic results, but is limited by its inflexibility, particularly in cases where the diagnosis is in doubt.

Technique

The skin is incised in a downward convex arch in a suprapubic skin crease 2–3 cm above the pubic symphysis. The anterior sheath is divided in the line of the incision (or just above in order to improve the cosmetic result). The anterior sheath is reflected superiorly and any vessels coagulated. The recti are then separated in the midline and retracted laterally. At this stage the operator may open the peritoneum or develop the extraperitoneal plane. Should more lateral exposure be required, it is possible to divide the belly of the rectus muscle and extend the incision into the oblique muscles. There is said to be a higher incidence of Spighelian and groin hernias after this extension, but no good evidence exists for this.

Rutherford–Morrison (Astley Cooper)

Definition

This is an oblique, slightly curved, muscle-cutting incision in the left or right iliac fossa.

Suitability

It is very similar to the transverse incision, but is usually more obliquely placed and, therefore, per-

mits a more extensive craniocaudal access. It is useful in the difficult appendicectomy, limited hemicolectomies or approaches to retroperitoneal structures.

Technique

The main difference between the Rutherford–Morrison and a straightforward transverse incision is that the external oblique muscle is split and the internal oblique and transversus muscles are cut. Extension medially into the rectus sheath and muscle further improves exposure.

Laparoscopic access to the abdomen

GENERAL TECHNIQUES

Pneumoperitoneum

The ability to perform safe and effective laparoscopic surgery is dependent primarily on the establishment of an uncomplicated pneumoperitoneum. The procedure should be performed under general anaesthetic, with the airway intubated, ventilation and full muscle relaxation. The patient should have voided or be catheterized prior to draping. The skin should be more extensively prepared than for open surgery as widely or laterally placed ports may be needed.

Insufflation is introduced through a Veress or disposable pneumoperitoneum needle which is inserted 'blindly' through the anterior abdominal wall after incising the skin and subcutaneous fat. The most popular site for placement is just below the umbilicus as it is claimed that this is the easiest and safest entry point, and also because this is the most oft-used position for the laparoscopic port. There is a growing trend to use alternative sites – particularly the left upper quadrant. It is suggested that here one obtains a better 'feel' for the needle passing through the various layers of the abdominal wall. In the presence of existing scars it is advisable to insert the needle in 'virginal' territory pointing away from the potential underlying adherent structures. If the infraumbilical site is to be used for the laparoscopic port it is sensible to make a transverse 'smile' incision (1–1.5 cm) just below the umbilicus. It is helpful to tent up the skin and underlying peritoneum, and this can be achieved either by grasping these by hand, or by using sturdy tissue-holding forceps.

The patient is put in the Trendelenburg (head down) position, and the needle is inserted at a downward angle of 30–40° to the perpendicular. Two 'clicks' are felt as the needle passes through the rectus sheath and peritoneum. Confirmation that the needle tip is correctly positioned can be gained in several ways. Free side-to-side movement of the needle usually implies full passage through the abdominal wall without snaring on any underlying structure. The 'hanging drop' saline technique, or the combination of free flow and low pressure insufflation, both also indicate that the needle tip is positioned freely within the peritoneal cavity. Some experienced laparoscopists prefer an open technique of pneumoperitoneum production. This can be achieved by performing a very small laparostomy incision. A purse string suture ensures that after the trocar has been introduced, an air-tight seal can be effected. This technique is particularly suitable for patients who have undergone previous abdominal surgery and in whom serious adhesion problems are anticipated.

Alternatively, a blind incision into a highly tented peritoneal recess (usually at the umbilicus) can be made, with the trocar then being directly introduced. These open techniques are said to be safer because they avoid the need to introduce the first trocar blindly, and they also permit a more rapid establishment of the pneumoperitoneum because insufflation proceeds at a much faster rate.

The pioneering laparoscopists used room air as their insufflation gas – utilizing a sigmoidoscope bellows. Nowadays carbon dioxide is the gas of choice as it can be conveniently stored, is readily absorbed by the peritoneal membranes as well as being relatively inert. Between 3 and 6 litres of gas may be required to fully distend the peritoneal cavity. The exact amount will depend on the body habitus of the patient and the degree of muscle relaxation. Whatever the volume required, it is important that the pneumoperitoneum is tense prior to insertion of the trocars – particularly the first. The intraperitoneal pressure is monitored and should be maintained at between 12 and 15 mmHg, although it is suggested that it should be intermittently released to permit recovery of the venous return to the heart and normal intra-abdominal blood flow. At the end of the procedure it is important to release all the gas from the abdomen as this reduces the amount of postoperative shoulder pain. Some operators leave a suction drain through one of the small port sites to help complete the gas removal, but this is not common practice.

Operating theatre set-up

To facilitate eye to hand coordination it is suggested that the operator is positioned on the contralateral side to the operation site. The primary monitor is then placed in an extension of a direct line from the operator's head through the operation site on the other side of the table. The surgeon should, therefore, be looking

'down the line' of the laparoscope. Two further ports are almost always required – an 'operating' (usually 10–11 mm) and a 'manipulating' (5 mm) port. The flexibility and efficiency of dissection is optimized if the line down which these two ports operate is close to 90° to the line of laparoscopic vision (Fig. 13.7). An extra one or two 'retraction' ports may be needed to achieve the necessary exposure.

Trocar insertion

Insertion of the first (laparoscope) trocar should be the only time when a trocar is not placed under direct vision. This is, therefore, the stage at which most of the potential complications of laparoscopy may occur. The most common site for placement of the first trocar is subumbilically and the patient is tilted 'head down' to allow the mobile abdominal contents to fall away cranially. The dominant hand should always be used to insert the first trocar. This is placed in the palm of the hand with the back of the trocar against the thenar eminence, and the middle or index finger placed along the shaft as a safety precaution against rapid overinsertion. Having confirmed that the pneumoperitoneum remains tense, the trocar is directed downwards at 45° through the linea alba towards the pelvis, but clear of its brim. Driving the trocar through the abdominal wall is achieved with a simultaneous combination of a steady pushing and screwing action. Confirmation of its position within the peritoneal cavity can be gained by opening the gas inlet valve and listening for the outrush of gas. The

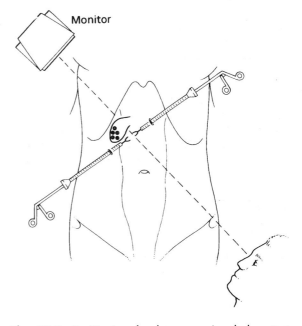

Fig. 13.7 Positioning for laparoscopic cholecystectomy.

warmed telescope is then introduced and a brief laparoscopy performed. The site of Veress needle and trocar insertion is inspected to exclude damage that may have been inadvertently caused in their introduction. The remaining trocars are then inserted in the direction in which they will be used, all under direct laparoscopic vision.

SPECIFIC LAPAROSCOPIC APPROACHES

Gall bladder

Access to the gall bladder and cystic duct relies on two principle manoeuvres. Firstly, upward retraction of the gall bladder and attached liver is produced by placing grasping forceps on the fundus and, second, by tilting the patient in reverse Trendelenburg and to the left. In this way the transverse colon, stomach and duodenum will fall away from the subhepatic space. Deflation and emptying of the stomach by placing a nasogastric tube further improves exposure and access but the tube should be removed at the end of the procedure.

Two main positions have been adopted to perform laparoscopic cholecystectomy. The first, most commonly used in the UK and USA, has the surgeon on the patient's left. The second, popular in continental Europe, has the patient in the 'Lloyd-Davies' position, with the operator between the legs looking up through the line of the laparoscope at the gall bladder area. The laparoscope port is usually placed infraumbilically but in larger, obese patients a supraumbilical port is better adopted. The operating port is inserted in the epigastrium a third of the distance from the xiphisternum to the umbilicus.

Appendix

The appendix and caecal pole are usually quite mobile and laparoscopic access and manipulation can be relatively straightforward. However, when the appendix is retrocaecal or inflamed, gaining access may prove very difficult. In general, the operator is on the patient's left with the laparoscope introduced through the umbilicus. A slight Trendelenburg and left-sided tilt, together with elevation and cranial retraction of the caecal port via a right upper quadrant port, all help to reveal the base of the appendix. Operating and manipulating ports can be placed according to the anatomical position of the appendix.

Oesophagus

Adequate exposure of the oesophagus and its hiatus can be difficult to produce at open surgery, even with the aid of a large incision and excellent retraction. It is an attractive idea, therefore, to try to gain access laparoscopically and antireflux surgery performed in this way is becoming increasingly popular. Some surgeons prefer to sit between the legs with the patient in the Lloyd-Davies position. In all cases 30–45° reverse Trendelenburg is needed to allow the abdominal viscera to fall away from the diaphragmatic recess. The laparoscopic port is introduced about 5 cm above the umbilicus in the midline, and operating and manipulating ports are inserted just below the xiphisternum and in the left subcostal region. It is helpful to insert two retracting ports. A fan retractor can be introduced through a right subcostal port to sweep the left lobe of the liver to the right. The stomach should be retracted downwards through a lateral left subcostal port.

Colon and pelvis

Access to the intra-abdominal and pelvic colon is relatively straightforward. In all cases a catheter should be placed to avoid bladder injury and to improve exposure. The laparoscope port is introduced through the umbilicus. For access to the left or right colon the patient should be tilted to the contralateral side and placed in the Trendelenburg position. Subcostal ports (left or right according to the side of the colon), provide access for grasping forceps which can then elevate and medially retract the colon to facilitate its mobilization. The operating port is most usually placed suprapubically, and additional ports placed as required.

For access to the pelvis more acute Trendelenburg tilt is required and all the ports are placed below the level of the umbilicus. The operating port can be suprapubic or in the left iliac fossa, and two further ports are placed just outside the line of the left and right linea semilunaris to allow retraction to either side.

References/further reading

1. Dudley H (ed.) *Rob and Smith's Operative Surgery. Alimentary Tract and Abdominal Wall. Volume 1 General Principles*, 4th edn. London: Butterworths, 1983.
2. Burnand KG, Young AE (eds) *The New Aird's Companion in Surgical Studies*. Edinburgh: Churchill Livingstone, 1992.
3. MacIntyre IMC (ed.) *Practical Laparoscopic Surgery for General Surgeons*. Oxford: Butterworth-Hennemann, 1994.
4. Rosin D (ed.) *Minimal Access General Surgery*. Oxford: Radcliffe Medical Press, 1994.

PART IV

Efficiency principles

CHAPTER 14

Design and safety of operating theatres

BRUCE P WAXMAN, ROBERT K WEBB

Introduction

The objectives of this chapter are to provide the information necessary to understand the principles involved in the design of operating theatres and to outline the responsibilites and duties of the surgeon, satisfying current standards of practice in the operating theatre environment that is safe for both the patient and health care workers. Aspects of design and safety emphasize mainly the role of a general surgeon operating on adult patients in a hospital with at least one operating theatre.

Sources of information are Australasian,[1] English[2] and Scandinavian[3] texts and the Australian Patient Safety Foundation, which has been managing an incident reporting system involving the collection of reports of problems occurring during anaesthethia in Australia for the past 5 years – the Anaesthetic Incident Monitoring Study (AIMS).[4] These data have provided many insights into what can go wrong in an operating theatre and what is necessary to prevent such problems occurring.[5] The data provide a strong case for a new approach to crisis management using algorithms with a well-rehearsed sequence of checks, rather than attempting logical analysis at a time of stress and distraction.[6] Most of the problems defined need a systems approach to solve them.[7]

Several documents provided by the Australian and New Zealand College of Anaesthetists are cited, but the standards recommended are internationally accepted.

For terminology of operating areas, we prefer the definitions of Brigden,[2] i.e. *operating department*: a unit of two or more operating suites and support accommodation; *operating suite*: comprises the operating theatre or operating room together with its immediate ancillary accommodation, anaesthetic room, preparation room, scrub-up area and utility room; and *operating theatre (room)*: in which surgical operations (tasks) and some diagnostic procedures are carried out. The chapter has two sections, one dealing with design, the other with safety, but there is considerable overlap.

Design of operating theatres

DESIGN BRIEF

In designing an operating department, preplanning using a system called *design brief* is necessary.[2] It is vital in the design brief for an operating department that clear identification of user requirements is sought. A well-constructed design briefing system is also important and includes a disciplined checklist approach, identifying the planning decisions which need to be made for every aspect of operating department design.

A project team responsible for the design brief needs to be multidisciplinary, keeping in mind that the facility needs to be designed both for patients and providers. There should be comfortable surroundings for the patients and the department should be not only efficient but also provide an enjoyable work environment for staff. It is vital that statutory regulations are adhered to.

The brief needs to take into account the functional content, size and location of the operating department including the scope of services, workload, any surgical specialities to be excluded and, in particular, whether laser surgery and endoscopy will be performed in the operating department.

The locality of the operating department is important, being on the same floor as the intensive care unit, and preferably also on the same floor as either the accident and emergency department or labour ward with easy access to the surgical wards, diagnostic laboratories and the imaging department.

The traditional concept of clean and dirty streams of traffic in the operating department has changed, and no longer are rigid restrictions on entry of personnel required.[8] The concept of four access zones has therefore developed[2] (see Fig. 14.1).

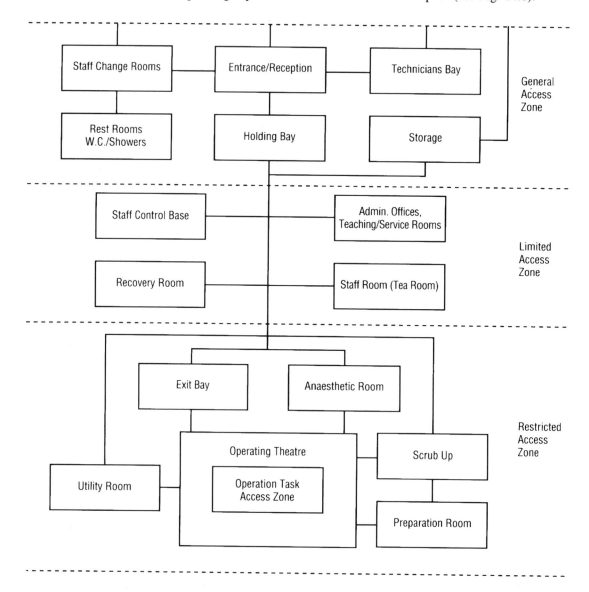

Fig. 14.1 Operating department access zones. (Adapted from ref. 8.)

1. *General access zone* where any authorized person entering the department is admitted; it includes the entrance, reception and patient transfer areas, and a general office area.

2. *Limited access zone* comprises the general circulation areas between the department entrance and operating suites, recovery staff base, staff rest rooms, storage areas and exit bays.

3. *Restricted access zone* is limited to persons appropriately attired and is directly related to activities in the operating suite.

4. *Operating zone* is defined as a zone which encompasses the operating area and the preparation room. The bacterial load can be reduced by reducing the number of persons in the operating zone and ensuring directed ventilatory air flow to the other access areas.

In addition to the access zones, it may be necessary to continue a 'red line policy', restricting flow of staff and patients between the different zones.

Transport to and from the operating department is most efficiently done on the patient's bed in preference to trolleys. This leads to a minimum number of transfers and reassures the patient, allaying anxiety being in one's own bed. This requires the need to provide sufficient doorway space throughout the operating department.

The provision for *supplies* needs to be considered including sterile supplies, pharmaceuticals, sutures, implantable devices, catering, clean linen and office equipment. A decision regarding the establishment of a theatre sterilizing servicing unit (TSSU), or relying on a central service (elsewhere in the hospital) is important. The latter is preferred. Sterilizing facilities within the operating department, including sterilizing of endoscopy equipment will be required in addition.

Consideration also needs to be given to: methods for disposal of 'sharps', dirty linen and other used equipment; facilities for administration and teaching (medical and nursing); catering services; provision of areas for cleaning, cleaners' rooms and associated plumbing; communication services with an efficient intercom or telephone system between operating theatres, and emergency alarm signals. A policy for the use of pagers, bleeps and mobile phones is necessary, but in general these are best kept at the reception desk. Direct telephone line service with outside line access is vital for all operating theatres.

Statutory regulations exist and design will need to comply with mandatory legislation. This particularly relates to fire safety regulations.

DESIGN SPECIFICATIONS AND CONSTRUCTION

General

The operating department is a unique part of the hospital and relatively expensive, involving approximately 6% of the hospital's budget; 60% of these costs relate to personnel, 30% to equipment and supplies.[3]

Determining the number of operating theatres is difficult and it should be remembered that a hospital with too few operating theatres is more efficient than one with too many. It is estimated that a hospital requires one operating theatre for every 25–50 general surgical beds and that approximately 0.1 operations are performed per bed per day. This is equivalent to approximately 1 hour of operating time per surgical bed per week, indicating that each operating theatre should perform approximately 65 operations per month. Mathematical models can be applied to make more accurate estimations of the requirements of operating theatres but this is beyond the scope of this text.[3]

All operating facilities in the hospital should ideally be centralized in the operating department, increasing efficiency and reducing costs with regard to staff, equipment and engineering.

Modern hospital design involves a low rise building of two to three storeys, which allows for better light, ventilation, internal courtyards or atria.

The operating department should be separate from the general traffic of the hospital, and from the air conditioning and ventilating plants to reduce airborne organisms and noise.

A recent concept in design is the modular operating suite, popular in Europe and the Middle East, designed to make maximum advantage of available space, and made from prefabricated sections on a hexagonal or square design (Fig 14.2).

Types of operating departments

Operating departments can be classed as one of three categories:

1. the single theatre suite with ancillary accommodation;
2. twin theatre suite with associated facilities;
3. operating department consisting of three or more operating suites with associated ancillary accommodation; in general, this would be best for most major teaching hospitals.

If there is a requirement for an operating department with eight or more theatres, serious consideration

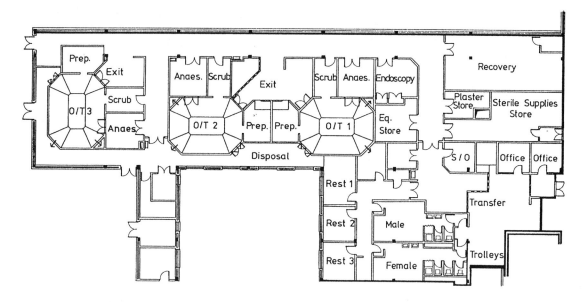

Fig. 14.2 A plan of a three operating theatre, pre-fabricated modular operating department (Haroldwood Hospital, North-East Thames Regional Health Authority). Medical Installations Co Ltd. (Adapted from ref. 2 with permission of the publisher and North-East Thames Regional Health Authority).

should be given to developing a separate operating department elsewhere in the hospital.

Construction and surfaces

This must be of a high standard of cleanliness, all surfaces being washable and all joins between walls, ceilings and floors curved to improve cleaning, with reinforced flooring to withstand considerable weight. Sprayed plastic skin or surfaces with epoxy resin paints are preferred. Ceramic tiles are porous and best avoided. A semi-matt finish is less reflective than gloss and light pale or pastel colours are preferred by the majority of staff.

Lighting

Where possible, daylight should be incorporated into the design with high level windows or borrowed light through corridors via glass doors. Windows should be triple glazed with the potential for blacking out. General lighting is provided by colour-corrected fluorescent lamps, giving even illumination of at least 500 lux, and requires the facility for dimming and complete blacking out (lux = an illumination of 1 lumen/m²; lumen (lm) = the luminous flux emitted within the solid angle at one steradian by a point source having a uniform intensity of one candela).

The choice of an operating luminaire ('theatre light') needs to take into account factors such as colour emitted, light intensity and pattern, shadow

reduction and the elimination of heat, and manoeuvrability.

Because the surgeon needs to differentiate between normal and diseased tissue and to perform tasks on materials with little colour contrast, the colour quality of the light must be in the region of 4000 kelvin (K). (Kelvin (K) = a unit of electrical energy equal to a kilowatt hour.) The density of light in the task area relates to the intensity of the light produced. The luminaire needs to have the capacity for 50 000–100 000 lux, being a metre from the task area, producing a light pattern of 20 cm diameter. The main reason for these high levels of brightness is that a large proportion of the light is simply absorbed and contributes little to visibility. The surgeon does not wish to work in shadows, but total shadow reduction is undesirable as the three-dimensional perception is lost. Shadow reduction is achieved by producing light at different angles. Heat is eliminated by dichroic reflectors (cold mirrors), absorbing reflectors and mirrors. As well as all this, the luminaire needs manoeuvrability to provide light from all sorts of angles.

Luminaires are either *multi-reflector* or *multi-lamp* types. The multi-reflector luminaires are either *scialytic*, a central lamp surrounded by a circle of glass mirrors which focuses the beam on to the task area, or metallic reflector type where the mirrors are metallic. The multi-lamp luminaires may either have a *cupola* housing (Fig. 14.3) or be separate on many *pode-mounted* supports.

Instrumental and head lights

The development of endoscopy and laparoscopy has involved the introduction of special light sources, necessary for this fibre optic equipment, for illumination and related video camera and monitors. A detailed discussion of this equipment is beyond the scope of this chapter.

An increasing number of surgeons are now using a headlight to produce better illumination of the task area and in some centres illuminated retractors with a similar light source to a head light producing a good quality of light deep in a body cavity.

Pendant services

Pipeline services in the operating theatre are best provided by ceiling-mounted pendants to minimize hazards of trailing leads, one for the surgical team and one for the anaesthetic team. The pendants ideally should be retractable, manoeuvrable and with lateral movement, and have shelf space for monitors

(Fig 14.3). The surgical pendant should include 10-bar medical compressed air, medical vacuum outlets, and at least four electrical socket outlets.

The anaesthetic pendant should include oxygen, nitrous oxide, 4-bar medical compressed air, medical vacuum and gas scavenging terminal outlets, and at least four electrical socket outlets[2].

Ventilation

The ventilation system provided in the operating department has three major functions:

1. to control temperature and humidity;
2. to dilute contamination by airborne micro-organisms and expired anaesthetic gases;
3. to provide air movement so that transfer of micro-organisms goes from clean areas to less clean areas.

This is achieved by the supply of heated or cooled, humidified, clean air to the operating suite with aero-

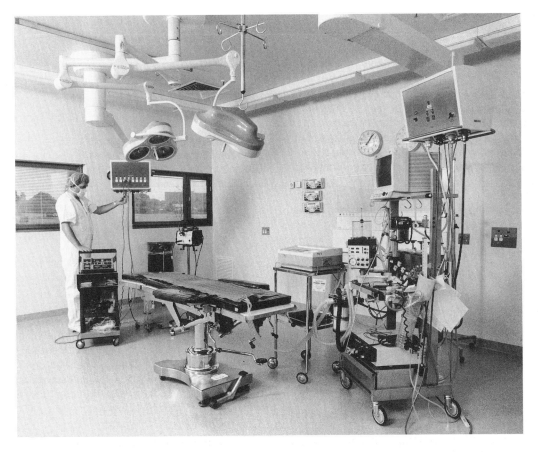

Fig. 14.3   A typical modern operating theatre featuring cupola luminaire system, ceiling-mounted pendant with elbow joint and natural lighting (Monash Medical Centre Operating Department, Clayton Campus, Australia).

bic counts less than 35 micro-organism carrying particles/mm^3. The optimal environment should be a compromise between staff comfort and patient needs. The patient is very susceptible to hypothermia as a consequence of the general anaesthetic which reduces muscle activity and causes vasodilatation and loss of body heat by ventilation, and also cooling by the influx of fluids and gases. The optimal temperature in the operating theatre is 20–22°C with a humidity of 40–60%.[8]

There are three types of ventilation systems installed in operating departments:

1. The *plenum turbulent airflow system* which is used in almost all non-orthopaedic operating theatres, involves air being drawn at the roof level by a series of fans and filters, humidified, cooled or heated and ducted into the operating suite through high level diffusers fitted into the walls or ceilings. The air pressure in the operating suite is always greater than the rest of the department, being highest in the preparation room (35Pa) and least in the utility and disposal area (−5 or 0 Pa). The air flows from the ceiling to the floor and through cracks around and under the doors to the different rooms, providing 20–30 air changes per hour (AC/h) at a velocity of 0.1–0.3 m/s.[8] Fifteen air changes per hour are necessary for the control of anaesthetic gas pollution. The operating theatre doors are best kept closed as open doors and movement of personnel, trolleys and beds in and out of theatre significantly disturb the air flow and the efficiency of the ventilation system. Although a well-maintained ventilation system can dilute atmospheric pollutants, a 'scavenging system' is recommended to remove expired anaesthetic gases and this is connected to the expiratory port of the anaesthetic breathing system to the scavenging connection on the anaesthetic pendant. Even so there is danger to female personnel, working within a metre of the anaesthetic equipment, of miscarriage during the first trimester of pregnancy.

   It is vital for quality checks to be maintained on the ventilation system by checking filters and by microbiological analysis of the operating suite air.

2. The *ultra clean ventilation (UCV) system* with 500–600 AC/h through laminar or unidirectional flow of air from an efficient filter removing inherent contamination, flowing at such a velocity to reduce eddies and turbulence. Air flow may either be vertical or horizontal. The advantage of this system is the reduction of bacterial contamination for joint replacement, high risk vascular surgery and in transplantation. The vertical system is preferred. The disadvantages of both types of this system are the noise and the high velocity of air.[9]

3. *High input/high exhaust enclosures* were developed by the orthopaedic surgeon Sir John Charnley in 1961[10,11] and later modified by an engineer, Howorth.[12] This method combines UCV with an enclosure that surrounds the operating team. Charnley also developed a body exhaust system (BES) to remove contaminated body convection currents, exhaled air and skin particles. Combined with prophylactic antibiotics, these systems have been shown to reduce wound and prosthesis infection significantly, but haematogenous seeding of prostheses remains a problem.[13]

Access zones (see Fig 14.1).

General access zones

Entrance

Operating departments should have a single main entrance with alternative access for staff change via an electrical security system with ID card entry. All patient movements should be visible from reception and additional space should be provided for a theatre technician (porter) base.

Reception

This is the central hub of the operating department and should contain the area for general clerical and administrative work, communication centre, and space for computer equipment and TV monitors.

Staff changing rooms

Changing rooms should be available for males and females, with sanitary facilities and lockers adequately ventilated. Toilets and showers should be separate from these changing facilities.

Disposal hold

An area set aside for the temporary holding of soiled dressings, linen and rubbish.

Limited access zone

Staff control base

This is separate but adjacent to reception and comprises the office of the nurse director/medical director of the operating department. There should be good visual access to reception and holding area, and preferably also to recovery. It includes a station for the alarms and must have communication with all the operating theatres by telephone and/or closed circuit television.

Recovery (post-anaesthetic recovery)

This is a mini operating suite in itself, whose importance has only been realized in recent years.

Two beds should be provided for each operating theatre and should be close to reception and the staff control base. Each bed should be provided with either wall-mounted or ceiling-mounted piped oxygen, medical vacuum, 4-bar medical compressed air, electrical sockets and nitrous oxide plus a gas scavenging system. Space should be provided for monitoring equipment, including ECG and pulse oximetry. The general lighting should be similar to the operating theatre and mobile spotlighting should be provided. There should be a staff base area, a utility room and disposal area, cleaning room and also space for extra monitoring equipment and resuscitation equipment.

Rest (tea) room

This area provides rest accommodation for staff and should have natural light and comfortable seating, with provision for minor short meal breaks with beverages and light snacks. Vending food and drink machines should be available and also access to the main kitchen for hot meals. A pantry is usually adjacent to the rest rooms. In North America, the 'surgeons' lounge' is very popular and is usually separate from the rest room provided for the nursing staff, and allows access for medical staff from the general hospital areas as well as the operating department.

Offices/seminar rooms/teaching facilities

These need to be provided for senior operating department nursing and medical staff as are facilities for teaching. A room for dictating should be available for medical staff.

The operating department needs to be seen as a teaching facility. Adequate rooms and appropriate teaching facilities are vital and may include provision for video transmission from the operating theatre to elsewhere in the operating department or hospital.

Storage

Space must be provided for sterile instruments and to pack equipment and gas bottles and also for cleaning. Most equipment is best stored on shelves rather than in cupboards.

Restricted access area

Anaesthetic room

This should be designed with a similar hygienic finish to the operating theatre, being at least 15 m^2 and with shelving for all the appropriate equipment. A pendant or wall-mounted pipeline for oxygen, compressed air and medical vacuum is necessary. This room serves many useful purposes: as a safe, quiet place for the patient to wait; for allowing increased patient turnover; and as an area to supervise trainees, perform local and regional anaesthesia, and insert lines without disturbing traffic flow into the operating theatre.[14]

Operating theatre

This should be at least 38 m^2 but should be larger where it is used for laparoscopic surgery. In addition to pendants, ventilation and lighting, other requirements include: shelving for writing notes, communications, and other clerical duties, X-ray boxes, and record boards for pack counts. Doors should be of adequate size to allow easy access of hospital beds and all equipment in the operating theatre should be made of stainless steel or aluminium for a hygienic finish and ease of clenaing.

Exit bay

There should be a separate route for the patient, other than the anaesthetic room, allowing rapid transfer of the patient to the recovery room.

Scrub up and gowning area

This should be immediately adjacent to the operating theatre but in a separate area. The troughs and taps should be hygienic with either elbow-operated taps or a light sensor activated system. The gowning area should be as far away as possible from the troughs.

Preparation room

This room should be of sufficient size to allow two staff and two trolleys. Ideally, sterile instruments, packs and drapes will arrive in pre-set tray packs from the sterilizing department. The doorway should be wide, allowing easy entry and egress. Shelving should be provided for easy storage of equipment. Separate trolleys may be set up with equipment relevant to the specialty of the surgeon and may include a book of likes and dislikes of each surgeon.

Utility room

This room should be directly adjacent to the operating theatre. It is an area for disposal of sharps, dirty linen and any other infectious material. Pathological and laboratory specimens may also be processed in this area.

Safety of operating theatres

STAFF RESPONSIBILITIES AND ORGANIZATION

Responsibilities

The majority of operations are performed under general anaesthesia and patients are unable to protect themselves. The onus, therefore, falls on all staff in the operating department to leave nothing to chance and to ensure that safety aspects of all tasks are continually kept in mind with ongoing evaluation and re-evaluation. Reducing the patient's anxiety should be a high priority.

The Australian and New Zealand College of Anaesthetists has produced a document which outlines the minimum facilities necessary for the safe conduct of anaesthesia in an operating department, addressing important issues such as staffing, equipment, infrastructure and process.[15]

The operating department is probably the most hazardous part of the hospital with a variable workload and staff working under stress requiring great concentration and little relaxation. The surgeon, however, is ultimately responsible for all aspects of the patient's care and related complications that may occur in the operating department.

The surgeon, therefore, needs to follow good principles in performing his or her craft:

1. Ensure appropriate senior qualification, recognized by the national specialist regulatory body and college.
2. Operate in an accredited hospital where staff and facilities are beyond reproach.
3. Be satisfied that the surgical team is efficient.
4. Only perform a procedure that is within the surgeon's capabilites, and elicit the help of surgical colleagues when there is any potential doubt or difficulty with a particular case.
5. Obtain appropriate informed consent from the patient.
6. Have adequate indemnity insurance cover.

It is the surgeon's responsibility with regard to any particular patient to:

1. Interview the patient preoperatively and ensure appropriate preoperative tests have been performed.
2. Be sure it is the right patient.
3. Be sure it is the correct operation.
4. Ensure that it is the correct side, limb or digit that is being operated upon.
5. Ensure blood and blood products are available if appropriate.
6. Arrange the availability of appropriate ancillary staff as necessary, e.g. radiological services.

The key to success is good preparation, good communication and no assumptions. This is particularly relevant to relationships between the anaesthetist and the surgeon, who should be in constant consultation throughout the perioperative period.

Organization

The operating department is administratively similar to any other hospital department, requiring a well-defined organizational structure with appropriate numbers of directors and subordinates. These numbers will depend upon the size and diversity of the department.

Ideally there is a Medical Director of the operating department, who is usually the Director of Anaesthesia, although there is an increasing trend towards the development of the position of Director of Theatre Services, who is usually an anaesthetist and often is a separate appointment to the Director of Anaesthesia.

The responsibilities of the director are to ensure prompt and efficient services, maintain safety standards and supervise the competence and appointment of staff, the purchase of new equipment and servicing routines.

The medical staff working in the operating department should possess appropriate training and skills in either anaesthesia[16,17] or surgery, and should have ongoing maintenance of those skills with appropriate continuing education.[18]

There needs to be clearly defined and publicized lines of communication between the staff working in the operating department and the director. Regular meetings should be scheduled to provide opportunities to discuss, in a non-threatening and informal manner, problems that have occurred within the work environment.[19]

There should be an established incident monitoring system to provide a mechanism for finding out what is going wrong within the system, and then mechanisms put in place to solve those problems.[4,20,21]

Operating theatre staff

The minimum staff required for any particular operation within the operating theatre should include the anaesthetist, an anaesthetic nurse who is soley responsible to the anaesthetist and able to assist in crises,[22] surgeon, surgical assistant, scrub nurse, scout nurse assisting the scrub nurse, and a theatre technician (orderly). All members of the operating theatre staff should be appropriately trained with facilities for further education. The technical staff should be experienced in all aspects of equipment used and any ancillary services such as gas supplies, electricity, suction and scavenging.[23]

There must be a mechanism for summoning extra experienced staff in the event of an emergency.

Maintenance of standards and quality assurance

As well as the *theatre subcommittee* responsible for the ongoing functions of the operating department, other committees need to be established, including a *credentials committee* to assess the qualifications and experience of anaesthetists and surgeons in performing new procedures, a *staff selection committee* and *electoral college committee* to elect new staff, an *accreditation committee* to ensure the standards of the operating department fit within statutory regulations and quality assurance, and an *audit committee* to monitor the ongoing performance and follow-up.

Staff numbers

Mathematical models can be used to estimate staff and theatre requirements based on the Godber Staffing Unit and the Erlang Unit of Traffic Intensity.[1] Taylor has used the queuing theory to estimate anaesthetic staff requirements for the emergency theatre.[24]

PATIENT HANDLING AND ASSESSMENT

Identification

The most efficient form of identification is a wrist band which should include the patient's surname, first name and initial, unit record number and date of birth.

Problems can arise: where there is failure to label the patient adequately on admission; if the wrong notes accompany the patient; if identification is attached to clothing and not to wrist; and when the order of the operating list is changed.

Correct side/limb

The surgeon should develop a routine when visiting the patient preoperatively, to mark the site of the operation with a permanent marker pen, indicate clearly in the notes and on the consent form the exact side by writing 'right' or 'left' *in full*, and with fingers to refer to these *by name*, e.g. index finger rather than number.

X-rays and scans

No assumption should be made regarding labelling of X-rays or scans and it is the surgeon's responsibility to check that the patient's name is adequately displayed and the correct side is interpreted appropriately.

Consent

It is the surgeon's responsibility to make sure the patient understands the principles involved in the operation and the common complications, and that this is also explained to a relative or guardian. Difficulty arises with unconscious patients and children. The surgeon should be aware of the difference between implied, verbal and written consent.

Preoperative assessment

This is the dual responsibility of the surgeon and anaesthetist. The surgeon will have, in most cases, seen the patient in the outpatient clinic or consulting room/office, performed a history, physical examination and ordered appropriate special investigations, and made an appropriate booking for the operation. Other preoperative precautions have been indicated above. The surgeon should also consider developing a series of illustrated brochures, or purchasing these from appropriate professional bodies, that explain the disease, the operation and the common complications to the patient. One should develop the habit of making notes that an explanation of the operation, complications and cost have been explained to the patient. A simple checklist is helpful.

With the move to a more efficient throughput of patients in the hospital setting, particularly in the environment of diagnostic-related groups (DRGs) and case-mix, increasing use is being made of *preoperative assessment clinics*, usually supervised by anaesthetists, and *preadmission clinics*, usually supervised by the surgical team with anaesthetic consultation. A combined preadmission clinic is ideal.[25] The patients are usually seen a week before their operation and all the documentation is completed, including any other tests felt necessary by the anaesthetist. Indeed, a full admission (clerking) can occur at this time, allowing the patient to be admitted on the day of surgery. Moreover, preparations can be made for postoperative care, including discharge planning, general practitioner follow-up, district nurse and community welfare services and relevant placement.

The preoperative visit is becoming redundant as a result of the above procedures. However, in some patients with complex medical problems, admission on the day before surgery is necessary. At the preoperative visit the anaesthetist can find out the particular concerns of the patient, discuss the various options available for general anaesthesia or regional anaesthesia, and decide upon the best technique that suits the needs of both patient and surgeon.

A standard preoperative checklist is completed by nursing staff on the ward and this is checked again by nursing staff when the patient arrives in the operating department.

Emergency admissions provide a challenge for the operating team, but the same principles apply.

Premedication

This is prescribed for a number of reasons, mainly to reduce anxiety, pain and secretions. There has been a trend in recent times away from the use of combined narcotic and drying and antivagal agents, to the use of oral sedatives. There is, however, a swing back to traditional premedication, particularly for day surgery.

Transport and handling

The majority of patients will be delivered to the operating department in their beds. The operating table is, however, a much harder and narrower surface than the bed and contains metallic appendages.

The physiological effects of general anaesthesia and muscle relaxation reduce the response to external stimuli and also cough reflexes and muscle tone, and the joints are much more mobile. The shivering response is lost and the patient is more susceptible to hypothermia and loss of vascular tone reduces the response to postural change. It is important to consider these changes when positioning the patient on the operating table.

Methods to overcome some of these problems include:

1. Monitor the vital functions of airway and breathing.
2. Provide a soft ripple mattress (Fig. 14.3).
3. Take care in transferring the patient from bed to operating table, avoiding excessive movements of joints, particularly shoulders and hips, especially when placing patients in the prone position.
4. Keep the patient either horizontal or head down.
5. Protect bony prominences from nerve entrapment.
6. Reduce heat loss by covering exposed limbs and by the routine use of a warming blanket (Fig. 14.3).

Transferring from bed to table

Many devices have been used for this process. For a conscious patient the simplest approach is simply to ask them to slide across on to the table. In other cases, roller slides and mechanical lifters are available. In moving the unconscious patient, at least three members of staff should be available to perform this task.

In general the operating table should have a stable base, be properly earthed, have wheels that move freely, be easily manoeuvrable and have a positive locking system.

The general principles which apply for positioning the patient on the operating table include:

1. Avoid pressure on joints, nerves, arteries and veins.
2. No metallic contact with the skin, especially the diathermy plate.
3. No forced movements of any joints after general anaesthetic induction.
4. Avoid rapid movements of limbs, and return the patient to normal anatomical position in a slow and steady manner.

5. After transfer, check all attachments to the patient remain intact.
6. Ensure adequate neck support during transfer and lifting.
7. Ensure patients have no sharp jewellery by removing or taping this preoperatively.

Specific positions

Supine (Fig.14.4)

The arms are best placed beside the body or, if on an arm board, at less than 90° at the shoulder joints. Pressure on the calves is avoided by placing a soft support under the ankles. When using a head screen, avoid contact with the shoulders and neck.

Trendelenburg (Fig 14.5)

In this position there is a tendency for the patient to slip off the table and brachial plexus injuries may occur from shoulder pads used to prevent the slip. The physiological changes of increased venous return, difficulty in ventilation, and tendency for the endotracheal tube to slip in the right main bronchus should be remembered.

Problems are reduced by: keeping the tilt to a minimum; using a corrugated mattress to reduce slipping; ensuring the shoulder rests are padded; and placing the arms by the side or over the chest. In the latter case avoid letting the elbows hang over the sides.

Prone jack-knife (Fig. 14.6)

The dangers of this position include compression of the chest and reduced respiration and ventilation, with fixity of the abdominal contents. In addition there is pressure on joints of the pelvis, back and neck, com-

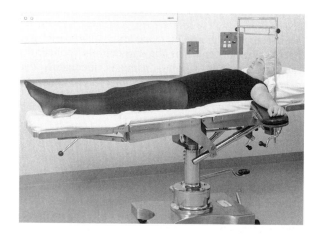

Fig. 14.4   Supine position on operating table.

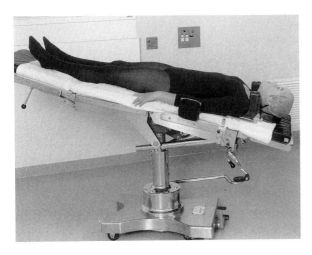

Fig 14.5 Trendelenburg position on operating table.

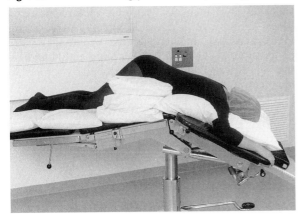

Fig. 14.6 Modified prone jack-knife position on operating table.

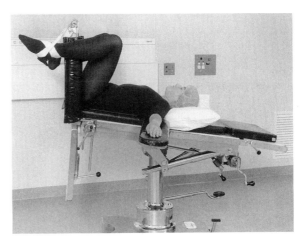

Fig. 14.7 Lithotomy position.

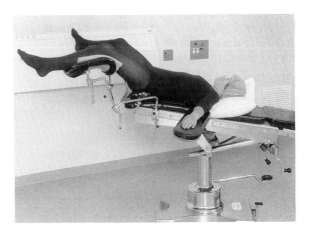

Fig. 14.8 Lloyd-Davies position for combined abdominoperineal procedures.

pression on the inferior vena cava and potential problems with the hands during the turning process.

These problems are avoided by controlled ventilation, use of an inverted U-sausage support, multiple pillows or a specially designed cylindrical plastic covered mattress roll. Furthermore, the body should be positioned with the head turned to one side and the hands and arms supported on arm boards with the patient in the so-called 'sunbathing' position. The body should then be strapped with adhesive tape to the operating table to avoid slipping.

Lithotomy/Lloyd-Davies[26] (Figs 14.7, 14.8)

The dangers of this position are: compression of the perineal nerve by the stirrups; compression of the medial aspect of the calf; strain on the sacroiliac joints; decreased vital capacity; together with decreased circulation to the legs and feet.

These problems can be avoided by placing the legs outside the lithotomy poles, using padding to protect the perineal nerve and to prevent contact of the limbs with the metal parts of the supports. The anterosuper-

ior iliac spine should be positioned at the level of the break of the table. The feet should then be fixed in straps, and during long colorectal cases, the exposed limbs covered with insulating sheets. After the procedure, the feet are returned to the anatomical position in a slow and controlled manner, the calves massaged, and pedal pulses checked to make sure there is adequate perfusion.

Lateral/kidney position (with bridge) (Fig. 14.9)

The dangers of this position are pressure on the underneath arm and the nerves of the top arm, a shift of the pelvis in relation to the body, reduced vital

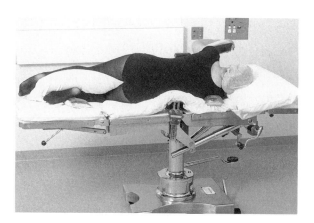

Fig. 14.9 Lateral or kidney position.

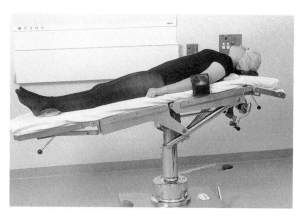

Fig. 14.10 Neck or thyroid position.

capacity with impaired ventilation:perfusion ratio in the lungs.

These problems can be avoided by placing the upper arm on a well padded support and by using a padded bridge over the operating table and a soft support in the axilla. The lower leg should be flexed and the upper leg extended and separated with a pillow.

Head/thyroid position (Fig. 14.10)

The danger of this position is excessive hyperextension of the neck. This is avoided by placing a sand bag under the shoulder and an adequate sized head ring under the head.

There are many other possible positions used in other surgical specialties, especially in neurosurgery and orthopaedics.

Care for other body parts

Eyes

The corneal reflex is lost and the eyes are best kept closed with tape or in prolonged procedures, particularly in neurosurgery, covered with a vaseline ointment.

Lips and teeth

The lips are best protected by vigilance and the teeth by the judicious removal of false teeth and bridge work in the operating theatre, documentation of any loose teeth, and the rapid recovery of any inhaled or dislodged teeth by bronchoscopy or oesophagoscopy.

Hypothermia/hyperthermia

Protocols and routines should be established in all operating departments to avoid these complications.

Hypothermia is reduced by the use of electric and water-diffused blankets, warming all infusions and gases, taking care to cover all exposed parts during long operations, maintaining the operating theatre temperature at 20–22°C and warming and humidifying all gases. Children are particularly prone to hypothermia.

It is the anaesthetist's responsibility to question the patient regarding family history of malignant hyperthermia and to be aware of the appropriate protocols for its management should it occur.

Deep venous thrombosis

Prevention has become routine in most operating departments with the use of Faradic calf stimulation and some form of anticoagulation, either low dose heparin, or oral warfarin. Both may be complemented by the use of graduated compression (TED) stockings.

Tourniquets

The danger with tourniquets is that they may be left on too long, leading to venous thrombosis, arterial ischaemia and gangrene. These may lead to subsequent shock and renal failure secondary to myoglobulin release into the circulation when the tourniquet is let down. When the tourniquet is too tight there may be associated skin, nerve and arterial damage at the site of the tourniquet.

These problems can be avoided by elevating the limbs to 90° or by the use of an Esmarch bandage to exsanguinate the limb. The skin under the tourniquet should be protected with a cotton wool circular bandage; and the tourniquet time never allowed to exceed 2 hours. The surgeon should reassure himself and his assistant at the end of the procedure that there has been adequate return of circulation and should document the tourniquet time. When a crepe bandage is applied after the release of the tourniquet, that part of the limb must be exposed to assess circulation subsequently.

Should the patient complain of pain, the bandage must be assumed to be too tight and must be removed.

Laboratory specimens

A policy for handling laboratory specimens is important as if these are lost or damaged this can lead to false diagnosis, delay in treatment, difficulty in assessing prognosis and the possibility of unnecessarily repeated surgery. Specimens should be appropriately documented in the operation register, in a specimen book provided in the operating department and also recorded in the operation notes.

Induction

Induction can be a particularly hazardous part of the anaesthetic. This would appear to be the time at which all equipment which had not been properly checked makes itself known. It is also the time at which problems with ventilation and intubation will be discovered.[27–29] A dedicated trolley is required, easily accessible, which contains all the appropriate equipment for difficult intubation. Plans for dealing with a patient who cannot be intubated or ventilated must be considered beforehand and appropriate equipment made available.[27] Monitoring equipment for oxygen and end-tidal CO_2 have become routine,[30,31] particularly the $EtCO_2$ monitor (capnograph) which ensures that the endotracheal tube is in the lungs and not the oesophagus. With the increasing trend towards pre-oxygenation, the patient can maintain a normal oxygen saturation for several minutes after oesophageal intubation,[28] and this complication is therefore less likely to be considered to be the cause of desaturation.

Local and regional anaesthesia

Although this is an alternative to general anaesthesia, it is important that patients should be worked up as if they might require a general anaesthetic as this may become necessary at any time during the regional procedure. It is also important to remember that the physiological trespass caused by a regional anaesthetic may be greater than that of general anaesthesia. It is a common misconception that if a patient is very ill, they can always withstand a local or regional anaesthetic.

Intraoperative care and monitoring

The minimum requirements for adequate monitoring of the circulation and respiratory system are well documented[32] and include an oxygen supply failure alarm, an oxygen analyser, pulse oximeter, alarm for breathing system disconnection or ventilatory failure, an ECG, together with monitoring of temperature, carbon dioxide and neuromuscular function. Other equipment as clinically indicated may also be required.

A protocol must be in place to govern the handling, replacement and filling of vaporizers. The AIMS together with other data have demonstrated that disconnection of the patient breathing circuit is a very common event during anaesthesia.[21,33,34] The consequences are obvious. Two independent monitors are needed to detect such a problem, the most common being the disconnection alarm and the capnograph. The pulse oximeter will eventually detect the disconnection by virtue of the fact that the patient becomes desaturated.

The ECG, though a traditional monitor, has proven of limited value in detecting problems early in their evolution, despite significant physiological trespass by the anaesthetist.[35]

Recovery

After completion of the operation, extubation and return to the bed, the monitoring and re-evaluation procedure continues in the recovery department.[23]

Instruments, packs and tubes

The surgeon is ultimately responsible for the counting of instruments, packs and drain tubes. The medico-legal aspects are obvious and the most common grounds for litigation by patients are either retained packs and instruments or operations performed on the wrong side.[1] With regard to the former, the most common is retained packs, followed by drainage tubes, then artery forceps. Most of these have been left in the peritoneal cavity. It is vital that there is a policy for an accounting system for packs and swabs, and that all these have radio-opaque markers. The surgeon should communicate closely with the scrub nurse during the counting procedure and assist the nurse at these times.

The problem of glove powder contamination of the peritoneal cavity has become recognized so that it has now become routine either to wash glove powder off before commencing surgery, or to use powderless gloves.

ACCIDENTS TO OPERATING DEPARTMENT STAFF

Although the most common accidents are musculo-skeletal injuries, the major concern amongst staff in the operating department is transfer of infection of blood-borne viruses, particularly human immunodeficiency virus (HIV), hepatitis B and hepatitis C.

It has become routine in the majority of operating departments to develop a policy of universal precautions with the use of eye protection and plastic aprons together with double gloving and plastic forearm protectors in known infected cases. Other routines include the development of a 'no-man's land' area on the operating table to avoid needlestick and sharp injuries; the routine use of a kidney dish lined with a pack containing either needles or scalpels; the abandonment of hand-held needles; and the introduction of blunted needles, particularly for fascial closure and the use of staples rather than needles for skin closure.

All operation department staff should receive active immunization for hepatitis B.

Accident prevention is an important principle in the operating department. Well-defined procedures, incident reporting with debriefing, safeguards against staff fatigue and regular maintenance of equipment are all important.[19]

TECHNICAL EQUIPMENT AND COMPLICATIONS

Electrical equipment

Electric current is either direct–unidirectional (DC) (e.g. battery) or alternating–oscillating at a fixed frequency (AC) (e.g. power lines). Most electrical equipment in the operating theatre is powered by AC but should have a DC back-up. AC supplies must comply with local regulations. AC current is much more harmful than DC, and should have isolated circuits.

In general, electric current should stay confined to the circuit in which it is intended to work. Leaks from that circuit may cause shock and ventricular fibrillation, interference with instruments, explosions when in contact with flammable gases and also burns.[36]

The electrosurgical unit (diathermy) has the greatest potential for electric mishap. The unipolar being more hazardous than the bipolar, as current returns via the patient and a wide surface of contact on the return pad is vital to prevent burns.[1]

Electrical failure

A back-up supply must be installed to provide adequate power supply in the event of failure at the main power service so that all essential equipment in the operating department can be kept functioning. This back-up system must be regularly tested to ensure appropriate operation when required. A plan must also be in place in the case of failure of the back-up system. All essential monitors should have inbuilt battery back-up.

Fire

A fire in the operating department can cause patient death, staff injuries and loss of equipment apart from legal damage for the hospital involved. The three most common ignition sources are lasers, electrical-corded equipment and high intensity power cords. The best method of fighting a fire is to avoid having one, and emphasis should be placed on prevention. Every operating department education programme should include elements of a fire plan that is consistent with the plan for that hospital.[37]

Operating theatre maintenance

To maintain a high standard of safety all operating theatres should be serviced on a monthly basis. The maintenance team should include an engineer, electrician, anaesthetic technician and plumber, fitter and turner, carpenter and microbiologist.

Summary

The operating department is a complex and potentially hazardous part of the hospital. The principles of good preparation, good communication and quality assurance are relevant to all aspects of operating deprtment design and safety to avoid any problems or complications in the provision of a high standard of health care for our patients.

References

1. Mainland JE, Dudley HAF (eds) *Safety in the Operating Theatre*. Melbourne: Edward Arnold/ The Royal Australasian College of Surgeons, 1976.
2. Brigden RJ (ed.) *Operating Theatre Technique*. Edinburgh: Churchill Livinstone, 1988.
3. Putsep E (ed.) Operation Department. In: *Modern Hospital: International Planning Practices*. London: Lloyd-Luke, 1981: 508–86.
4. Webb RK, Currie M, Morgan CA *et al*. The Australian Incident Monitoring Study: an analysis of 2000 incident reports. *Anaesthes Intens Care* 1993; **21**: 520–8.
5. Runciman WB, Sellen A, Webb RK *et al*. Errors, incidents and accidents in anaesthetic practice, *Anaesthes Intens Care* 1993; **21**: 506–19.
6. Holland R. Symposium – The Australian Incident Motoring Study. *Anaesthes Intens Care* 1993; **21**: 501–5.
7. Runciman WB, Webb RK, Lee R, Holland R. System failure: an analysis of 2000 incident reports. *Anaesthes Intens Care* 1993; **21**: 684–95.

8. Humphreys H. Infection control and the design of a new operating suite. *J Hosp Infec* 1993; **23**: 61–70.

9. Department of Health and Social Security (UK). *Requirements for Ultra-Clean Ventilation (UCV) Systems for Operating Departments*. London: HMSO, 1986.

10. Charnley J. A clean-air operating enclosure. *Br J Surg* 1964; **51**: 202–5.

11. Lidwell O. Sir John Charnley, Surgeon (1911–81): the control of infection after total joint replacement. *J Hosp Infec* 1993; **23**: 5–15.

12. Howorth FH. Prevention of airborne infection in operating rooms. *J Med Eng Technol* 1987; **11**: 263–6.

13. Lidwell OM, Elson RA, Lowbury EJL. Ultraclean air and antibiotics for prevention of postoperative infection. *Acta Orthop Scand* 1987; **58**: 4–13.

14. Meyer-Witting M, Wilkinson DJ. A safe haven or a dangerous place – should we keep the anaesthetic room? *Anaesthesia* 1992; **47**: 1021–2.

15. Australian and New Zealand College of Anaesthetists. *Recommended Minimum Facilities for Safe Anaesthetic Practice*, Policy Document Review T1. Melbourne: ANZCA, 1995.

16. Australian and New Zealand College of Anaesthetists. *The Supervision of Trainees in Anaesthesia*, Policy Document Review E3. Melbourne: ANZCA, 1994.

17. Faculty of Anaesthetists, RACS. *Privileges in Anaesthesia*, Faculty Policy Review P2. Melbourne: FARACS, 1991.

18. Australian and New Zealand College of Anaesthetists. *Maintenance of Standards: Programme Guidelines Bulletin*, Vol. 3, August. Melbourne: ANZCA, 1994: 10–11.

19. Runciman WB. Audit and quality assurance. In: Aitkenhead AR, Jones RM (eds) *Anaesthesia in Clinical Practice*. London: Churchill Livingstone, 1993.

20. Flanagan JC. The critical incident technique. *Psychol Bull* 1954; **51**: 327–58.

21. Cooper JB, Newbower RS, Long CD, McPeek R. Preventable anaesthesia mishaps: a study of human factors. *Anesthesiology* 1978; **49**: 399–406.

22. Australian and New Zealand College of Anaesthetists. *Minimum Assistance for the Safe Conduct of Anaesthesia*, Policy Document Review P8. Melbourne: ANZCA, 1993.

23. Australian and New Zealand College of Anaesthetists. *Guidelines for the Care of Patients Recovering from Anaesthesia in the Recovery Area*, Policy Document Review P4. Melbourne: ANZCA, 1995.

24. Taylor TH, Jennings AMC, Nightingale DA *et al.* A study of anaesthetic emergency work IV. The practical application of queuing theory to staffing arrangements. *Br J Anaesthes* 1969; **41**: 357–62.

25. Livingstone JI, Harvey M, Kitchin N *et al.* Role of pre-admission clinics in a general surgical unit: a 6-month audit. *Ann Roy Coll Surg Engl* 1993; **75**: 211–12.

26. Lloyd-Davies IV. Lithotomy–Trendelenburg position for resection of the rectum and lower pelvic colon. *Lancet* 1939; **2**: 74–6.

27. Williamson JA, Webb RK, Szekely S *et al.* Difficult intubation: an analysis of 2000 incident reports. *Anaesthes Intens Care* 1993; **21**: 602–7.

28. Holland R, Webb RK, Runciman WB. Oesophageal intubation: an analysis of 2000 incident reports. *Anaesthes Intens Care* 1993; **21**: 608–10.

29. Szekely SM, Webb RK, Williamson JA, Russell WJ. Problems related to the endotracheal tube: an analysis of 2000 incident reports. *Anaesthes Intens Care* 1993; **21**: 611–16.

30. Runciman WB, Webb RK, Barker L, Currie M. The pulse oximeter: applications and limitations – an analysis of 2000 incident reports. *Anaesthes Intens Care* 1993; **21**: 543–50.

31. Williamson JA, Webb RK, Cockings J, Morgan C. The capnograph: applications and limitations – an analysis of 2000 incident reports. *Anaesthes Intens Care* 1993; **21**: 551–7.

32. Australian and New Zealand College of Anaesthetists. *Monitoring During Anaesthesia*, Policy Document Review P18. Melbourne: ANZCA, 1995.

33. Webb RK, Van Der Walt JH, Runciman WB *et al.* Which monitor? An analysis of 2000 incident reports. *Anaesthes Intens Care* 1993; **21**: 529–42.

34. Caplan RA, Posner KL, Ward RJ, Cheney FW. Adverse respiratory events in anesthesia: a closed claims analysis. *Anesthesiology* 1990; **72**: 828–33.

35. Ludbrook GL, Russell WJ, Webb RK *et al.* The electrocardiograph: applications and limitations – an analysis of 2000 incident reports. *Anaesthes Intens Care* 1993; **21**: 558–64.

36. Buczko DB, McKay WPS. Electrical safety in the operating room. *Can J Anaesth* 1985; **34**: 315–22.

37. Norris J. Fire safety in the operating room. *Today's OR Nurse* 1992; **14**: 8–10.

CHAPTER 15

Modern surgical instrumentation

JEA WICKHAM, MS NATHAN

Introduction

Surgery can be defined as 'curative mechanistic intervention to correct or modify any pathological process in the body amenable to manual manipulation'.

To implement the surgical process there are two prime desiderata:

- good visualization of the area of activity;
- adequate manipulatory mechanisms to achieve the requisite modification of the pathological process

For several centuries these objectives have been achieved by the somewhat simplistic concept of:

1. displaying the affected area of the body through open access incisions often of an incongruously gross degree for the indicated task;
2. using manipulation of the hands within the body to power basic instrumentation which has changed little in design for many decades – namely the scalpel, the haemostat, the grasping forceps and the scissors.

It has also been the experience of many surgeons over the last 50 years that when a circumspect and gentle use of even these somewhat basic mechanisms was invoked the results of surgical intervention both in terms of morbidity and mortality was vastly improved. It was always taught by one's more thinking mentors that gentleness in the manipulation of tissues was one of the greatest secrets of surgical success.

Over the last 100 years increasing sophistication in instrumentation has resulted in the lessening of interventional trauma in many areas. For example, the advent of lithotripsy resulted in a fall in mortality of treatment of the bladder stone from 40 to 1%. More recently, the treatment of gall stone obstruction of the bile duct by endoscopic retrograde choledopancreatography has vastly reduced the morbidity of this procedure.[1] The difference in the results of extracorporeal lithotripsy and endoscopic stone extraction for renal calculi when compared with open renal surgery is perhaps the most striking example.[2] Endoscopic cholecystectomy is the latest example of this progressive trend that has penetrated all areas of interventional therapy.[3]

Evaluation of these changes in the mid-1980s gave rise to the concept of 'minimally invasive therapy'[4,5] with its primary aim of reducing trauma in all areas of interventional medicine. It was also the realization that most of these outstanding advances have been due almost entirely to the advent and application of newer and more complex instrumental technology – the lithotripter is an excellent example. Such thinking encouraged the establishment of the Society of Minimally Invasive Surgery in 1989, later to become the Society for Minimally Invasive Therapy, to encompass the interventional radiologists already forming a covert branch of interventional medicine. Other similar societies have subsequently evolved.

Probably the most important thrust that has permitted these profound changes in the interventional attitude has been the evolution of instrumentation which has developed along two main paths.

- imaging and methods of visualizing the target of pathology;

- manipulation – sophisticated manipulatory mechanisms that have permitted refinement in organ handling and the avoidance of unnecessary tissue trauma.

Imaging and methods of visualization

- Endoscopy
- Scanning systems: computerized tomography (CT), nuclear magnetic resonance (NMR) and ultrasound.

ENDOSCOPY

The long history of the endoscope has been well documented, commencing with the development of the Lichtleiter by Bozzini (Fig. 15.1) in the late nineteenth century, passing through the incandescent bulb endoscopes introduced by Nitze, to the current solid rod lens system (Fig. 15.2) devized by Hopkins in the 1950s and 1960s and fibre optic endoscopes (Fig. 15.3). It is interesting to remark that nearly all the systems have been pioneered in clinical use by the

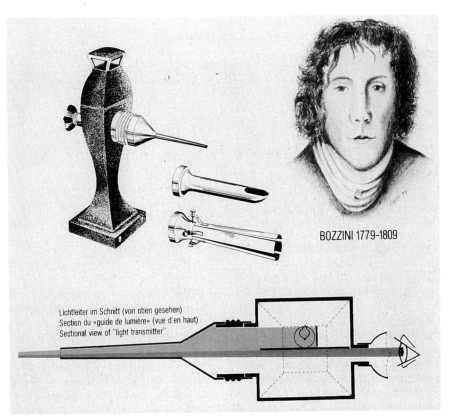

Fig. 15.1 First primitive endoscope (cytoscope) by Bozzini.

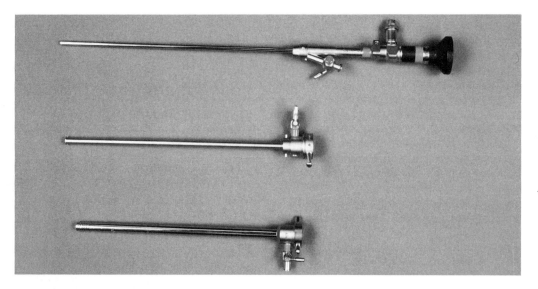

Fig. 15.2 Typical solid rod lens endoscopes (cystoscope) developed by Professor Hopkins 1969, Reading University, UK.

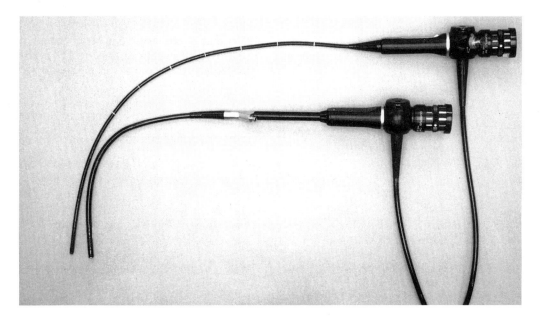

Fig. 15.3 Fibre optic flexible endoscopes (choledochoscope and bronchoscope).

specialist surgeons, notably the urologist, gynaecologist, ear, nose and throat (ENT) and orthopaedic surgeons.

Endoscopes enable the detailed examination of the area of surgical interest to be undertaken, frequently under magnification, but most importantly they allow close inspection of areas of the body inaccessible to the naked eye. Finally, and probably most importantly, they permit visualization to be achieved through very small instruments of only a few millimetres in diameter thus obviating the need for vastly

traumatic intrusion into the body purely as a means of obtaining adequate visualization of the operative area.

Until about 10 years ago it was customary to place the eye to the optic of the endoscope to view the area of interest (Fig. 15.4). With the introduction of the small chip cameras in the mid-1980s it is now almost unusual to place the eye to the endoscope. The imaged picture is projected on one or two television monitors so that not only the operator, but also the rest of the staff in the operating theatre can see the area of activity (Fig. 15.5).

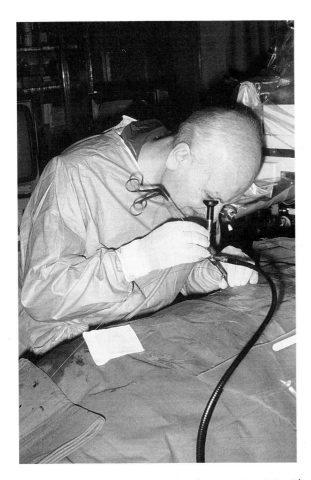

Fig. 15.4 Previous method of endoscopy (1960s) with the unsterile eye to the endoscope.

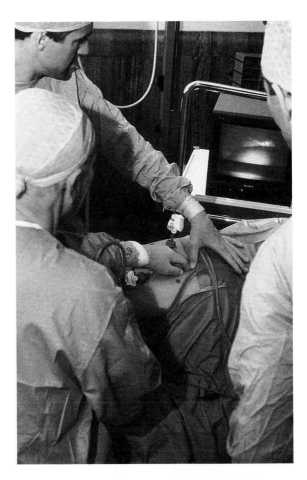

Fig. 15.5 Current, 1990s configuration of endoscopy with camera and images displayed on high resolution televisions.

Endoscopes may be used by way of artificially constructed channels made into the operative area or they may be introduced through the natural apertures of the body – the mouth, nose, ears, urethra, anus and vagina. Endoscopes may be simply classified into solid rod and flexible systems (Fig. 15.6).

SOLID ROD ENDOSCOPES

These instruments have a hollow steel shaft into which a series of small glass rod lenses is inserted. These lens systems transmit excellent images with little loss of clarity. They are made in a wide variety of sizes usually measured in millimetre circumference known as the Charier or French scale, although there is now a tendency for the manufacturers to quote instrument size in millimetres of diameter rather than this old scale. The smallest range from 2–3 mm diameter up to extremely large instruments of 28 mm but the most commonly used are those in the 7–10 mm range. The optics are arranged to give

either a 0° straight ahead view or an oblique viewing angle ranging from 5° to 70°. The field of view subtended is also variable from a wide to narrow angle of spread. Illumination is provided by glass fibre bundles arranged alongside the viewing optic and powered from a high intensity external light source connected by a flexible cable to the proximal end of the instrument. These instruments are usually quite robust and can be chemically or heat sterilized and vary considerably in length from 2 to >30 cm. They are in common use in:

1. urology as cystoscopes, resectoscopes, nephroscopes and ureteroscopes;
2. gynaecology as laparoscopes, hysteroscopes and resectoscopes;
3. orthopaedics as arthroscopes;
4. in general surgery as laparoscopes and transanal resectoscopes;
5. in ENT as sinus endoscopes and laryngoscopes.

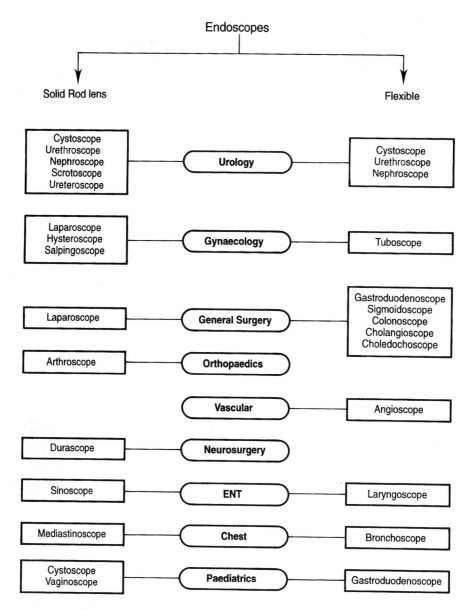

Fig. 15.6 Classification of endoscopes.

Less commonly rod lens systems are coming into use in vascular surgery and neurosurgery. Magnifying systems are used external to the body as operating microscopes in ENT, ophthalmology, neurosurgery and microvascular surgery.

FLEXIBLE ENDOSCOPES

These are much more delicate instruments and are built of coherent bundles of glass fibres that transmit a good image but with less clarity than the solid rod systems. Flexibility of the fibre bundle allows these endoscopes to be deflected away from straight lines so they may be used to negotiate deviations in direction particularly when used intraluminally in the bowel or bronchus and, moreover, to negotiate intraperitoneal structures when used laparoscopically. They are in common use in the following areas:

1. gastroenterology – oesophagoscopes, gastroscopes, duodenoscopes, colonoscopes and choledochoscopes;
2. thoracic surgery – bronchoscopes;
3. urology – ureteroscopes, urethroscopes, cystoscopes and nephroscopes;
4. gynaecology – salpingoscopes;
5. ENT – sinus and laryngoscopes.

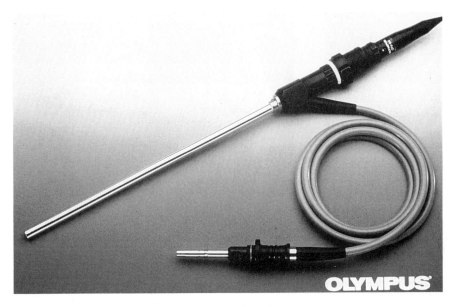

Fig. 15.7 A typical laparoscope (30 cm) with a chip camera.

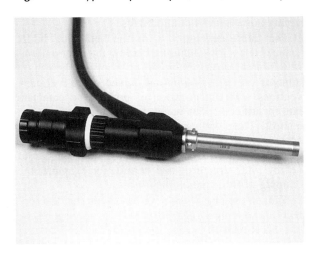

Fig. 15.8 The new short (10 cm) zoom laparoscope.

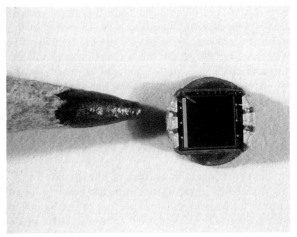

Fig. 15.9 A miniature camera chip in real size comparison with a pencil point.

With this armamentarium of endoscopes most areas of the body have become accessible to optical visualization. Further developments in endoscope design that are already being marketed are three-dimensional (3-D) systems that allow multidimensional assessment of areas of interest which obviously provide an aid to manipulations by secondary, ancillary instruments. Zoom and autofocus endoscopes (Figs 15.7 and 15.8) are also coming into production that will enable the operator to focus closely on the area of optimum interest and then revert to a panoramic view of the whole area of operation to gain orientation of the position of associated manipulatory instruments. Such zoom systems may well become voice activated in the near future so the surgeon need not move his or her hands away from the primary instrumentation to change optical focus.

Probably the next most important development will be the advent of high definition television systems. These give pictures of superb detail of the operative field under magnification such that the operator can have the impression of viewing the abdominal contents as being totally exposed as in laparotomy. Unfortunately, such systems are at present unduly expensive but as with most electronic apparatus the price will, in due course, be reduced.

The chip cameras which transmit the optical image into the digital electronic form are also undergoing modification and miniaturization (Fig. 15.9) so that

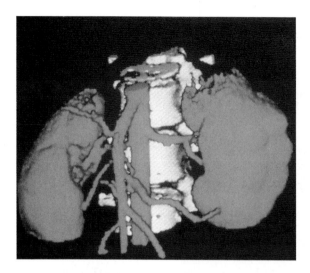

Fig. 15.10 Reconstructed 3-D images of the kidneys and their vasculature from 2-D scanning images.

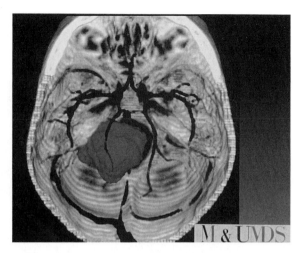

Fig. 15.11 Three-dimensional reconstruction of an acoustic neuroma within the cranial fossae showing its relation to the vital structures.

instead of being mounted in the instrumental probe at its proximal end outside the body the chips will be distally placed, thus diminishing the diameter of the probe and reducing the need for optical transmission systems along the probe; the connection between the chip and electronic control box will be made simply by wires and will also enable the instrument to become totally flexible.

SCANNING SYSTEMS

The newer scanning modalities of ultrasound, CT X-ray and NMR imaging are already being applied directly to the interventional process rather than as a purely diagnostic tool. Initially these systems were used to demonstrate transverse sectional images of the body. The next step was the ability to develop multiplanar images by NMR and finally we have the reconstructed 3-D computer images of all body areas from these primary scans (Fig. 15.10). Such systems have until quite recently been used in a diagnostic mode so that the interventionist could remotely assess the pathology concerned.

More recently, such systems are being looked at in a more interventionist manner by both radiologists and neurosurgeons. For example, CT or NMR images of the patient's head and brain are initially constructed. Underlying pathological processes can be identified within the brain substance, their detailed relationships determined and a 3-D reconstruction of the organ developed (Fig. 15.11). This developed image can then be projected on to the head of the patient at the time of surgery and the best trajectories and paths of access determined through small access tracks and

burr holes to avoid the necessity for the construction of large osteoplastic craniotomies.

The latest development of the split ring NMR scanner (Fig. 15.12) can now allow the interventionist to not only scan and visualize lesions such as brain tumours but will also permit guided operative interventions with the insertion of probes and catheters into identified lesions under direct real-time scanning control. They will also enable the identification of access trajectories for optical endoscopes to be inserted into areas of interest without damage to nearby vital structures and permit, for example, the clipping of intracranial aneurysms.

Thus in the last 5 years we have seen the development of imaging systems that will not only supersede our direct optical visualization of the area of surgical interest but will also provide facilities for more detailed manipulations in the operative area. Our areas of activity will thus be vastly expanded by the facilities already being offered by the techniques and manipulations of these scanning systems which, more and more, will invoke the expertise of the interventional radiologist.

In effect, the modern endoscopes and scanning systems that are being offered will be the eyes at the tips of our fingers which can see round corners, see through solid structures and provide us with extraordinary clarity of detail in a way that we have never been able to achieve with open surgery. For instance, instead of viewing the cystic/bile duct junction at a distance of 2 feet we are now able to visualize the anatomy under magnification at a distance of a few millimetres with the resultant implications for greater safety in any interventional procedures.

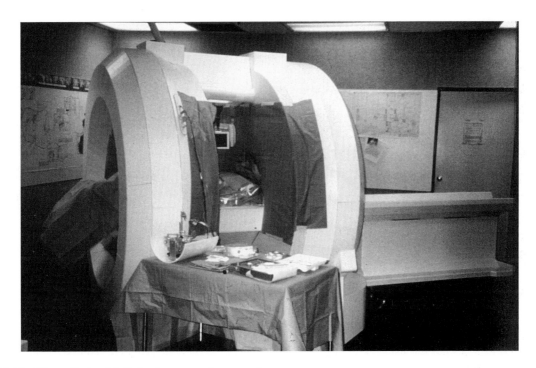

Fig. 15.12 The split ring NMR for intraoperative scanning.

Manipulation

Now that endoscopic and other imaging techniques have permitted astonishingly good visual access to practically all areas of the body through minimal access sites, we are entering a new phase in the evolution of manipulatory instrumentation. The requirement for vast access incisions for visualization being negated, a similar need has arisen to modify and reduce the size of ancillary manipulatory instrumentation.

The basic surgical armamentarium of scalpel, grasping forceps, haemostat, scissors and needle and thread permitted incision, dissection, haemostasis, resection and anastomosis of tissues. Obviously these conventional hand-held instruments have become unsuitable for manipulations down fine access tracks and thus instrumentation is rapidly becoming modified to accept these new challenges. The initial endoscopic procedures such as prostatic resection, arthroscopy and endoscopic nephrolithotomy substituted high frequency cutting currents in place of the scalpel by introducing ancillary instrumentation down operating and irrigation channels which were integral with the endoscope. Grasping was still achieved by long shafted modifications of conventional dissecting forceps and haemostats but there was a marked deficiency in the ability to achieve reconstruction by suturing and anastomosis of divided tissues. Haemostasis, as in open surgery, could still be achieved by diathermy coagulation.

It was probably the advent of interventional laparoscopic surgery in the mid-1980s, particularly by the gynaecologist, Semm, in Germany that led to the new generation of manipulatory instruments (Fig. 15.13). Such instruments have been specially configured so that they may be passed through small secondary access tracks of a few millimetres and the access ports down which they are placed for laparoscopic surgery have been well publicized in this field and will not be independently itemized (Fig. 15.14). The main surgical manoeuvres described above can now be achieved by these newer instruments, for instance:

1. Cutting and dissection of tissue is now achieved by high frequency diathermy utilizing needles, hooks, forceps and activated scissors.
2. Grasping is produced by means of elongated narrow-bladed forceps.
3. Haemostasis is achieved by diathermy coagulation or by stapling.
4. Conjunction of tissues is now more frequently performed by stapling devices. Suturing at a distance through small access channels has proved unduly laborious and would seem doomed, to be gradually excluded from the manipulatory repertoire.
5. Clearance of blood clot and debris from the operative area is by means of fine irrigation and suction devices rather than by swabbing with absorbent cotton fibres.

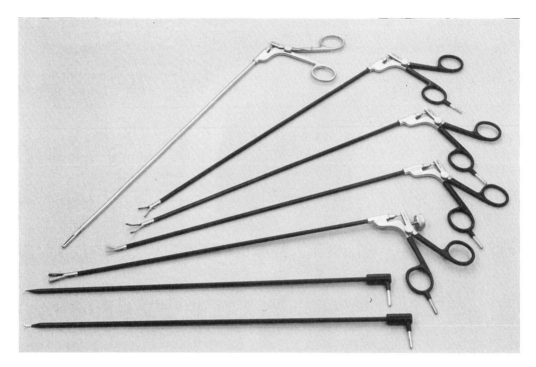

Fig. 15.13 Laparoscopic ancillary instruments.

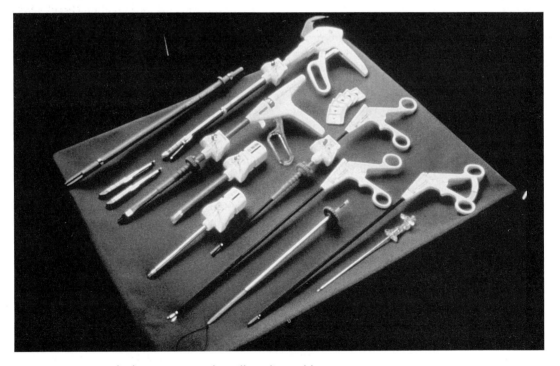

Fig. 15.14 Access ports for laparoscopy and ancillary disposables.

All these instruments were initially produced in a 'non-disposable' mode but in the last 5 years many have become available as 'disposables'. These are in general costly and there is now a swing back to the reusable configuration. It is true, however, that these types of surgical instruments are increasingly proving less than adequate for the newer interventional tasks that are being undertaken.

Magnification of the target tissues has demonstrated the relative crudity of the current devices and has highlighted the clumsiness of manually coupled and manipulated instrumentation. The length of these instruments, usually of the order of 30 cm, originated with the gynaecologists who operated on the pelvic organs from umbilical level. There is, of course, little need for such elongated and clumsy instrumentation. The area of surgical interest directly targeted with shorter and more delicate instrumentation would be more beneficial and such instruments are being slowly developed. The stupidity of the 'Harley Davidson' position needed to use these instruments is immediately apparent.

It is thus almost inevitable that much more sophisticated methodologies will be evolved in the next few years. It is entirely possible that some form of mechanical or robotic assistance will be required to control and guide the manipulatory end effector of the future. Such mechanisms have already been introduced into the areas of ophthalmology, neurosurgery and ENT surgery.

Two shortcomings of current laparoscopic instruments are immediately apparent:

- The movements are restricted to an area with limited degrees of freedom based around the access point of the instrument through the body wall, such that the end of the effector cannot move fully and freely in space as in an open surgical approach.
- When viewed endoscopically the end effector cannot be moved intuitively as in open surgery because of the restriction of movement of the instrument at the point of entry into the body. For example, a downward movement of the forceps appears as an upward movement on a television monitor and can prove to be disastrously confusing to the endoscopically inexperienced.

To overcome this disability it would seem that in time we are going to need articulated effectors with six degrees of freedom, such as with the human hand, to enable the end effector to be placed accurately and orientated in space. How, therefore, can an end effector be suitably coupled at a distance to the surgeon's hand to produce the desired movements? One solution would be to have a robotic glove-like device but this would obviously be very clumsy. Developments in the aviation and computer industries have already made such devices available and terminal mechanisms can be controlled by space mice, joysticks, trackers or immersion probes.

Work at the Fraunhoffer Institute in Stuttgart,[6,7,8] among others, has already addressed this problem and has demonstrated that the immersion probe mechanism coupled with an articulated endoscope is probably going to be the most useful. A hand-held stylus that is connected to an electromagnetic arm is gripped by the surgeon like a pen. Movement of the point of the stylus is tracked and reduplicated by slave instruments passed into the body through an access port. This slave instrument is visualized on a television monitor and its movements can be initiated and controlled by movements of the stylus in the surgeon's hand. These movements are seen under magnification and the stylus is activated and suitably stabilized by the tracking arm. This stabilization also eliminates the commonly observed manual unsteadiness seen if the instrument is held free by the surgeon (Fig. 15.15). Such stylus-tracking mechanisms could be mounted with appropriate end effectors such as scissors, forceps and hooks and the arms could be programmed not to move outside preset dimensions thus avoiding instrumental trauma to surrounding vital structures. Mechanisms such as NMR scanners and endoscopes coupled to the robotic arm will enable the surgeon to operate upon the patient remotely from a work station. This distance between surgeon and patient is

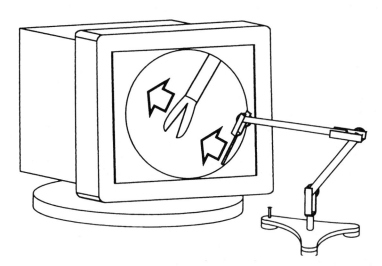

Fig. 15.15 The immersion probe stylus after Wapler M, Fraunhoffer Institute, Stuttgart.

then determined purely by the electronic connections between the two. Thus a surgeon could theoretically operate upon a patient in another hospital or even in another city or country by satellite linkage.

The future

TRAINING

The concept of minimally invasiveness is inevitably leading surgical instrumentation into a more mechanistic and possibly robotic area of manipulative control. We are currently in a half-way situation between free hand-held instrumentation and robot-assisted control. There is obviously much work to be done in the next few years to perfect this newer instrumentation and refining it to our needs. Whilst simple grasping, cutting and haemostasis can be easily achieved, the next large hurdle is the development of more sophisticated anastomotic and stapling systems to allow conjunction and reconstruction of divided tissues. Ablation of large tissue masses such as tumours and their removal through small access ports is a further problem that will be addressed with tissue macerators and diathermy and laser vaporizers.

A further consequence of the development of these newer instrumental systems is the need for surgeons to train and undergo retraining to encompass these skills. Much has been written in the medical and lay press on this topic in the last year or so. Clearly for those unused to the endoscope and the dissociation of visualization from manipulation it is of vital importance to develop training systems to encourage accurate hand–eye coordination. Such skills can usually be achieved by simple 'lunch box simulation' using inanimate objects for practice such as the peeling of grapes or the dissection of animal entrails. The next step would be to practise on anaesthetized live animals but, quite rightly, such systems are banned in the United Kingdom.

In order to progress from a simple simulation to more advanced systems the computer industry has been hard at work attempting to recreate the whole of the intra-abdominal contents coupled with simulated manipulatory instruments with tactile feedback to produce a 'virtual reality' abdomen. At the time of writing such systems are unduly simplistic and unconvincing and the next logical step in training is surely for the trainee to assist an experienced operator at a number of clinical procedures and then to carry out simple procedures under conditions of strict proctoring. It should be pointed out that most of these training systems are directed at laparoscopic interventions which, in reality, constitute only a modest area of activity when the whole of the surgical spectra of

ENT, orthopaedics, urology, neurosurgery and vasculary are considered.

THE INTERVENTIONAL RADIOLOGIST

It must have become apparent to the most casual surgical observer that the interventional radiologists have over the last decade begun to move more and more into the area of therapy rather than merely diagnosis. This trend started in the late 1970s with the development of angiographic techniques for visualization of arterial lesions and progressed into therapy with the inception of intraluminal balloon dilatation of obstructed vessels. Since that time radiologists have become even more active in their ability to ream, dilate and stent obstructive vessels and to embolize arteriovenous malformations and even whole organs such as the kidney. Their instruments are, in general, simple – in comprising guidewires and catheters – but there is now progression into more sophisticated devices such as expandable arterial stents, mechanical reamers and intraluminal lasers.

In gastroenterology the ability to pass an endoscope into the duodenum and intubate the bile duct through the ampulla has allowed the radiologist or medical gastroenterologist to remove bile duct stones with baskets and fragment them if necessary with electrohydraulic, ultrasound or laser disintegrators. Direct hepatic puncture has allowed the radiologist to insert expandable mesh stents for treatment of bile duct strictures, both benign and malignant, with reasonable long-term results.

In urology, percutaneous puncture of the kidney to provide drainage and extract stones is being performed without the need for surgical intervention – and prostatic stenting instead of transurethral resection is ideal for treatment of acute retention in the fragile patient.

Fine-needle biopsy of lesions in any organ such as the liver, lymph nodes or the prostate is now commonplace and is usually done under ultrasound guidance. Radiological microdiscectomy is now possible for the treatment of prolapsed spinal discs by needle puncture of the appropriate area and either mechanical or chemical dissolution of the nucleus pulposus, followed by aspiration without any need for surgical intervention.

The advent of the split ring NMR scanner is obviously going to open up potential areas for the radiologist to display his interventional skills, for example, direct needling of liver metastases, followed by the passage of a laser fibre into the tumour with laser disintegration of all malignant cells which can now be done entirely by the radiologist without any surgical input. The advent of the technique of extracorporeal focused ultrasound is being rapidly developed and will probably come into use for treatment of bladder carcinoma and benign hypertrophy of the prostate, metastatic lesions of the liver and, possibly, intracerebral lesions.

It must again be emphasized that most of these advances in interventional radiology have emanated from the increasingly sophisticated instrumentation that has been developed in the last few years. This process is inevitably set to continue and rather than adopt a confrontational attitude it is essential to enter into a symbiotic partnership with our interventional radiologists. I have personally experienced the valuable input of my radiological colleagues into the management of renal calculi by various methods and I am sure that radiologists should become part of any standard interventional team within most specialities.

CONCLUSION

Currently, there is a concerted swing away from conventional methods of achieving surgical intervention spurred on by the well-documented benefits of a less traumatic approach to interventional therapy. Much of the success in this area in the last 20 years has been due to increasingly sophisticated instrumentation that is still very much in the development phase. The pace of change is quite often dictated by the wishes of our patients, in this case to be exposed to the least possible bodily trauma to cure their condition. This constitutes a driving force in a situation that provides ongoing scope for interventional innovation particularly in the area of new instrumentation.

Computer-assisted and robotic surgery

High failure and morbidity rates exist in operations requiring precision or repeated mechanical actions. This is well exemplified in operations on the spine, base of skull and the intracranium. Complicated anatomy with closely related vital structures make these procedures technically demanding and even a small human error can lead to tragic complications. The present availability of modern imaging systems where the images are digitally enhanced with a computer or generate 3-D models can give accurate and vivid pictures of the complicated operating field and even go as far as to simulate the consequences of a surgeon's action. In situations where precise human action is required, or a trajectory with minimal access is needed, robots have been developed to assist the surgeon.

DEFINITION

The Robotic Institute of America defines a robot as 'A reprogrammable multifunctional manipulator designed to move material, parts, tools, or specialised devices through variable programmed motions for the performance of a variety of tasks.'

A robot is not a hard automaton that cannot vary its task nor is it intuitive as a human. It is a flexible programmable machine, primitive in comparison with the five senses, power of judgement or manual dexterity of a human. Thus a robot falls between human labour and hard automation.

Historical review

The term robot first appeared in Karel Capek's play RUR (*Rossum's Universal Robot*) in 1923. In Czech the word *robota* means 'a worker (slave)' to relieve the master from his or her toils. The first robotic process was implemented in the die casting industry in 1961 to protect workers from the hostile work environment. The great motor industries of Japan and America soon incorporated robots into their assembly lines. Although these robots are multifunctional they could not sense and intuitively vary their tasks. American and Soviet space programmes in the late 1960s led to the development of robots with sensors that could react to various situations.

The 1970s saw the first use of robots in medicine to rehabilitate physically handicapped patients. They were autonomous wheelchairs with a stair-climbing facility and simple arms for feeding, drinking and other manipulative tasks. In the late 1980s passive robots for stereotactic neurosurgery and an active robot to transurethrally resect the prostate gland were developed. The first active robotic surgery in the world was performed in April 1991 to remove quantities of prostatic tissue from a patient.[9]

The structure of a robot

Robots can be easily compared with humans in their structure and, depending upon their use, they may incorporate few or all the systems of the human body. The mechanical design forms the skeleton of the robot and this varies widely depending on its function. Designing a robot to perform a wide range of tasks is costly and very complicated, thus most robots are designed for a specific task.

The skeleton or the framework is moved by actuators that are the muscles of the robot. These actuators may be pneumatic, hydraulic or powered by electric motors. Hydraulic forces are commonly used when gross movements with great force but minimal accuracy are required. For precise, delicate movements with accuracy, electrical actuators such as AC or DC servomotors are used. With the recent development of micromotors (microactuators), very delicate and accurate motions in tiny, confined spaces can be achieved.

The actuators are usually controlled by a motion controller which forms the pyramidal and extrapyramidal systems of the robot. The motion controller makes the system inherently faster but more complicated. The motion controller is in turn controlled by a computer which forms the brain of the robot.

Sensors are incorporated into a robot to give information of the robot's position and its surrounding environment. These sensors can be positional, force or visual. Positional sensors are essentially potentiometers that sense the position of the robot or its effectors within the given working space. Force sensors delineate the consistency of the tissues and are especially useful in orthopaedic surgery where the torque of the drill needs to be altered depending on the density of the bone. Visual sensors are used to analyse various imaging modalities like CT, NMR and ultrasound scans. Thus the sensors can inform the computer of a varying environment that can appropriately change the commands to the actuators and adjust the movement of the frame much like the human animal but in a primitive form.

Robots in medicine

In medicine, robots are available for health care to assist physically handicapped patients at their homes and offices; for paramedical services to transport patients; for medical laboratories to do various tasks such as tissue typing and DNA sequencing; also for diagnostic medicine and to assist in surgery. Figure 15.16 shows the classification of the various robots developed in medicine.

Robots used in surgical practice may be active or passive depending on their function. Active robots perform a part or most of the operative procedure while passive robots aid in guiding trajectory, matching prosthesis, giving information about the depth and position of tools and simulating operations.

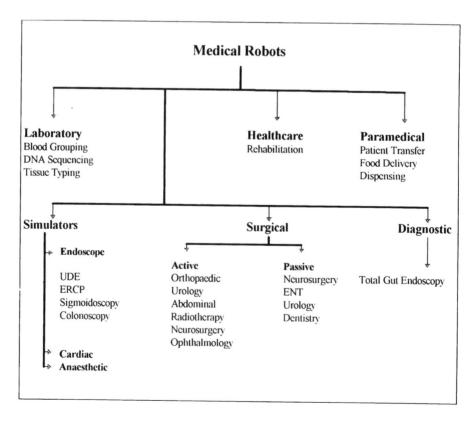

Fig. 15.16 Classification of medical robots.
UDE: Upper digestive endoscopy; ERCP: Endoscopic retrograde choledopancreatography.

Table 15.1 Glossary

Simulation
A participatory experience with significant aspects of a given procedure, which must faithfully reproduce the reality of the procedure as closely as possible.

Seamless images
Images realistically linked without any gaps or visual jumps between images.

Real-time
Images that appear and change in response to the user's action and appear seamless.

Interactive video technology (IVT)
A simulation system that uses actual images stored on video disc player and later displayed in real-time.

Computer graphics simulation (CGS)
A simulation system that uses computer-generated graphics instead of the actual images as in IVT.

Video graphic tool technology (VGTT)
A simulation system that uses a hybrid of IVT and CGS to portray movement of devices in several planes over the actual endoscopic pictures in real-time.

Variable resistance devices (VRD)
It gives variable tactile feedback resembling closely the varying human tissue consistency.

Calibration
To spatially configure a robot to the human body so its stored images of landmarks and anatomy accurately correspond to the operating field.

ROBOTIC SIMULATION DEVICES

Following great success in the military and aviation industries, robotic simulators have been gradually introduced into medicine. The demand for speciality training in medicine is growing exponentially, requiring the training of increasing numbers of specialists and allied health professionals. It is difficult, time consuming and potentially hazardous to patients to train health staff in actual situations like the operating theatres or cardiac resuscitation units. These circumstances would benefit from robotic simulations in standardizing learning, shortening of the learning curve, establishing the criteria of competency, the ability of regulatory agencies to certify and recertify surgeons and a possible rapid dispersal of new techniques.[10]

The first interactive simulator was the Sim Aid Medical simulator which was a realistically configured human body developed at the University of Southern California in 1980 to interact with medical students. In 1982 a cardiopulmonary resuscitation simulator was developed by the American Heart Association that forms an integral part of cardiac training in medicine. In 1984 a shock trauma simulator was developed which requires instantaneous response to developing patient situations which

would in turn change its response to the user's actions. Recently, an anaesthetic simulator incorporating a complete anaesthetic machine with all the monitors and a patient surrogate has been developed. It has been programmed to present normal, unusual and emergency situations and responds according to the user's actions.[11]

Endoscopic simulators for upper and lower gastrointestinal tracts (GIT) have been developed. A system to teach upper GIT endoscopy has been developed which consists of a standard non-instant jump video disc player, a computer with a touch screen monitor and IVT connected to a moulded mannequin. Optical sensors and potentiometers relate the position of the endoscope in the mannequin so that as it is moved, real-time pictures of the digestive tract appear and seamlessly change with the user's actions. A similar ERCP simulator has been developed which uses an endoscope with VRD. The original model of this simulator allowed only cannulation and movement within the duodenum but recent improvements with CGS and VGTT allow straightening manoeuvres and the performance of a pancreatogram or cholangiogram. Similar devices have been developed for flexible sigmoidoscopy and colonoscopy.[10,11]

Presently, simulators using VRD and CGS real-time seamless images are being developed for laparoscopic cholecystectomy, bronchoscopy, angioscopy and angioplasty. The next logical and futuristic step will be the development of intelligent endoscopes. These will be capable of automatic steering and guidance if requested and could recognize pathology or present information from a visual database for comparison.

Orthopaedic surgery

In the prosthetic surgery of bones a major consequence of imprecise surface or cavity preparation is inadequate contact between bone and prosthesis. The resulting gaps lead to micromotion between bone and prosthesis affecting the quality and quantity of bony ingrowth. This leads to persistent thigh pain in hip surgery and radiologically visible failure. It is thus desirable to have a perfect 3-D fit between bone and prosthesis. This desire has led to the development of robots in this field.

PROSTHETIC HIP SURGERY

A purpose-built robot has been developed to mill the femoral canal accurately for a variety of selected prosthesis. It consists of a milling machine, the movements of which are controlled by a computer. Preoperatively three fine-calibration pins are driven under local anaesthesia, one each into the greater trochanter and the two femoral condyles. The hip is CT scanned and a 3-D model generated to select a prosthesis.[12]

After exposing the hip, the femur is immobilized using an external fixator which is attached to the base of the robot. A ball attached to the robot arm is moved over the three calibration pins to spatially configure the robot so it knows where its drill is in relation to the bone. Under the surgeon's supervision the femoral canal is milled accurately.

Studies on human cadavers and dogs showed that by the traditional hammer and broach method the cavity was oversized by 33% while the robot had a submillimetric accuracy. A pilot study on ten patients was safely carried out with a success rate of 70% at a year's follow-up. Presently a large series of 300 patients is undergoing clinical trials.[13,14]

A similar robot is being developed not only to mill the femoral canal but also to prepare the acetabulum for total hip replacement allowing early mobilization and placement of stress on the joint.

PROSTHETIC KNEE SURGERY

Success in knee replacement crucially depends on accurate placement of the prostheses on the ends of the femur and tibia to achieve perfect alignment. Systems similar to the active robot for hip surgery are in development for robotic total knee replacement.

ANTERIOR CRUCIATE LIGAMENT RECONSTRUCTION

Plastic reconstruction of the anterior cruciate ligament (ACR) involves making two tunnels, one each in the femoral notch and the tibia, and then inserting and fixing the patellar tendon. The success of the procedure depends on the tunnel–tendon position and the initial tension selected. Ideally the graft should be isometric and remain constant in length during extension and flexion. To achieve this a computerized optical localizer using infrared emitters and charge couple device (CCD) cameras has been developed to optimize the placement of the tunnels. A clinical trial on 12 patients has been reported with a good success rate.[15]

LOWER LIMB DEFORMITY CORRECTION BY ILIZAROV'S METHOD

In this procedure multiple osteotomies are done and the bony pieces connected to an external fixator. By gradually adjusting the fixator the angle or the length of the bone can be corrected. The success of the procedure depends on accurate three-dimensional alignment of the pieces per- and postoperatively. Computer-assisted 3-D models are first generated from CT scans. Using these models, simulation exercises are done that would indicate the best osteotomy placement sites and position of the external fixator hinges. Postoperative rate and duration of the bone adjustments can also be simulated and the best surgical plan drawn.[16]

SPINE

Insertion of spinal screws is a delicate operation with a great potential hazard of driving a screw into the spinal cord or nerve roots and causing paralysis or damaging abdominal and intercostal vessels. The operation requires accurate placement of a fine screw through the lamina with careful consideration of the depth, angle and torque. A purpose-built active robot has been developed to drive a screw precisely guided by 3-D CT scan and magnetic resonance (MRI) images. A clinical trial on six patients has demonstrated the robot to be extremely accurate and safe.[17]

Neurosurgery

For decades mechanical stereotactic frames have been used in neurosurgery to guide the surgeon towards a deep-seated lesion through burr holes to avoid a formal craniotomy. The frames are cumbersome to use and often cause postoperative pain at their fixation sites to the skull. Moreover, they have the disadvantage that the surgeon operates only by feel without visual orientation. Based on this principle a passive robotic arm has been developed and clinically tried with success in intracranial surgery. It consists of an aluminium arm with joints allowing six axes of movements. High precision digital encoders within the joints accurately reflect its position in space. It has a versatile final segment that can accommodate various end effectors like blunt needle pointers, endoscopes, biopsy forceps and ultrasound transducers with their central axes and tips coinciding in the same position.

Using CT scan and MRI images, 3-D models are generated preoperatively and the arm is calibrated and positioned. The computer then superimposes the CT scan or MRI pictures on the operating field so that the surgeon can plan an accurate and least traumatizing trajectory. The arm has been successfully used in intracranial biopsy, draining haematomas, endoscopy and fenestrating cysts. In all the cases a small burr hole was accurately placed and the trajectory formed with the help of the robotic arm thus avoiding a formal craniotomy.[18]

A similar arm has been motorized to make it an active robot. This robot is preprogrammed to move the end effector automatically to selected sites with submillimetric accuracy. A similar active robot has been developed with which the operation can be preoperatively simulated, perfected and stored in memory to be used later during the actual procedure. Clinical reports are awaited.

Abdominal surgery

Passive and active robotic arms have been developed as assistants in laparoscopic surgery. The arms are similar in their mechanical design and consist of joints that can be independently moved and fixed during surgery. Pneumatic or servomotors are used to move the joints. In most of the designs the arms are controlled manually, while two models employ a head gear which controls the motions of the arm by movement of the surgeon's head. One model using voice commands has been recently developed and clinically tried with success. The arms have been built to hold and move laparoscopic cameras, instruments and retractors. The major advantage of these arms is that up to six memory positions can be stored and with a single command the camera can be made to focus on a port entry site or back to the target area.[19,20]

Radiosurgery

The aim of conformal radiotherapy is to deliver a specific dose of radiotherapy on a target volume with high precision, concurrently irradiating little healthy tissue and organs. Ablation of intracranial tumours using a gamma knife requires accurate delivery to avoid radiating normal brain tissue. With the help of computers, 3-D models of the brain and the lesion are generated from CT scan and MRI images. With the head fixed in a ring, these images are used to target the gamma knife accurately on to the lesion. Trials have revealed a high success rate.

A similar system using CT and MRI images has been developed to generate a 3-D image of the prostate. During therapy, transrectal ultrasound images are used to calibrate the patient to the preoperative 3-D images and accurate targeting of the radiation beam achieved. This avoids unnecessary irradiation of the bladder and rectum preventing distressing post-irradiation symptoms. Clinical trials are yet to be reported.[21]

Otolaryngologic surgery

Surgical localization of infected or deformed mastoid antrum, sigmoid sinus and tegmen mastoideum can be difficult even for the seasoned otologist. Furthermore, many surgeons routinely perform a mastoidectomy to identify the superior semicircular canal and internal auditory canal. Computerized imaging and robotic surgery would be advantageous to perform these operations. A passive robot similar to the neurosurgical one has been developed and tried on cadavers with a high success rate.[22]

During stapedectomy a fine hole needs to be drilled in the footplate of the stapes to attach the prosthetic piston. This requires delicate and precise manoeuvres as the inner ear can be easily damaged. A computer-assisted drill has been developed and tried with success on cadavers. This indicates the breakthrough point and the position of the tip of the drill so that rapid retraction can be achieved after maximum and precise drilling.[23]

Urology

SEMI-AUTOMATIC RESECTION OF THE PROSTATE

It was in this field that the world's first active robot was used successfully on patients. Transurethral resection of the prostate (TURP) forms the major workload of urologists and requires considerable time and experience to learn. Despite its high success rate it has a morbidity of nearly 18%. The chief causes of the morbidity are haemorrhage and transurethral resection syndrome, both of which are directly related to the resecting time. These factors clearly indicate the advantage of a shorter operating time to avoid not only surgical, but also anaesthetic, complications.

A feasibility study using a five axes industrial Unimate Puma robot revealed that automated resections were possible but the working envelope had to be restricted for maximum safety. This led to the development of a safety frame. Manual transurethral resections of the prostate using the frame were successful on 40 patients. The frame was motorized and using transrectal ultrasound images of the prostate a pattern-directed robot was developed.[24] Clinical trials (Fig. 15.17) have proved it to be safe.[25] A current model using transurethral ultrasound images and faster software is under clinical trial (Fig. 15.18).

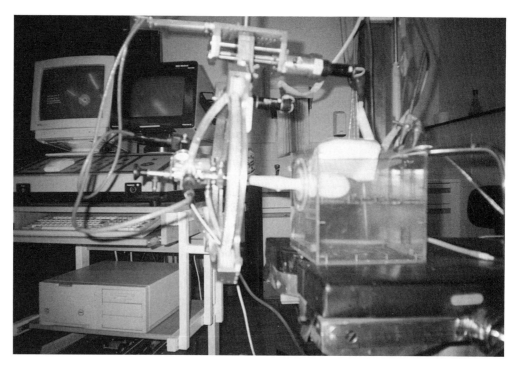

Fig. 15.17   Bench trial on potatoes with the new transurethral prostatectomy robot.

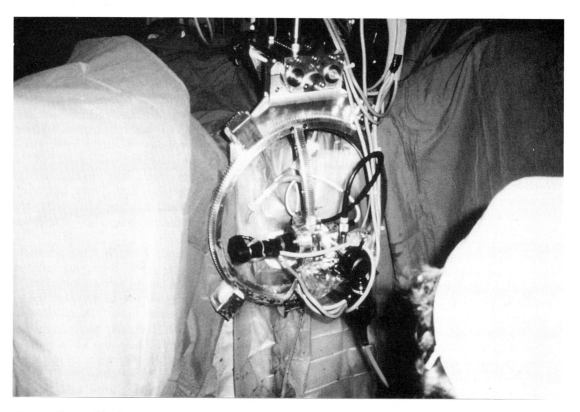

Fig. 15.18   The world's first active robotic surgery (April 1991) to remove prostatic tissue transurethrally.

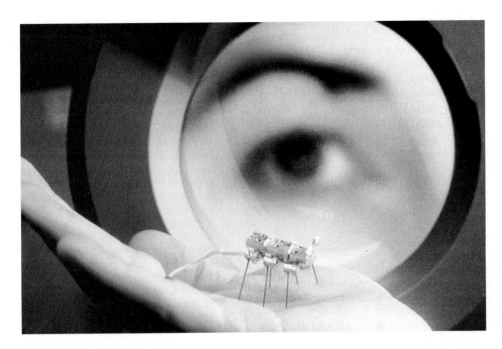

Fig. 15.19 Total gut endoscopic robots.

IMAGE-GUIDED NEPHROSTOMY

Renal biopsies and percutaneous nephrostomies rarely lead to major complications but minor complications like persistent haematuria and capsular haematomas causing loin pain are frequently worrying. Three-dimensional orientation using two-dimensional images is difficult to learn and master. A passive robotic arm has been developed to guide a nephrostomy needle accurately into a specific point within the kidney using images from an X-ray C arm. This would be useful for creating nephrostomy tracts, draining the kidneys or for accurate biopsy of renal lesions. Cadaveric trials are to be reported.[26]

Total intestinal endoscopy

Miniature robots with diameters less than the size of a 1 cm coin have been developed to travel through the entire gut from the mouth to the anus and relay normal or 3-D pictures of the gastrointestinal tract. Two models, one using tank wheel tracks and the other using spider legs, have been developed. They are moved by microactuators and at present require a very thin flex to supply power (Fig. 15.19). Developments are underway to power this magnetically from an external source so that these robots can be made active totally by remote control.

Dentistry

Prosthetic tooth fillings require accurate preparation of the jaw bone so that the angle and position align well with that of the implant. A passive robot has been developed using CT scans which identify the optimal axis and trajectory to drill the jaw bone. A clinical trial on one patient has been done successfully and the system is being upgraded to an active robot.[27]

Ophthalmology

Microcannulation of the retinal vessels to inject dye to study the vasculature, or inject thrombolytic agents to clear emboli, requires accuracy and precision. A purpose-built active robot has been developed which allows the surgeon to enter the sclera with a hypodermic needle through which it inserts a micropipette into a selected vessel. Animal trials have been done successfully and a new model is being developed for clinical trials.[28]

Conclusion

In many areas the application of robotics to clinical surgery is progressing rapidly. In the next decade miniaturization and more sophisticated intraoperative imaging systems will increasingly aid the surgeon in tasks requiring the delicate and accurate manipulation of interventional instrumentation. Whilst obviously not replacing the manipulatory capabilities of the surgeon, robotic instrumentation will undoubtedly become a vitally important assistant and aid in the areas of surgery requiring meticulous accuracy that cannot be obtained by the free motion of the human hand. It is of clear importance that the surgeon of the twenty-first century should familiarize him- or herself with these early developments.

References

1. Neoptolmos JP, Carr-Locke DL, Fossard DP. Prospective randomised study of preoperative endoscopic sphincterotomy versus surgery alone for common duct stones. *Br Med J* 1987; **294**: 470–4.
2. Charig C, Webb DR, Payne SR, Wickham JEA. Comparison of treatment of renal calculi by open surgery, percutaneous nephrolithotomy and extracorporeal shockwave lithotripsy. *Br Med J* 1986; **292**: 879–83.
3. Cuschieri A. Laparoscopic treatment of gall bladder disease. *J Min Inv Ther* 1992; **1**: 115–23.
4. Wickham JEA. Editorial. *Br Med Bull* 1986; **42**: 221–2.
5. Wickham JEA. 'The New Surgery'. *Br Med J* 1987; **295**: 1581–2.
6. Daum W, Endohard A. Manipulation for minimally invasive therapy. *VI International Meeting for the Society for Minimally Invasive Therapy* 1994; **3**: (Suppl 1): 27.
7. Flaig T, Neugebauer JG, Wapler M. Virtual reality for improved man-machine interactions in robotics. *'ORIA' 94 From Telepresence towards Virtual Reality*. Marseille, 1994: 141–7.
8. Satava RM, Simon IB. Teleoperation, telerobotics and telepresence in surgery. *Endoscop Surg Allied Technologies* 1993: 285.
9. Davies BL, Hibberd RD, Ng WS *et al*. The development of a surgeon robot for prostatectomies. *J Eng Med* 1991; **3**: 172–9.
10. Noar MD, Soehendra N. Endoscopy simulation training devices. *Endoscopy* 1992; **24**: 159–66.
11. Noar MD. Robotics interactive endoscopy simulation of ERCP/sphincterotomy and EGD. *Endoscopy* 1992; **24** (Suppl 2): 539–41.
12. Goldsmith MF. For better hip replacement results, surgeon's best friend may be a robot (News). *JAMA* 1992; **267**: 613–14.
13. Taylor KS. Robodoc: study tests robot's use in hip surgery. *Hospitals* 1993; **67**: 46.
14. Paul HA, Bargar WL, Mittlestadt B *et al*. Development of a surgical robot for cementless total hip arthroplasty. *Clin Orthopaed Rel Res* 1992: 57–66.
15. Lavallee S, Orti R, Julliard R *et al*. Computer assisted knee anterior cruciate ligament reconstruction: first clinical tests. *Proceedings First International Symposium on Medical Robotics and Computer Assisted Surgery*, Pittsburgh, Sept 1994; **1**: 11–16.
16. Lin H, Birch JG, Samchukov ML, Ashman RB. Computer assisted surgery planning for lower extremity deformity correction by the Ilizarov method. *Proceedings First International Symposium on Medical Robotics and Computer Assisted Surgery*, Pittsburgh, Sept 1994; **1**: 126–38.
17. Nolte LP, Zamorano LJ, Jiang Z, Want G. A novel approach to computer assisted spine surgery. *Proceedings First International Symposium on Medical Robotics and Computer Assisted Surgery*, Pittsburgh, Sept 1994; **2**: 323–8.
18. Koivukangas J, Louhisalmi Y, Alakuijala J, Oikarinen J. Ultrasound-controlled neuronavigator-guided brain surgery. *J Neurosurg* 1993; **79**: 36–42.
19. Moran ME, Bonnell L. Robotic arm assistant for urologic laparoscopy. *J Min Inv Ther* 1993; **2**: 103–4.
20. Sackier JM, Wang Y. Robotically assisted laproscopic surgery: from concept to development. *Surg Endoscopy* 1994; **8**: 63–6.
21. Trocca Z, Menguy Y, BOlla M, Cinquin P. Conformal external radiotherapy of prostatic carcinoma: requirements and experimental results. *Radiother Oncol* 1993; **29**: 176–83.
22. Kavanagh KT. Applications of image-directed robotics in otolaryngologic surgery. *Laryngoscope* 1994; **104**: 283–93.
23. Bret PN, Baldwin D, Stone RS, Reyes L. Automated tool for microdrilling a flexible stapes footplate. *Proceedings First International Symposium on Medical Robotics and Computer Assisted Surgery*, Pittsburgh, Sept 1994; **2**: 245–9.
24. Davies BL, Hibberd RD, Ng WS *et al*. Mechanical constraints: the answer to safe robotic surgery. *Innov Tech Biol Med* 1992; **13**: 425–36.
25. Nathan MS, Davies BL, Hibberd R, Wickham JEA. Devices for automated resection of the prostate. *Proceedings First International Symposium on Medical Robotics and Computer Assisted Surgery*, Pittsburgh, Sept 1994; **2**: 342–4.
26. Potamianos P, Davies BL, Hibberd RD. Intraoperative imaging guidance for keyhole surgery. *Proceedings First International Symposium on Medical Robotics and Computer Assisted Surgery*, Pittsburgh, Sept 1994; **1**: 98–105.
27. Fortin T, Loup Coudert J, Lavallee S, Champleboux G. Computer assisted dental implant surgery. *Proceedings First International Symposium on Medical Robotics and Computer Assisted Surgery*, Pittsburgh, Sept 1994; **2**: 329–33.
28. Jensen PS, Glucksberg MR, Colgate JE, Grace KW. Robotic micromanipulator for ophthalmic surgery. *Proceedings First International Symposium on Medical Robotics and Computer Assisted Surgery*, Pittsburgh, Sept 1994; **2**: 204–11.

CHAPTER 16

Clinical audit in surgical practice

DA TOMALIN, AW CLARK

In order, therefore, to procure this valuable collection, I humbly propose, first of all, that three or four persons should be employed in the hospitals (and that without any ways interfering with the gentlemen now concerned), to set down the cases of the patients there from day to day, candidly and judiciously, without any regard to private opinions or public systems, and at the year's end publish these facts just as they are, leaving every one to make the best use he can for himself.

Francis Clifton, 1732

Introduction

If you were asked what you would most like to improve in the way you care for patients you could probably come up with a number of suggestions. You would perhaps be less sure of the benefits of each change without some review of current practice, activity levels and effectiveness. Clinical audit provides evidence of what needs to change whilst highlighting what that change should be.

Development of quality assurance in the NHS

In the past there has been little formalized attention to quality. The term audit is not new; it is of Latin derivation meaning 'hearing', but was not referred to officially. It was undertaken on a sporadic, haphazard basis for many years.[1] Some of the earliest examples include the work undertaken by Florence Nightingale during the Crimean War, the requirement of the American College of Surgeons in 1912 that applicants for fellowship submit 50 records for inspection and again in the USA in 1917, the establishment of a national programme of hospital inspections to check that certain minimum standards were adhered to.

In the UK, the 1950s heralded the Confidential Enquiries into maternal and perinatal mortality. The 1980s witnessed many changes in health care structures, financing and management (e.g. purchaser/provider scenario, trust status, regional reorganizations, the Griffiths Report) coupled to increasing public accountability but still without formal attention to quality of medical care. The National Confidential

Enquiry into Perioperative Deaths (NCEPOD) was established to examine deaths occurring in hospitals after surgery throughout the UK.

Then in 1989, the Department of Health (DOH) introduced medical audit as a national requirement for all doctors in their White Paper *'Working for Patients'*.[2] Medical audit was defined as 'the systematic, critical analysis of the quality of medical care, including the procedures used for diagnoses and treatment, use of resources and the resulting outcome and quality of life for the patient'. Ringfenced monies were devolved through regional health authorities to set up medical audit programmes in provider units. These monies were to be used to provide audit support facilities, although precisely what the monies should be spent on was not specified.

'Working for Patients' stated that every doctor should participate in regular, systematic audit which should form part of their routine clinical practice; that audit should be professionally led and that managers needed to contribute to the consideration of the overall form of audit. Medical audit was to be a contractual requirement and medical audit committees were to be established in every trust or hospital board. Then, in 1991, a three-year programme to enable a widespread take-up of audit by the nursing and therapy professions was initiated by the DOH.

Medical audit is now well established in the NHS. For the majority of doctors, audit is now part of their clinical practice, leading to significant improvements in standards of care, use of resources and stimulation of cultural change in the medical profession.[3] And although audit is now widely regarded as a key element of postgraduate education, these achievements are only the beginning. In 1993, the NHS Management Executive (NHSME) shifted the strategic direction of audit from unidisciplinary to multidisciplinary 'clinical' audit to reflect the growing involvement of other clinical professionals in medical audit whilst placing strong emphasis on assuring the quality of care and measuring clinical outcomes.[4] This will mean that the scope and impact of audit should increase in the future.

The NHSME definition of clinical audit is:

Clinical audit is the systematic and critical analysis of the quality of clinical care, including the procedures used for diagnosis, treatment and care, the associated use of resources and the resulting outcome and quality of life for the patient.[4]

However, we find a more useful working definition in Brighton Health Care to be that:

Clinical audit involves systematically reviewing, maintaining and improving the quality of patient care.

Between 1989/90 and 1993/4, the DOH invested £221 million in 'ringfenced monies' to support audit.

Today, all health care providers have audit staff and resources although there is huge variation.[3] However, in most places, audit staff are working with clinicians on a variety of audit projects. The ringfenced monies have now finished and to maintain audit providers have to negotiate with their purchasers, both for the finance to support the staff and the types of project undertaken.

Clinical audit can be represented diagrammatically by a spiral (Fig. 16.1) or circle (Fig. 16.2) to emphasis that audit is an ongoing, continuous activity, organized in a systematic way to bring about improvement in the quality of care given to patients. It examines what is being done, compares it with best practice derived from external sources or the audit itself, shows ways to improve what is being done, and through this structure, allows re-evaluation ('closing the audit loop') and the beginning of a new cycle of improvement.

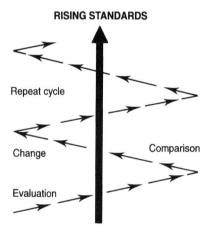

Fig 16.1   Audit spirals. Rising standards.[5]

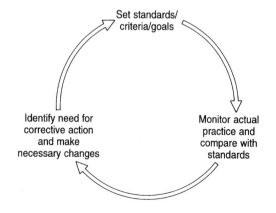

Fig 16.2   Audit cycle.

Types of audit

There are different types of audit depending on who is involved and how or where it is carried out. Unidisciplinary audit usually involves just one professional group, e.g. medical audit (doctors), nursing audit (nurses). Multidisciplinary audit involves the whole multidisciplinary team including clinical and non-clinical staff. Either of these types of audit can be divided up into speciality – medical, surgical – or interdepartmental – obstetric anaesthesia. Then there is interface audit such as those set up between GPs and hospital consultants to audit the quality of hospital discharge letters and GP referral letters; the more broadly based regional audits (where a project will involve a number of sites throughout a health region) or national audit projects such as those led by the Royal Colleges (e.g. annual National Comparative Audit of the Royal College of Surgeons: National Confidential Enquiry into Stillbirths and Deaths in Infancy (CESDI) or the DOH. The National Comparative Audit allows surgeons to compare their clinical performance anonymously, based on their own audit data, with that of other surgeons throughout the country participating in the study. Audit data are gathered by proforma, written by steering groups representing the different discipline groups. The results are fed back to individual surgeons in the form of a ranking relative to the database for different procedures. To date, the service has been used by general, ear, nose and throat, orthopaedic and paediatric surgeons and urologists.

Benefits of quality assurance

The most significant benefit of properly managed quality assurance is that it produces improvements in care. Examples from Brighton Health Care include improved access to accident and emergency (A&E) facilities through a triage nurse, open access booking for urgent breast lump assessment and better patient information booklets. On the clinical side, proformas and guidelines for head injury care have been developed and guidelines for cholangiography have reduced unnecessary exposure to X-rays and saved operating time. NCEPOD conclusions have improved the availability of operating theatres for daytime emergencies, and are enhancing the skills and experience of surgeons and anaesthetists for the sick patient.

Irvine and Irvine[6] neatly summarize the benefits of undertaking audit from the professional's point of view. Audit brings about change; reduction in frustration; reduction in organizational and clinical error;

improves efficiency and effectiveness; demonstrates good care; meets the patient needs and expectations; stimulates education; promotes higher standards of hospital and community care for patients; provides the means to bid for resources; and secures effective medical defence through risk avoidance. We believe that another essential benefit of clinical audit is that it allows one to set or determine if guidelines of clinical practice are being met. Such guidelines obviously need to be well researched and based on sound scientific evidence and previous audits. Further, they need to be coordinated at a national level because this is more likely to produce valid and reliable guidelines at a local level. This in turn will help avoid duplication of effort.

As an example of the usefulness of audit we can review the effect of auditing practice in a tide of technological change, in relation to both therapeutic endoscopy and surgical practice. In 1985, our population in Brighton (300 000) underwent 230 cholecystectomies, with a further 22 common bile duct explorations with cholecystectomy. Endoscopy was used to treat the bile duct stones of another 24 patients, making a total of 276 cases. We set a guideline based on published papers of identifying all common duct stones by history and tests, and treating them primarily by endoscopy. Furthermore, those who were elderly and had remaining gall bladders with stones would not have surgery unless the gall bladder gave further symptoms. By 1990, reaudit showed cholecystectomies reduced to 164 for the same population, with 15 surgical explorations of the common duct and 78 endoscopic. This reduction in open surgery and almost complete abandonment of ritual on-table cholangiography produced estimated net savings of 52 hernia equivalents of activity per annum, which were devoted to other needier patients.

Audit is not a 'witch hunt', it is not about apportioning blame, and it is not a negative activity. It is a method of highlighting aspects of the service which would benefit from change and helping to direct what that change should be. Once the benefits of systematic audit become apparent, it is ethically inescapable for clinicians, and its deployment becomes a central requirement of patients through their agents, the purchasers, and of training supervisory bodies – royal colleges, including nursing and professions allied to medicine, universities, regional postgraduate deans and undergraduate degree programmes. In addition, the financial pressures on health care providers to ensure cost-effective and cost-efficient care requires purchasers to seek evidence that providers are monitoring and continually improving the quality of service they offer. All these needs can be met through careful, thought-out, clinical audit.

Audit and research

The key difference between audit and research is that research seeks to identify what is best practice whilst audit looks to see if best practice is being met. For example, clinical research is conducted to determine whether treatment A is better than treatment B. The findings indicate that treatment B is the more clinically efficacious. An audit is therefore undertaken to see whether treatment B is actually being carried out in practice.

As another example, 250 years ago James Lind demonstrated the value of fresh lemon juice in preventing scurvy among seamen. This excellent research was partly wasted for lack of audit – scurvy continued, since it was wrongly assumed that the juice would keep its effect if kept in barrels.

However, confusion continues as to the differences between research and audit partly because the boundaries between the two are not always distinct. The main differences between research and audit are highlighted in Fig. 16.3.

It must be accepted that research and audit do have much in common. In particular, they share a rigorous approach to methodology in terms of design, procedure, analysis and interpretation of data. Both also depend on the spirit of inquiry, must be 'bottom-up' to be fully effective and use the appropriate quantitative and qualitative research methods.

How is audit done?

Audits are most effective when they are planned as complete projects. A structured approach needs to be taken to selecting, planning, implementing and evaluating projects to ensure all parts of the audit cycle are completed. Brighton Health Care[11] has produced some useful guidelines just for this purpose which are linked to a set of audit project record forms. These help ensure the audit project is 'right first time' by providing prompts and checklists, enabling progress to be monitored, timescales to be maintained and information to be aggregated and analysed simply.[12]

Thus, there are four clearly identifiable stages to each complete audit project – selection of the topic,

Audit	Research
• Is a systematic approach to peer review of clinical care in order to identify possible improvements and to provide a mechanism for bringing them about.	• Is a systematic investigation which aims to increase the sum of knowledge. It usually involves hypothesis testing.
• Raises questions to be answered by research.	• Generates the knowledge to be used by audit.
• Is a test of whether things are being done the way it has been agreed they should be done; it compares care provided against agreed standards in order to identify whether best practice is being applied locally.	• Is concerned with discovering the right thing to do, identifying the most effective form of treatment and establishing what constitutes best clinical practice.
• Never involves allocating patients randomly to different treatment groups.	• May involve allocating patients randomly to different treatment groups.
• Never involves a placebo treatment.	• May involve administration of a placebo.
• Never involves a completely new treatment, and usually focuses on treatments where there is some consensus about what constitutes best clinical practice.	• May involve a completely new treatment, and usually focuses on treatments where knowledge about what is best clinical practice does not exist.
• Examines particular types of care given over a particular period of time, in a particular location and the results apply only to the population examined.	• Results can be generalized.
• Involves the voluntary participation of specialities and departments; data recorded and analysed relates to the participating clinician's own work.	• Chooses clinicians and patients to participate because they are representative so that results can be generalized.
• Is an ongoing and continuous process.	• Usually has an endpoint which is often when an adequate sample size has been obtained.
• Results are fed in a timely manner back into a discussion about peer performance; changes in practice are made as appropriate.	• Results are usually published so that all relevant clinicians can learn from the research.

Fig. 16.3 Key differences between audit and research.[1, 7–10]

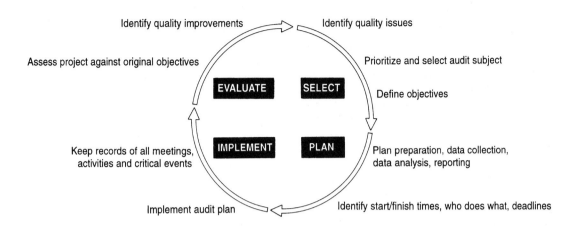

Fig. 16.4 Four stages of an audit project.

planning of the project, implementation of the project plan and evaluation of the project (see Fig. 16.4).

PROJECT SELECTION

Audit topics vary from the simplest to the grandest. The best way to decide how you are going to join in is to remember that audit is for you. Success, however, will only come if others share your suggested changes. Thus, the first audits in a young doctor's life concern their world – unnecessary bleeps, broken microwaves, empty food cabinets. Progressing into a speciality such as surgery invites audits into inappropriate minor and intermediate surgery, asking questions about analgesia, wound infection, multiple operations for simple conditions such as ingrowing toe nail or pilonidal sinus. Eventually the consultant seeks reviews of satisfactory outcome in non-malignant conditions such as biliary pain or antireflux surgery and complication rates and survival in bowel resection, breast cancer or arterial reconstruction. Often there is little to be gained from grander plans other than the discovery of the energy required to carry them through. Smaller schemes, often with the patients viewpoint in mind, give greater dividend.

An audit topic may be identified from problems going on within your area of practice at the present time. Possible sources for selecting an audit topic include:

- standards/guidelines, e.g. Are they being met? Do they exist?
- informal and formal complaints;
- risk management data, e.g. drug errors, property damage, falls;
- informal comments, e.g. suggestions box, voiced frustrations;

- staff turnover, absence and morale;
- multidisciplinary team when each team member can see a situation from a different point of view and an audit enables a consensus to be reached through standard setting;
- data on clinical and management computer systems;
- national initiatives, e.g. Health of the Nation, League Tables, Patient's Charter;
- quality frameworks, e.g. Donabedian,[13] Maxwell;[14]
- examining research and literature, e.g. trust/directorate forward plans, health authority contracts.

Ideally, an audit topic is best selected within the multidisciplinary team and should reflect professional, managerial, provider, purchaser and national priorities. Prioritization of audit topics and forward planning are essential to ensure a directorate/clinician-led plan of topics reflecting a balance between the vast number of interests. If a project team launches straight into the first audit topic which comes to mind there is the risk that there is a more

Table 16.1 Criteria to select an audit project

1. Does the project address a known quality issue?
2. Does the project address an important area of practice?
3. Is there an achievable quality improvement?
4. Does the project address an area of clinical certainty and consensus?
5. Will the project test, use or set explicit standards?
6. Does the project have clinical support?
7. Does the project involve self-audit?
8. Is the project multidisciplinary?

important or more relevant subject that should be addressed first, or indeed that an uncomfortable problem is being passed over. You should therefore agree your selected topic for audit with your department audit lead.

We use eight criteria[11] to help us determine whether it is worth pursuing an audit project. These criteria are listed in Table 16.1. We would also add to these criteria that a literature review should be undertaken to establish what best practice is, if a need for change is identified. Since we think these criteria are important, each criterion is stated in more detail below, and the rationale for its use is explained. The project which can answer each question positively is more likely to succeed than one which gets negative answers.

- Does the project address a known quality issue?
  Is it focused on something which is known to present quality problems – an area of practice where substandard care is acknowledged to exist, for whatever reason?
  In most clinical departments, there are plenty of known and acknowledged quality problems waiting to be addressed. Audits which focus on an area where everyone thinks they are probably doing quite well may do more to comfort and reassure clinicians than to actually produce quality improvements.
- Does the project address an important area of practice?
  Is the topic important because it involves a high volume of patients, or because it covers areas of especially high cost, or because it addresses practices or procedures known to be of high risk to patients?
  Since you can do only a limited number of audits and there will always be more topics than time and resources allow, you will want to maximize the overall improvement in quality you produce. This is done by focusing on high volume, high cost or high risk areas because these are the places where changes will have the most effect.
- Is there an achievable quality improvement?
  Are there grounds for believing that the quality problems addressed by the project are actually soluble – do practical, potential solutions exist?
  Every department has problems which it cannot solve itself – either because it lacks the resources or because they lie outside the department's control. Audits which focus on areas where the department itself cannot make the necessary changes (and cannot persuade anyone else to do so) are likely to fail.
- Does the project address an area of clinical certainty/consensus?
  Is there agreement among clinicians about what good quality/practice is, or is there a lack of consensus/knowledge and a need for research rather than audit?
  Audit is much more pragmatic, down to earth and basic than most research. It is about applying existing knowledge (making sure that what we do measures up to best practice) rather than about establishing what best practice is – that is research. In every department, there are many topics where clinical consensus exists, and audit should be focused on these areas.
- Will the project test, use or set explicit standards?
  Are there agreed standards which will be used in the project, or will standards and/or clinical protocols or guidelines emerge from the project?
  Experience suggests that standards and protocols are useful both in documenting what people expect to happen, and in identifying whether those things actually happen. They also help to make changes in practice take place, because the agreed approach to practice is clearly defined in writing. Audits which use standards are therefore more likely to result in real and lasting quality improvements.
- Does the project have clinical support?
  Is the project the ' baby' of a single clinician, or is it supported by all or most clinicians in the speciality/department?
  If people are going to change their practice, they need to support the audit from the start. A lone voice among clinicians may be right, but he or she needs to get their colleagues signed up to the audit project before it starts. Simply presenting the results to them at the end is unlikely to produce any worthwhile quality improvements. You need to ensure that your audit lead and senior clinicians are signed up to the proposed audit topic as a priority.
- Does the project involve self-audit?
  Is the purpose of the project to audit the practice of the clinicians proposing it, or does it effectively involve auditing the practice of other departments or specialities?
  If the audit looks at the practice of other departments, it needs to involve them. For example, audits of the communication between departments, or of the service received by one department or another, are of little use if both sides are not involved. Sometimes, auditing the services received from other departments is mistakenly used as a substitute for auditing your own practice.
- Is the project multidisciplinary?
  Does the project solely involve one professional group, such as medical staff, or is it truly multidisciplinary, involving several disciplines at all stages of the project (not just data collection)?
  While some audit topics relate solely to a single profession, they are really in the minority. As soon

as you start to examine the processes or systems of care, you usually find that other professions are involved or have a legitimate interest in the topic. Certainly, when you start to plan quality improvements, it is hard to do so without affecting other professions or groups. Again, it is better to involve these people before the start of the project than to simply present them with the results.

PROJECT PLANNING

Having a written plan for your audit project is important for five main reasons – knowing who is doing what (and by when); meeting deadlines and identifying critical events; managing your workload and balancing priorities; identifying and resolving potential problems; and keeping track of how projects are progressing.

The plan needs to start with clear, specific, realistic objectives indicating the aim of the audit project. An audit method is then selected, the methods and practical issues of data collection are addressed, plans for data analysis are made and the costs of the project are estimated. Areas of work within the project are assigned to individuals and a timetable is planned.

The choice of audit method is largely implied by the nature of your project: focused studies with a criterion-based approach, occurrence screening (i.e. adverse event screening), case reviews, mortality and morbidity assessment meetings, measures of quality, workload analysis, organizational audit and patient satisfaction.

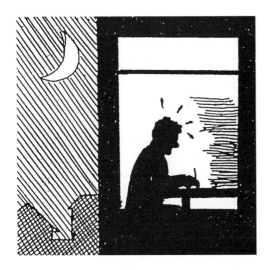

Fig. 16.5 'Audit can easily be fitted in to the clinical routine'.

A choice has to be made about data collection. Will it be by case note screening, observation, interview, questionnaire, extracting from the hospital information system, or a combination of these? Will it come from patients, relatives or staff? Data handling needs to be addressed before collection begins. The advice of experienced audit personnel should be sought – they know the problems and pitfalls and can help with advice, facilities and even time!

Whichever method is used, a sample is more likely to be analysed than a whole population. Care should be taken to ensure that the sample resembles the population it is drawn from as closely as possible.

Finally, the resources required should be estimated. The main one may well be your own time (see Fig. 16.5). Discuss this with your team. Audit is work, and they will want to know the answer and help out accordingly. Consider eventually how you will write up, present or even publish your audit. Put it in your CV.

PROJECT IMPLEMENTATION

Data collection and analysis takes place and a record of all meetings, critical decisions, activities and phone conversations should be kept. The results of the audit are then taken back to the project group and discussed. Results are compared with objectives and the original standard/guideline being assessed. If the standard or objectives have not been met, appropriate changes in practice are identified using brainstorming or problem analysis techniques involving all staff whose work is touched by these changes. The suggested changes are then prioritized either using a pros and cons list or by scoring solutions. The change(s) decided on are then facilitated. Action plans or documentation of procedures as guidelines or standards can assist this process. Practice is then monitored to assess whether the agreed changes have taken place, perhaps through repeating or continuing with the data collection process.

PROJECT EVALUATION

The audit should be evaluated against its objectives, the costs of undertaking it, the resulting quality improvements and problems encountered, to establish and quantify the success of the project and learn lessons for the future. It is important to remember that you can always learn from results. Understanding reasons for success and failure makes each project a learning experience for all involved. Ensure you evaluate the project before moving on to the next project despite the great temptation to leap straight into the new project.

There are a number of key questions to ask to assist this evaluation process:[11]

- Were the objectives met?
- What stopped the objectives being met?
- What quality improvements were made?
- What problems were encountered?
- What resources were used?
- Does the project need to be revisited?

In addition, there are three other important questions that we would add:

- Was there a cost saving?
- Was there an improved outcome in care?
- How will the new guidelines be retained in practice in the unit?

Confidentiality for the patient, system and staff

This is obviously a concern for all practising clinicians which is rising ever more to the fore with the developing interest of purchasers in clinical audit.

Members of staff who participate in clinical audit have a right to expect that the details of the process and its outcome will remain confidential, and that access to information which identifies individual members of staff should be appropriately controlled and restricted.[15] The results of an audit are intended to be fed back to just those involved. Nobody outside the group need see the findings, although the identified improvements can be publicized in a general form.

Walshe and Bennett[15] suggest key principles to ensure that material identifying individual patients is kept to an absolute minimum:

- members of staff may only be identified in audit documentation if absolutely necessary;
- where it is not possible to avoid identifying patients or members of staff, steps must be taken to anonymize those records and any related documentation;
- minutes or notes of audit meetings should refrain from identifying individual patients or members of staff, or include any information which could be used to identify individuals;
- all audit documentation should be clearly labelled to show that it is part of the audit process, and that it is confidential;
- the sender of any audit information should ensure its circulation is controlled as tightly as possible;
- the recipient of any audit documentation should

accept full responsibility for ensuring its storage, handling and eventual destruction.

Individual patients have a right to expect that the confidentiality of their medical records is respected by all those who have access. Furthermore, access to these records should be restricted to personnel who are involved in the provision, evaluation or support of patient care.[15] The clinical audit process should respect patient confidentiality by ensuring that access to information identifiable to individual patients is appropriately controlled and restricted.

The pitfall of routine data collection

Audit does not mean routine data collection through clinical information systems whether departmental or hospital based. There are five principles of good practice to govern the collection, management and analysis of information in clinical audit:

1. *Audit-driven information needs.* The information to be collected or used in clinical audit should be clearly and definitely determined by the quality measures being used in the audit process rather than on the basis of the data available in existing information systems.
2. *Limited role of information in audit.* Information collection, management and analysis are only a limited and relatively small part of the clinical audit process. Many data gathered by existing information systems are extraneous to the needs of clinical audit being concerned rather with workload, activity and resource utilization. There is a common but mistaken belief that large quantities of data in such systems will inevitably inform the clinical audit process.
3. *Use of byproduct data when relevant.* Clinical audit should make use of relevant and meaningful data already available from existing information systems whenever it can, and access to this information therefore needs to be widely available to avoid clinical audit collecting it all over again. Hospitals collect excellent data on their admitted patients but too often it is either unavailable to clinicians or ignored by them.
4. *Data collected specifically for audit.* When data are collected specifically for audit, the quantity should be carefully limited, relate specifically to the project's objectives and be gathered over

a fixed time period. Very often sampling is required. Projects that require large data sets, or which demand the continuous collection of data for long periods of time should be reviewed and the relevance to clinical audit carefully considered.

5. *Information systems in an audit.* It is generally not appropriate to install information systems solely to collect data for clinical audit, since the information needs of clinical audit are better served by small, focused, fixed-term data collection exercises.

Too often the drudgery of routine data collection and entry in a departmental microcomputer has deflected the attention of consultants from other quality issues, while making audit a psychonoxious word for junior doctors.

Way forward

The development of clinical audit will have increasing relevance to the interrelationships of clinicians, managers, providers and purchasers. The interaction between purchasers, management and clinical audit is increasingly in focus because of the changes in funding of audit. The emphasis on funding of clinical audit is now through the purchasing process.[16] Managers are increasingly looking towards clinical audit as a tool to inform the business planning process and improve delivery of health care. They and purchasers are looking to share general information from clinical audit. In addition, purchasers expect to see established clinical audit programmes in all provider units with which they contract, as supporting evidence of the efficacy of care that they are purchasing for their population. Both as buyers of health care services and in their public health capacity, they need to assess whether and how services they buy are benefiting patients, and are interested in cost-effective methods of improving services. Thus, the principles of cost–benefit are coming to the fore but have been little addressed to date. Those who make measurable changes through audit need to make clear the economic effect of their improvements and give credit to the audit system to ensure its virtues are recognized in times of economic pressure.

Audit is better known in North America and in industry generally as 'quality assurance' and we should probably begin to drop the term audit, useful though it has been, and focus our energies on the broader term 'quality', which can be assured via a number of quality improvement techniques including utilization review of facilities, incident-reporting systems, morbidity and mortality meetings, patient satisfaction, claims analysis, risk management and most of all through clinical audit.

Audit was initially seen as an 'extra' in clinical life, but royal colleges and postgraduate deans now expect active participation in audit as evidence of educational activity by both trainers and trainees.

References

1. University of Dundee. *Moving to Audit – What Every Doctor Needs to Know about Medical Audit.* Dundee: The Postgraduate Office, Ninewells Hospital, 1992.
2. Department of Health. *Working for Patients.* Medical audit, Working paper 6. London: HMSO, 1989.
3. Buttery Y, Walshe K, Coles J, Bennett J. *The Development of Audit. Findings of a National Survey of Healthcare Provider Units in England.* London: CASPE Research, 1994.
4. NHS Management Executive. *Clinical Audit: Meeting and Improving Standards in Healthcare.* London: Department of Health, July 1993; EL(93)**59**: 4.
5. Vasanthakamur V, Brown P. *Qual Health Care* 1992; **1**: 142.
6. Irvine D, Irvine S (eds). *Making Sense of Audit.* Oxford: Radcliffe Medical Press, 1991.
7. Jacyna MR, de Lacey G, Chapman J. 3. How does medical audit differ from research? How necessary are computers? *Hosp Update* 1992; **18**: 592–6.
8. *Making Medical Audit Effective.* London: Joint Centre for Education in Medicine, 1992.
9. Madden AP. Research or audit? *Network* 1991; **1**: 1.
10. Smith R. Audit and research. *Br Med J* 1992; **305**: 905–6.
11. Walshe K. *Making audit work – guidelines on selecting, planning, implementing and evaluating audit projects.* CASPE Research and Brighton Health Care Department of Clinical Audit. Brighton Health Care NHS Trust, Department of Clinical Audit, 1993.
12. Walshe K, Tomalin DA. Raincheck. *Health Serv J* 1993; 29 April: 28–9.
13. Donabedian A. Evaluating the quality of medical care. *Milbank Mem Fund Quart* 1966; **44**(3): 166–206.
14. Maxwell RJ. Quality assessment in health. *Br Med J* 1984; **288**: 1470–2.
15. Walshe K, Bennett J. *Guidelines on Medical Audit and Confidentiality.* Brighton Health Authority and

South East Thames Regional Health Authority, January, 1991.

16. NHS Management Executive. *Clinical Audit in* *HCHS: Funding for 1994/95 and Beyond.* London: Department of Health, 1993. November. EL(93)104.

For further information regarding surgical audit undertaken by the Royal College of Surgeons contact: The Surgical Audit Unit, The Royal College of Surgeons of England, 35/43 Lincolns Inn Fields, London WC2A 3PN.

CHAPTER 17

Clinical information technology and clinical information science

FT DE DOMBAL†, SE CLAMP

Introduction

One of the most important developments in clinical medicine in the second half of the twentieth century has concerned clinical information. Medicine is not alone in this. The society in which we live is driven by information – its generation, its access, its use, and the difficulties in general of 'keeping up' in an ever more complicated world.

In many areas of human activity (such as banking and airlines) the so-called information revolution has already taken place – necessarily so, since information is generated in the course of these activities in vastly greater quantities that could ever have been imagined a few decades ago. Medicine, however, is different – a fact often overstated by doctors and underappreciated by computer scientists and information technologists. Nonetheless, physicians and surgeons cannot sit idly by while the information revolution gathers pace; it has become increasingly

relevant to include basic information science and technology in the 'core knowledge' which every physician and surgeon possesses. Indeed, such was the recommendation contained in the recent document *Tomorrow's Doctors* produced by the General Medical Council of the UK.[1]

The problem is that the medical profession is understandably reluctant to take on board yet another discipline – particularly since most young people qualify as doctors with the idea of dealing with people not machines. Thus, a vicious circle is set up in which the average physician or surgeon is unable to benefit from the information revolution, largely from a lack of familiarity with the technology, the science and its implementation.

The purpose of this chapter is to attempt to achieve a remedy for this situation – not so much by didactic teaching (for informatics in medicine is still a very young science) but by a discussion of the issues. Hopefully, the reader may thereby better appreciate

† It is with great regret that we note that Professor FT de Dombal died suddenly on 31 December 1995. He will be sadly missed.

the prospects and problems related to clinical information, and in turn be better able to address specific practical problems from a position of some basic understanding. In this chapter, therefore, we shall consider such fundamental issues as the nature of clinical information, how one assesses it, how information flows around the hospital or between different locations, what role is potentially available for information systems and technology (in both the medium and short term), how clinicians currently perceive their role; and finally (and most important) what all of us need to do to achieve a situation where the benefits of information technology are obtained without the undoubted problems.

Some basic definitions

Perhaps the most fundamental stumbling block to the understanding of clinical information is embodied in the title of this section. Unfortunately, in relation to information science, terms are often used interchangeably and confusingly. Clinical information is no exception. It is therefore necessary to begin with some basic definitions. (More detailed definitions are set out elsewhere, see Appendix.[2])

DATA, INFORMATION AND KNOWLEDGE

These terms are often used interchangeably, but they are not synonymous. Data (pl.) and information differ from one another in one significant respect. Data are observations made and recorded as such. Information implies that an observation has been made, and the datum (sing.) has been in some way interpreted.

Thus, straightforward observations (the time is 4pm; the patient's haemoglobin level is 14.1 g/dl, and so on) would be regarded as data. No significant interpretation has been made. They are merely observations.

On the other hand, most of what a clinician receives amounts to information rather than simple data, because it implies that an interpretation has already been made. For example, a statement such as 'the patient has ulcerative colitis' may or may

not be true – but either way, data have been interpreted and thus the statement consists of information.

The difference between 'information' and 'knowledge' is again fundamental. In an ideal world, the mere transmission of information would guarantee its accurate reception. In the real world this is not so. Everyone is familiar with the way in which transmitted information such as 'Send reinforcements, we're going to advance' becomes (erroneously) translated by the recipient of this information as knowledge 'send three and fourpence we're going to a dance.'

It is all too easy to dismiss this silly example as being of no consequence. In practice, the distinction between information and knowledge is crucial. Consider a (1-hour) surgical lecture. In the average lecture of this type upwards of 1000 'facts' (information) are imparted. Research shows that the knowledge received amounts to just nine 'facts' per hour. As in science, so in medicine therefore. Information (1000 facts) is what is transmitted; knowledge (nine facts) is what is received.

CLINICAL INFORMATION SCIENCE AND TECHNOLOGY

Another fundamental problem in the minds of many clinicians concerns the difference between information science and information technology. Often these are perceived as synonymous. In effect they are completely different, as Table 17.1 demonstrates.

In Table 17.1 we consider some parallels between surgery, and information science and technology, and the distinction between these two latter subjects becomes more clear. In surgery, the surgeon uses hardware (the instruments and implements found in the operating theatre). Surgeons do not, however, use these empirically – but rely on an operating code of practice (surgical manual, or something similar). By this means the surgeon learns to conduct specific operations in a particular sequence found to be most appropriate. The operating implements and manuals are both made available by commercial companies. Underlying this, however, are several layers of surgical science without which operating procedures would be empirical, dangerous and potentially harmful to the patient.

Table 17.1 Some basic definitions and comparisons.

Aspect	Drug therapy	Surgery	Information
Hardware	Drugs	Instruments	Computer technology
Development	Pharmaceutical industry	Equipment manufacturers	Computer companies
Modus operandi	Therapeutics/regimen	Surgical technique/manuals	Computer programs
Underpinning science	Pharmacology	Surgical research	Information science

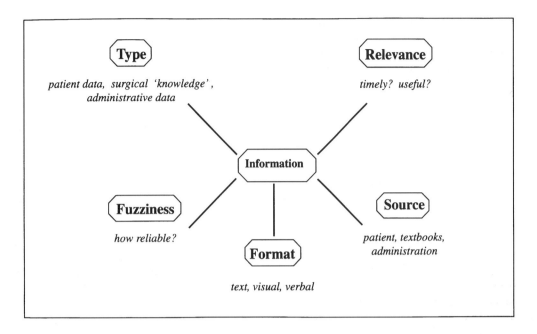

Fig. 17.1 The dimensions of information. Every item of clinical information has a number of attributes. These are just some of them.

It is exactly the same in the world of information. What is used are not surgical instruments but a different form of hardware (the computer usually). This is often referred to as 'information technology'. It is used with a particular code of practice – a sequence which has been found to be optimal (the software). Commercial companies manufacture both of these. Underlying both, however, is layer after layer of 'information science', without which any use of computers would be empirical and potentially dangerous.

Of course it is possible to take this analogy too far. For example, could the surgeon, following a set of operating instructions taught to him by his or her peers be referred to (as some contend) as simply working through an algorithm? There are, nevertheless, intriguing parallels between the computing world and the world of the surgeon which enable us to understand both worlds a little better.

TELEMATICS AND THE SUPER HIGHWAY

These two further terms have recently emerged and it may be helpful to mention them here. Both have caused confusion but both in essence represent simple concepts. 'Telematics' is a corruption of two words: 'telecommunications' and 'informatics'. The concept of telematics implies a fusion of these two topics – telecommunications allowing information to be transmitted in great profusion over whatever distance is desired, and informatics allowing an appropriate use of the information provided at the distant location. The allied term 'health care telematics' has thus been coined to encompass the fusion of telecommunications and informatics in a variety of applications relating to health care.

The 'super highway' represents a concept rather than being a technical term. In the field of telecommunications, such has been the pace of advance that the capacity to exchange and access data between remote locations is now almost unlimited – at least for all practical purposes, since our ability to transmit and exchange information now exceeds our ability to know what to do with the information that has been transmitted or received.

So the implications of the super highway are that nowadays, at minimal cost, a network of communication facilities has sprung up which can, to all intents and purposes, be accessed by any individual user on the planet. Again, this has implications for health care and clinical medicine – in terms of remote 'conferencing' and also (as we shall discuss later) in terms of access to clinical information by a wide variety of non-medically qualified persons.

What makes clinical information special?

Much of the information generated in relation to health care is relatively unremarkable. There is no difference in principle between the information related to the administrative running of a hospital (hours worked by cleaners, number of employees on the pay roll, etc.) and comparable data from other walks of life. This is not what makes clinical information special.

What makes clinical information special, and also so difficult to assess and analyse, is that it is not homogeneous. It comes in a variety of guises and situations (Fig. 17.1). Indeed, the different forms of clinical information are so numerous as to be almost bewildering.

Some examples of these different characteristics are:

- the type of information – visual, verbal, written, etc;
- the format – textual, numeric or pictorial;
- The apparent confusion regarding 'hard' vs 'soft' information.

This last aspect (perhaps more than any other) is what distinguishes clinical information from other types of information. The surgeon (or for that matter the physician) is constantly bombarded by all sorts of information (visual, verbal, textual, numeric) on all sorts of topics (medical, administrative or whatever) and of varying reliability (ranging from 'this patient's haemoglobin level is 14.1 g/dl' to 'I was reading something about porphyria the other day') – and in ever increasing quantity and frequency. Small wonder that surgeons have become increasingly overwhelmed with clinical information – and that there has been increasing interest in the last few decades in the way they deal with it, and how they can be helped do so more effectively.

Information in surgical practice

We have seen that the types of information in clinical practice are bewildering in their complexity. It may be helpful to consider a standard clinical situation in which the individual surgeon faces an individual patient with a particular surgical problem. To deal with this the surgeon needs clinical information under three broad headings:

- information about the particular patient;
- surgical knowledge base;
- knowledge of the working environment.

Lacking any one of these three categories of information, the surgeon cannot proceed with patient management in an effective manner. It may, therefore, be helpful to consider each separately.

PATIENT INFORMATION

Most surgeons will recall an introductory course which they attended as a student, and will have from that time been familiar with the litany of information to be secured from the patient (Table 17.2). Such a scheme (from the Leeds third year undergraduate course) has been around for many years; and is probably rather close to the clinical method which most surgeons were taught in their early days as a student.

It came as something of a surprise, therefore, to researchers 30 or 40 years ago when simple studies of the type known as 'process tracing' indicated great variety in behaviour patterns of individual surgeons.[3] Some surgeons pursue an inflexible (or algorithmic) approach – particularly junior surgeons who tend to collect a large amount of information and analyse it later. Others (particularly more experienced surgeons) adopt a more flexible goal-seeking or heuristic behaviour (often referred to as pattern matching). In this they ask a few questions, form a hypothesis or working diagnosis and then attempt to seek further information to either confirm or refute the initial hypothesis.

There is thus no uniform manner by which surgeons assimilate information from patients. There is a type of behaviour (flexible, goal seeking and pattern matching) which is typical of senior surgeons – but this is the very antithesis of what we teach medical students and junior surgeons!

THE SURGICAL KNOWLEDGE BASE

If a surgeon is to manage an individual patient appropriately, that surgeon must possess a sound knowledge of what has traditionally been referred to as surgical practice, but what in information science terms would be referred to as the surgical knowledge base.

Some examples of this are shown in Fig. 17.2. The figure merely lists some of the aspects of a particular surgical problem with which the surgeon must be familiar in order to manage a patient effectively. As illustrated, these aspects include basic definitions, disease criteria, criteria for extent and severity of a particular disease, the minimum data set of items to be elicited from the patient – along with their definitions – together with the appropriate indication for high technological investigation and the indications for operative intervention.[4]

This list is by no means exhaustive, but it is exclusive – in the sense that failure to possess the

Table 17.2 Information from a patient with acute abdominal pain. Note that the volume of information vastly exceeds the capacity of the individual surgeon to handle it

Category of information	No. of items
Interview presenting complaint, associated symptoms, past history, etc.	50+
Examination general, abdominal inspection, palpation, percussion, auscultation	40+
Investigation haematology, biochemistry, radiology, imaging, etc.	Possibility unlimited

appropriate information about any one of the aspects listed may well lead to an inappropriate form of management for the individual patient concerned.

WORKING ENVIRONMENT

Nowadays the surgeon is part of a working team. Consequently, the surgeon clearly needs a great deal of further information concerning the working environment not merely, as previously, about the theatre and wards in which he or she works. Today, information concerning the local, regional and national administration of the health care delivery system in which the surgeon is occupied is equally important. Indeed, with the increasing blurring of the distinction between primary and secondary care, the surgeon's information base concerning many aspects of administrative work has expanded dramatically.

Resultant problems

It is not difficult to predict from the above section that the surgeon – provided with an increasing wealth of incoming information from a variety of sources – is likely to encounter problems in dealing with this clinical information. Any surgeon who questions this premise would do well to read a paper by Miller[5] entitled 'The magic number 7 – plus or minus 2', in which he argues cogently that the average

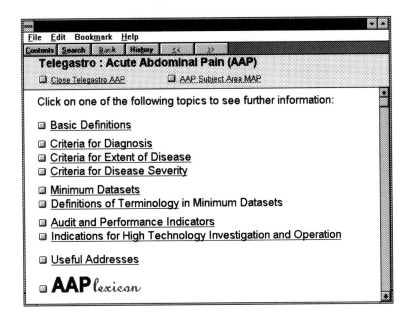

Fig. 17.2 Examples of aspects of the surgical knowledge base with which the surgeon must be familiar in order to manage a patient effectively.

human being cannot cope with more than half a dozen or so incoming facts at once.

PATIENT INFORMATION

It might also be argued that the information overload encountered by the surgeon in day-to-day life is of little practical value. Unfortunately, the reverse is true. A number of careful studies have been carried out over the years which demonstrate the problems of information overload for the surgeon.

Studies in the last 20 or 30 years have demonstrated repeatedly that surgeons – like other doctors – do not elicit information at all well from patients. They ask large numbers of irrelevant questions[6] often at the expense of those which would be relevant[7] with the advantage of hindsight. Surgeons, like other doctors, ignore obvious clues to diagnosis and/or management[8] and obtain much relatively useless data (see Table 17.2) of which they utilize less than 5%.[9, 10]

This leads in turn to poor diagnosis and decision-making. Studies in this field of acute abdominal pain have shown again and again that diagnostic accuracy at initial patient contact is less than 50%. In many centres perforation rates in appendicitis patients have exceeded 25%, whilst negative appendicectomy rates have also exceeded 25%.[11] Moreover, despite the cosy theory that 'things are getting better', the most recent studies from the north western region of the UK show that if anything performance levels are declining, with bad surgical error rates and perforated appendix rates exceeding 30% in some centres.[12]

SURGICAL KNOWLEDGE BASE

The problems which arise from the explosion of information about the progress and practice of surgery are harder to document – even though the gap between the knowledge base of the average surgeon and the potential knowledge base concerning practice is growing day by day. Moreover, this problem (in contrast with the problem concerning patient information) is more likely to affect more experienced surgeons.[13]

Interestingly, the most serious of these effects are two-fold. At one end of the spectrum is a widely recognized danger which might be termed 'intellectual atherosclerosis'. In this condition, a surgeon thus afflicted reacts to the avalanche of new data concerning surgical practice by ignoring it. Whilst it is easy to sneer at such a practice, this condition in practical terms is more rational and less harmful than the alternative. Such surgeons, by ignoring new developments, continue to practise their profession up to the

standard when they stopped taking in new data – and often these standards are very high indeed.

Far more serious (but sadly also far more prevalent) is the alternative – namely uncritical evaluation of new surgical techniques. It is unfortunately true that many surgical 'advances' in wide practical use have not been critically evaluated and would not have been adopted at all had this happened at an early stage.

The problem is far from academic, and it is central to this discussion. The list of surgical advances which have come into fashion, enjoyed a brief vogue, proved worthless and been abandoned is long and depressing. Why have surgeons, the vast majority with great integrity and high intelligence, so readily followed these false pathways?

Various answers (often denigrating surgeons' intellectual ability – or even honesty) have been proposed but here dealing with the information explosion the answer is obvious. Deprived of conclusive scientific evidence and faced with a sensory overload the surgeon, who is only human, will sometimes opt for what is glossy and well-presented rather than what is worthy but dull. Thus surgical 'fashion' – profligate of time, resources and patients' lives – has been recognized for many years. What the study of information science contributes to the problem is the realization that in these circumstances surgical 'fashion' is not only prevalent, but inevitable.

WORKING ENVIRONMENT

Finally, in this section, we need to note briefly the problems of the working environment and what the surgeon needs to know about it. Some problems already described will not be repeated – except to observe that some surgeons (possibly wise ones) respond to the increasing complexity of the working environment by delegating much of this complex activity to their more junior staff (or to the increasing number of managers employed in surgical departments these days).

Possible solutions

In this final section we consider some of the solutions which have been proposed to deal with information explosion in clinical medicine. These solutions can be divided into three groups: those which are clearly not appropriate, those which might possibly assist to some extent and, finally, those which appear to offer the best hope (Table 17.3).

Table 17.3 Potential solutions to the information explosion grouped according to likelihood that the proposed solution will work in practice

Unlikely to work	May work	Best prospects
Longer medical curriculum	Altered selection	Definition of objectives
More intelligent students	Recertification	Change to problem solving
Super-specialization	Job sharing	Education re teamwork
Better administration	Delegation tasks	Core curriculum
Arbitrary target setting	Public education	Paramedical staff
		Sensible audit
		Use information technology

PROPOSED SITUATIONS OF MINIMAL POTENTIAL VALUE

At the undergraduate level, increasing the length of the medical curriculum and selecting 'cleverer' medical students would seem to be of minimal value. Simple mathematics indicate the medical curriculum would have to be extended to over 200 years to learn the whole of clinical medicine. Such solutions therefore are clearly impractical.

At the graduate level, the proposed solution has in the past been ever more super-specialization. Clearly, this is an increasingly unworkable solution. Quite apart from the dangers of a super-specialist making inappropriate judgements in a field with which he or she is not familiar, there is a limit to the degree of specialization; and it is clear, that even in a particular field, a specialist is going to have difficulty keeping up to date. (In gastroenterology approximately 25 000 relevant papers are published a year; one every 4 minutes of the working week.)

At the national and public health level, a number of facile proposals have been made – none of which do more than scratch the surface of the problem. Proposals such as 'better administration' are now widely seen as political slogans rather than sensible remedies. The idea of 'setting targets' and 'maintaining standards' constitutes an almost laughably simplistic solution. At present, the standards which exist in some areas of clinical surgery are woefully inadequate, and to actively seek to maintain the status quo constitutes an abrogation of responsibility.

PROPOSED SOLUTIONS OF POSSIBLE VALUE

At the undergraduate level, the proposal widely made recently concerns more appropriate selection to the profession. This is clearly long overdue – in that the current situation (selection to the profession dependent upon the ability to retain and recite fact) is clearly inappropriate. Any trend towards more appropriate selection would be welcome – with the proviso that 'more appropriate' can be defined.

At the graduate level, two possible proposed solutions may also have something to offer. The first concerns recertification. There currently exists an impetus to require a certain amount of postgraduate (continuing) medical education every year from qualified doctors – whether house surgeons or consultants – and the logical step from this is a requirement for recertification after so many years' clinical practice. Such a solution may have something to offer, but it will clearly not solve, by itself, all the problems.

At the national and public health level, developments which may have something to offer (in terms of sharing the information load) include the formation of health care teams, job sharing and also public education. One of the current problems in clinical medicine is increasing public expectations, often to a point where they are totally unrealistic, followed by medico-legal action in the event of a patient's treatment being less than entirely successful. Public education *per se* and public education concerning surgeons' abilities and practices would be a useful, partial solution.

POTENTIALLY APPROPRIATE SOLUTIONS

At the undergraduate level there needs to be much more careful definition of educational objectives than at present – in particular a change in the educational format from fact acquisition towards problem-solving ability – and especially towards education about team work in the National Health Service.

At both undergraduate and postgraduate levels the core curriculum thus needs to be defined more carefully than at present – and at postgraduate level it would seem reasonable to explore the use of paramedical staff in order to reduce the workload for relatively trivial matters of the average practising surgeon.

At the national and public health level, sensible audit and quality assessment procedures are clearly beneficial – again with the proviso that 'sensible' has to be defined in such a way as to be acceptable, not merely to the administration of the National Health Service, but also to those who practise surgery within it.

The use of information technology

So far in this chapter we have not discussed the use of information technology, or its potential role in solving problems which the information explosion has brought about. This has been deliberate, for two reasons.

First, the medical profession has lagged some way behind other professions such as banking, airlines and so on in the introduction of information technology. As such, there has until relatively recently been little experience upon which to draw.

Second, in the last few years two developments have occurred which have changed the situation very considerably. The first of these concerns the development of networking. Readers will be familiar with the term super highway but may be less familiar with the option which this opens up in clinical surgery. The science fiction writer Arthur C Clarke has proposed a simple dictum 'don't commute, communicate!' All very well, but since most clinical information is complex, often verbal, often visual and frequently requiring moving images it was (until recently) impossible to transmit. Networking now makes this possible. The other development which is relevant is the ability to store and transmit vast amounts of information cheaply (e.g. the CD-ROM). A single CD-ROM will hold the equivalent of 300 000 pages of A4 typescript and has been welcomed with open arms. What this offers the surgeon, however, is the option known as 'multimedia', i.e. information accessed from a computer which at the same time provides textual, verbal and visual information about a patient.

These two developments, networking and multimedia, taken together have therefore revolutionized the information technology field – and opened up to surgeons a number of opportunities. Some of these will be described briefly below.

REMOTE TELECONFERENCING

The development of large-scale computer networks in which information can flow combined with the telecommunications revolution already described, clearly offers opportunities for the surgeon. One major problem in surgery is that the surgeon is continually being consulted about patients who (although seriously ill and warranting personal attention) are not in the same place as the surgeon concerned. In the past it has often been difficult to do very much for such patients; but with the development of telecommunications (and the ability to send and retrieve visual, verbal and textual data) it is now possible for surgeons to give an opinion from a remote location – or more often *to* a remote location. This ability is called remote teleconferencing. It is clear that although this topic is in its infancy, it is important, and has potential; considerable development may be anticipated in the very near future.

DECISION SUPPORT

It has been shown that decision support by simple computer packages has led to improvement in clinical care, particularly from relatively inexperienced surgeons. The best known work in this regard concerns acute abdominal pain where such improvements were registered as long ago as 1972.[14] In the UK the best known study is that of Adams *et al.* in 1986[15] where tangible improvement in diagnosis and decision-making were noted. More recently, these improvements have been reproduced in 64 hospitals around the European Union (Fig. 17.3).[16]

It is, nevertheless, also clear that surgeons will not readily accept such computer support even in an ancillary capacity. Far more acceptable, however, is the use of information technology to store a basic up-to-date compendium of colleagues' views on such matters as criteria and standards or diagnosis, severity and extent of disease, minimum data sets and their definitions, performance indicators and indications for high technology investigation and even for surgery. Such a package is exemplified in the European Union's Telegastro package (Figs 17.4 and 17.5).[17]

INFORMATION TECHNOLOGY AND EDUCATION

This leads naturally to what is perhaps becoming the main use of information technology in the immediate future in surgery – namely its use for computer-assisted education. At undergraduate level, a number of packages are now available – these are widely

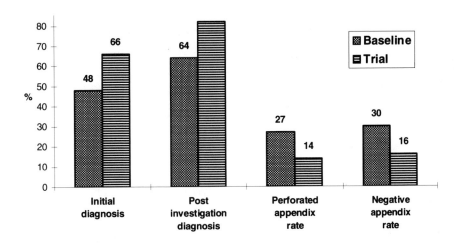

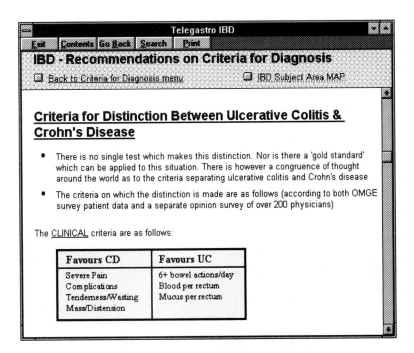

Fig. 17.3 Results from the EU Concerted Action on Acute Abdominal Pain showing improvements in diagnosis and decision-making in 14 963 cases, from 64 hospitals.

Fig. 17.4 Computer screen from Telegastro package showing information concerning inflammatory bowel disease and the criteria for diagnosis based on real life, patient data and a compendium of clinicians' views.

known, but it is worth mentioning in passing that the use of multimedia techniques has revolutionized the attraction of using such packages (Fig. 17.6). At postgraduate level, a further exciting prospect at the present time is the rapid development of 'virtual reality' techniques, so that surgical procedures

(especially minimally invasive or laparoscopic surgical procedures) can be practised repeatedly by neophytes – to try and avoid the sort of problems which have occurred with widespread, rapid (and possibly overambitious) introduction of this new surgical specialty.

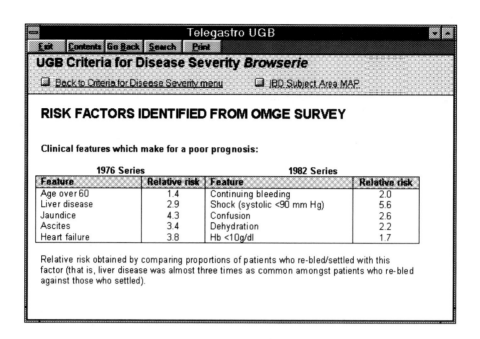

Fig. 17.5 Computer screen from Telegastro package showing information concerning upper gastrointestinal bleeding and the criteria for disease severity.

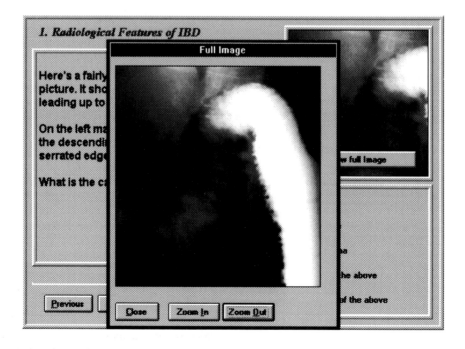

Fig.17.6 Example of the use of multimedia techniques to enhance undergraduate computer-assisted teaching.

Conclusion

We have seen that the information explosion which has occurred in clinical medicine over the last two or three decades has been of unprecedented proportion, and has had serious impact on the practice of clinical medicine and surgery. It is clear from this discussion that the problem, as well as being of considerable magnitude, is likely to become far worse in the medium term.

Many and varied are the proposals which have been made in order to address this problem. A number of them are extremely unlikely to be beneficial; though, on the other hand, some proposals listed will be of at least partial benefit. The role of information technology in addressing the problems of information has been discussed. Already, it is clear from existing experience that information technology–based solutions may become increasingly relevant in the future.

A FINAL CAVEAT

However, there is one danger concerning information and the use of information technology which needs to be in the forefront of the mind of every surgeon. This concerns the use not simply of information technology, but of 'unfettered' information technology. For 20 or 30 years' experience with information technologists teaches us that their agenda is not the same as that of the practising surgeon.

Used wisely and well, information technology may have a real role to play in helping surgeons cope with the information explosion. However, it is important to ensure that the technology is used wisely and well, and this is unlikely to be the case unless surgeons themselves pay very close attention to its development.

The final lesson which the short history of 'surgical informatics' teaches us, therefore, is that if information technology is to assist the surgeon of the future, then the surgeon of today must assist the information technology field by providing (1) input as to what is desired, (2) input as to what is unacceptable and (3) input concerning evaluation of systems which emerge – so that these emerging systems may benefit both future surgeons and future patients undergoing surgery.

Appendix: some further definitions

(with acknowledgment to G de Moor *et al.*)[2]

Multimedia
The simultaneous use of text, sound, images, colour and motion.

Interactivity
The possibility of controlling, without a noticeable delay, what is transmitted.

Broadband
A feature of a telecommunications network. Bandwidth is a way of expressing the maximum flow of information that a link can carry.

Digitization
The capacity to represent any kind of information with an 'alphabet' of only two 'digits'. It is the basis of multimedia.

Bits and bytes
The bit is the unit used for measuring the quantity (or volume) of digitized information. Its multiples are the kilobit (kb = 1024 bits), the megabit (Mb = 1024 kilobits) and the gigabit (Gb = 1024 megabits). A byte is a group of bits, usually 8 bits. Printable characters are coded with 1 byte. A page of text contains between 1 and 2 kilobytes (8–16 kilobits).

Bits per second
The bit per second (b/s or bps) is the unit used for measuring the flow of digitized information through a communications link.

E-mail
E-mail stands for electronic mail. It is a service allowing different computer users to communicate through a network.

File(s)
This is a group of digital data, with a name.

Database(s)
Any 'collection of data or information' stored in digitized electronic form and with a suitable indexing mechanism for quick access to relevant parts of the information.

Parallel computing
One method of increasing computing power by sharing the work between communicating processors.

Neural networks
A special case of parallel computing based on a simplified model of brain cell interactions.

References

1. General Medical Council. Recommendations on undergraduate medical education. *Tomorrow's Doctors*, December, 1993.
2. De Moor G, Lacombe J, Noothoven van Goor J, Thayer C. *Telematics for Health Care*. ACOSTA for the Commission of the European Union, the Telematics programme of DGXIII/C and its health care domain (AIM).
3. Leaper DJ, Gill PW, Staniland JR *et al.* Clinical diagnosis process: an analysis. *Br Med J* 1973; **3**: 569–74.
4. de Dombal FT, Winding O, Ohmann C. Quality assurance in gastroenterology: the joint OMGE/EC study. *Gastroent Int* 1992; **5**: 262–7.
5. Miller GA. The magic number 7 – plus or minus 2: some limits on our capacity for processing information. *Psychol Rev* 1966; **63**: 81.
6. Taylor TR. Computers in medicine in the decade of the 1970s. *Scot Med J* 1970; **125**: 353.
7. de Dombal FT. Picking the best test in acute abdominal pain. *J Roy Coll Phys Lond* 1979; **13**: 203–8.
8. Gruver RG, Fries ED. A study of diagnostic errors. *Ann Intern Med* 1957; **47**: 108.
9. Dixon RH, Lazlo J. Utilisation of clinical chemistry services by medical house staff. *Arch Intern Med* 1974; **134**: 1064.
10. Durbridge TC, Edwards F, Edwards RG, Atkinson M. Evaluation of benefits of screening tests done immediately on admission to hospital. *Clin Chem* 1976; **22**: 968.
11. McAdam WAF, Brock BM, Armitage T *et al.* Twelve years' experience of computer-aided diagnosis in a district general hospital. *Ann Roy Coll Surg* 1990; **72**: 140–6.
12. Rowsell KV, Johnson AD, Annis SE. The application of knowledge based decision support: computer-aided diagnosis of abdominal pain at Ormskirk and District General Hospital 1988–1993. *South Lanc Med J* 1995; **1**: 12–15.
13. de Dombal FT. How do surgeons assimilate information? *Theor Surg* 1986; **1**: 47–54.
14. de Dombal FT, Leaper DJ, Staniland IR *et al.* Computer aided diagnosis of acute abdominal pain. *Br Med J* 1972; **II**: 9–13.
15. Adams ID, Chan M, Clifford PC *et al.* Computer-aided diagnosis of abdominal pain: a multi-centre study. *Br Med J* 1986; **293**: 800–4.
16. de Dombal FT *et al.* Objective medical decision making – acute abdominal pain. In: Beneken JEW, Thevenin V (eds) *Advances in Biomedical Engineering*. Amsterdam, Oxford, Washington and Tokyo: IOS, 1993: 65.
17. Ohmann C, de Dombal FT, Winding O and the International Evaluation Panel. Evaluation procedures in the TELEGASTRO project. *Theor Surg* 1994; **9**: 90–103.

INDEX